Innovation and Evidence for Achieving TB Elimination in the Asia–Pacific Region

Innovation and Evidence for Achieving TB Elimination in the Asia–Pacific Region

Editors

Philipp DuCros
Hamidah Hussain
Kerri Viney

MDPI • Basel • Beijing • Wuhan • Barcelona • Belgrade • Manchester • Tokyo • Cluj • Tianjin

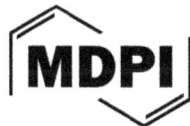

Editors

Philipp DuCros
Tuberculosis Elimination and
Implementation Science
Burnet Institute
Melbourne
Australia

Hamidah Hussain
IRD Global
Singapore
Singapore

Kerri Viney
Research School of Population
Health
Australian National University
Canberra
Australia

Editorial Office
MDPI
St. Alban-Anlage 66
4052 Basel, Switzerland

This is a reprint of articles from the Special Issue published online in the open access journal *Tropical Medicine and Infectious Disease* (ISSN 2414-6366) (available at: www.mdpi.com/journal/tropicalmed/special_issues/TB_elimination).

For citation purposes, cite each article independently as indicated on the article page online and as indicated below:

LastName, A.A.; LastName, B.B.; LastName, C.C. Article Title. *Journal Name* **Year**, *Volume Number*, Page Range.

ISBN 978-3-0365-2551-8 (Hbk)
ISBN 978-3-0365-2550-1 (PDF)

© 2022 by the authors. Articles in this book are Open Access and distributed under the Creative Commons Attribution (CC BY) license, which allows users to download, copy and build upon published articles, as long as the author and publisher are properly credited, which ensures maximum dissemination and a wider impact of our publications.

The book as a whole is distributed by MDPI under the terms and conditions of the Creative Commons license CC BY-NC-ND.

Contents

About the Editors vii

Philipp du Cros, Hamidah Hussain and Kerri Viney
Special Issue "Innovation and Evidence for Achieving TB Elimination in the Asia-Pacific Region"
Reprinted from: *Trop. Med. Infect. Dis.* **2021**, 6, 114, doi:10.3390/tropicalmed6030114 1

Lan Huu Nguyen, Andrew J. Codlin, Luan Nguyen Quang Vo, Thang Dao, Duc Tran, Rachel J. Forse, Thanh Nguyen Vu, Giang Truong Le, Tuan Luu, Giang Chau Do, Vinh Van Truong, Ha Dang Thi Minh, Hung Huu Nguyen, Jacob Creswell, Maxine Caws, Hoa Binh Nguyen and Nhung Viet Nguyen
An Evaluation of Programmatic Community-Based Chest X-ray Screening for Tuberculosis in Ho Chi Minh City, Vietnam
Reprinted from: *Trop. Med. Infect. Dis.* **2020**, 5, 185, doi:10.3390/tropicalmed5040185 5

Tuan Huy Mac, Thuc Huy Phan, Van Van Nguyen, Thuy Thu Thi Dong, Hoi Van Le, Quan Duc Nguyen, Tho Duc Nguyen, Andrew James Codlin, Thuy Doan To Mai, Rachel Jeanette Forse, Lan Phuong Nguyen, Tuan Ho Thanh Luu, Hoa Binh Nguyen, Nhung Viet Nguyen, Xanh Thu Pham, Phap Ngoc Tran, Amera Khan, Luan Nguyen Quang Vo and Jacob Creswell
Optimizing Active Tuberculosis Case Finding: Evaluating the Impact of Community Referral for Chest X-ray Screening and Xpert Testing on Case Notifications in Two Cities in Viet Nam
Reprinted from: *Trop. Med. Infect. Dis.* **2020**, 5, 181, doi:10.3390/tropicalmed5040181 17

Elvi S. Siahaan, Mirjam I. Bakker, Ratna Pasaribu, Amera Khan, Tripti Pande, Alwi Mujahit Hasibuan and Jacob Creswell
Islands of Tuberculosis Elimination: An Evaluation of Community-Based Active Case Finding in North Sumatra, Indonesia
Reprinted from: *Trop. Med. Infect. Dis.* **2020**, 5, 163, doi:10.3390/tropicalmed5040163 33

Jacob Creswell, Amera Khan, Mirjam I Bakker, Miranda Brouwer, Vishnu Vardhan Kamineni, Christina Mergenthaler, Marina Smelyanskaya, Zhi Zhen Qin, Oriol Ramis, Robert Stevens, K Srikanth Reddy and Lucie Blok
The TB REACH Initiative: Supporting TB Elimination Efforts in the Asia-Pacific
Reprinted from: *Trop. Med. Infect. Dis.* **2020**, 5, 164, doi:10.3390/tropicalmed5040164 45

Luan Nguyen Quang Vo, Andrew James Codlin, Huy Ba Huynh, Thuy Doan To Mai, Rachel Jeanette Forse, Vinh Van Truong, Ha Minh Thi Dang, Bang Duc Nguyen, Lan Huu Nguyen, Tuan Dinh Nguyen, Hoa Binh Nguyen, Nhung Viet Nguyen, Maxine Caws, Knut Lonnroth and Jacob Creswell
Enhanced Private Sector Engagement for Tuberculosis Diagnosis and Reporting through an Intermediary Agency in Ho Chi Minh City, Viet Nam
Reprinted from: *Trop. Med. Infect. Dis.* **2020**, 5, 143, doi:10.3390/tropicalmed5030143 57

Sheelu Lohiya, Jaya Prasad Tripathy, Karuna Sagili, Vishal Khanna, Ravinder Kumar, Arun Ojha, Anuj Bhatnagar and Ashwani Khanna
Does Drug-Resistant Extrapulmonary Tuberculosis Hinder TB Elimination Plans? A Case from Delhi, India
Reprinted from: *Trop. Med. Infect. Dis.* **2020**, 5, 109, doi:10.3390/tropicalmed5030109 71

Nyi-Nyi Zayar, Rassamee Sangthong, Saw Saw, Si Thu Aung and Virasakdi Chongsuvivatwong
Combined Tuberculosis and Diabetes Mellitus Screening and Assessment of Glycaemic Control among Household Contacts of Tuberculosis Patients in Yangon, Myanmar
Reprinted from: *Trop. Med. Infect. Dis.* 2020, 5, 107, doi:10.3390/tropicalmed5030107 85

Srinath Satyanarayana, Pruthu Thekkur, Ajay M. V. Kumar, Yan Lin, Riitta A. Dlodlo, Mohammed Khogali, Rony Zachariah and Anthony David Harries
An Opportunity to END TB: Using the Sustainable Development Goals for Action on Socio-Economic Determinants of TB in High Burden Countries in WHO South-East Asia and the Western Pacific Regions
Reprinted from: *Trop. Med. Infect. Dis.* 2020, 5, 101, doi:10.3390/tropicalmed5020101 99

Roma Haresh Paryani, Vivek Gupta, Pramila Singh, Madhur Verma, Sabira Sheikh, Reeta Yadav, Homa Mansoor, Stobdan Kalon, Sriram Selvaraju, Mrinalini Das, Chinmay Laxmeshwar, Gabriella Ferlazzo and Petros Isaakidis
Yield of Systematic Longitudinal Screening of Household Contacts of Pre-Extensively Drug Resistant (PreXDR) and Extensively Drug Resistant (XDR) Tuberculosis Patients in Mumbai, India
Reprinted from: *Trop. Med. Infect. Dis.* 2020, 5, 83, doi:10.3390/tropicalmed5020083 119

Anthony D. Harries, Ajay M.V. Kumar, Srinath Satyanarayana, Pruthu Thekkur, Yan Lin, Riitta A. Dlodlo, Mohammed Khogali and Rony Zachariah
The Growing Importance of Tuberculosis Preventive Therapy and How Research and Innovation Can Enhance Its Implementation on the Ground
Reprinted from: *Trop. Med. Infect. Dis.* 2020, 5, 61, doi:10.3390/tropicalmed5020061 129

Le T. N. Anh, Ajay M. V. Kumar, Gomathi Ramaswamy, Thurain Htun, Thuy Thanh Hoang Thi, Giang Hoai Nguyen, Mamel Quelapio, Agnes Gebhard, Hoa Binh Nguyen and Nhung Viet Nguyen
High Levels of Treatment Success and Zero Relapse in Multidrug-Resistant Tuberculosis Patients Receiving a Levofloxacin-Based Shorter Treatment Regimen in Vietnam
Reprinted from: *Trop. Med. Infect. Dis.* 2020, 5, 43, doi:10.3390/tropicalmed5010043 145

Monyrath Chry, Marina Smelyanskaya, Mom Ky, Andrew J Codlin, Danielle Cazabon, Mao Tan Eang and Jacob Creswell
Can the High Sensitivity of Xpert MTB/RIF Ultra Be Harnessed to Save Cartridge Costs? Results from a Pooled Sputum Evaluation in Cambodia
Reprinted from: *Trop. Med. Infect. Dis.* 2020, 5, 27, doi:10.3390/tropicalmed5010027 157

Thuong Do Thu, Ajay M. V. Kumar, Gomathi Ramaswamy, Thurain Htun, Hoi Le Van, Luan Nguyen Quang Vo, Thuy Thi Thu Dong, Andrew Codlin, Rachel Forse, Jacob Crewsell, Hoi Nguyen Thanh, Hai Nguyen Viet, Huy Bui Van, Hoa Nguyen Binh and Nhung Nguyen Viet
An Innovative Public–Private Mix Model for Improving Tuberculosis Care in Vietnam: How Well Are We Doing?
Reprinted from: *Trop. Med. Infect. Dis.* 2020, 5, 26, doi:10.3390/tropicalmed5010026 167

Aye Mon Phyo, Ajay M. V. Kumar, Kyaw Thu Soe, Khine Wut Yee Kyaw, Aung Si Thu, Pyae Phyo Wai, Sandar Aye, Saw Saw, Htet Myet Win Maung and Si Thu Aung
Contact Investigation of Multidrug-Resistant Tuberculosis Patients: A Mixed-Methods Study from Myanmar
Reprinted from: *Trop. Med. Infect. Dis.* 2019, 5, 3, doi:10.3390/tropicalmed5010003 181

Nang Thu Thu Kyaw, Aung Sithu, Srinath Satyanarayana, Ajay M. V. Kumar, Saw Thein, Aye Myat Thi, Pyae Phyo Wai, Yan Naing Lin, Khine Wut Yee Kyaw, Moe Myint Theingi Tun, Myo Minn Oo, Si Thu Aung and Anthony D. Harries
Outcomes of Community-Based Systematic Screening of Household Contacts of Patients with Multidrug-Resistant Tuberculosis in Myanmar
Reprinted from: *Trop. Med. Infect. Dis.* **2019**, 5, 2, doi:10.3390/tropicalmed5010002 . . . . **197**

Mrinalini Das, Dileep Pasupuleti, Srinivasa Rao, Stacy Sloan, Homa Mansoor, Stobdan Kalon, Farah Naz Hossain, Gabriella Ferlazzo and Petros Isaakidis
GeneXpert and Community Health Workers Supported Patient Tracing for Tuberculosis Diagnosis in Conflict-Affected Border Areas in India
Reprinted from: *Trop. Med. Infect. Dis.* **2019**, 5, 1, doi:10.3390/tropicalmed5010001 . . . . **209**

Amyn A. Malik, Hamidah Hussain, Jacob Creswell, Sara Siddiqui, Junaid F. Ahmed, Falak Madhani, Ali Habib, Aamir J. Khan and Farhana Amanullah
The Impact of Funding on Childhood TB Case Detection in Pakistan
Reprinted from: *Trop. Med. Infect. Dis.* **2019**, 4, 146, doi:10.3390/tropicalmed4040146 . . . . **217**

About the Editors

Philipp DuCros

Dr. Philipp du Cros is an infectious disease specialist with a Master's degree in Clinical Epidemiology and more than 15 years of clinical and public health experience in the management of TB/HIV programs in Africa, Central Asia, South East Asia, and the Pacific. He is the co-Head of the Burnet Institute's Tuberculosis Elimination and Implementation Science working group. His work has a strong focus on research improving diagnosis and treatment of drug-resistant TB and leads grants supporting field testing of novel TB diagnostic tests and improved models of care for TB active case finding. He is a member of the steering committee for the MSF-sponsored TB-PRACTECAL MDR-TB randomized controlled trial. He is a member of the World Health Organisation rGLC for the Programmatic Management of Drug-Resistant TB (WPRO region).

Hamidah Hussain

Hamidah Hussain is a Director at IRD Global and a public health professional with over two decades of experience in designing, implementing, and evaluating global health service delivery programs and epidemiological research in Pakistan, Bangladesh, Tajikistan, Indonesia, Philippines, and South Africa. Her portfolio includes work on active case finding for susceptible and drug-resistant TB, childhood TB, TB preventive services, childhood vaccines, and preventable diseases, Malaria control programs along with costing and cost-effectiveness of these interventions. Previously, Dr. Hussain worked at the Johns Hopkins Bloomberg School of Public Health in Baltimore and BRAC in Bangladesh. Dr. Hussain received her medical degree from The Aga Khan University, a Master in Health Policy, Planning, and Financing from the London School of Hygiene and Tropical Medicine, and a Ph.D. in health economics from the University of Bergen, Norway.

Kerri Viney

Kerri Viney is a Team Lead at the Global Tuberculosis Programme, WHO. She leads the Global TB Programme's work on TB-HIV, TB-comorbidities, and TB in vulnerable populations, including in children and adolescents. She is a senior international public health scientist with expertise in the programmatic management of TB, public health capacity building, development of global infectious diseases policies, and the translation of research into policy. She is an adjunct Associate Professor at the University of Sydney's School of Public Health and an affiliated researcher at the Department of Global Public Health, Karolinska Institutet. She did her public health training at the New South Wales Ministry of Health and has a Ph.D. in TB epidemiology from Australian National University.

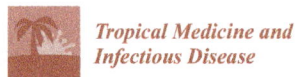

Editorial

Special Issue "Innovation and Evidence for Achieving TB Elimination in the Asia-Pacific Region"

Philipp du Cros [1],*, Hamidah Hussain [2] and Kerri Viney [3,4]

1. International Development, Burnet Institute, Melbourne 3000, Australia
2. Interactive Research and Development (IRD), Global IRD, 583 Orchard Road, #06-01 Forum, Singapore 238884, Singapore; hamidah.hussain@ird.global
3. Department of Global Public Health, Karolinska Institutet, 171 77 Stockholm, Sweden; vineyk@who.int
4. Research School of Population Health, Australian National University, Canberra 2600, Australia
* Correspondence: philipp.ducros@burnet.edu.au

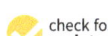

Citation: du Cros, P.; Hussain, H.; Viney, K. Special Issue "Innovation and Evidence for Achieving TB Elimination in the Asia-Pacific Region". *Trop. Med. Infect. Dis.* **2021**, *6*, 114. https://doi.org/10.3390/tropicalmed6030114

Received: 22 June 2021
Accepted: 24 June 2021
Published: 28 June 2021

Publisher's Note: MDPI stays neutral with regard to jurisdictional claims in published maps and institutional affiliations.

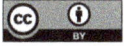

Copyright: © 2021 by the authors. Licensee MDPI, Basel, Switzerland. This article is an open access article distributed under the terms and conditions of the Creative Commons Attribution (CC BY) license (https://creativecommons.org/licenses/by/4.0/).

The World Health Organization's (WHO) END-TB strategy has set the world on course to climb the highest of medical mountains by 2035, with a targeted peak of reductions in TB deaths by 95%, TB cases by 90%, and no burden of catastrophic expenses on families due to TB [1]. Eliminating TB in the Asia-Pacific region, which has 62% of all estimated TB patients globally, will require innovation, rigorous research, and sustained investment. The Lancet series "How to Eliminate Tuberculosis" outlines an evidence-based approach to ending TB based on four key areas: rethinking data management to target hotspots, active case finding (ACF) and prompt treatment, treating TB infection, and employing a biosocial approach [2]. However, there is still much to learn and improve if this approach is to be effectively implemented. This special issue connects original research and viewpoints on pertinent approaches for improving TB care and prevention in the Asia-Pacific region.

There are multiple components to ACF, and innovation and improvement in all aspects of ACF are required if its contribution to TB elimination is to be maximized. However, evidence that ACF makes a difference at a population level remains limited and the importance of well-conducted evaluations has been highlighted [3]. In this special issue, three studies evaluate ACF interventions conducted in the community. Nguyen et al. reported that community-based, mobile chest X-ray (CXR) screening, regardless of symptoms, followed by Xpert MTB/RIF testing for patients screening positive, had high yields [4]. Half of patients diagnosed had subclinical TB with no or minimal symptoms which is unlikely to be detected with TB symptom screening alone [4]. In a controlled intervention study in Vietnam, Mac et al. reported on an evaluation of community health workers (CHWs) and their ability to refer household contacts (HHCs) and people with symptoms of TB for CXR screening. They reported an 18.3% increase in notifications of all forms of TB [5]. Siahaan et al. evaluated a multicomponent community-based ACF intervention, which included laboratory strengthening and community awareness in two locations in Indonesia. Results from the same intervention differed considerably between the two intervention sites, with a 22% increase in bacteriologically confirmed patients on Nias Island, while there was almost no change in notifications on mainland North Sumatra. They also noted how ACF can place an increased burden on screening and diagnostic cascades, including in the laboratory, which highlights the importance of investments in health system strengthening [6].

In this special issue, three approaches to ACF within health facilities are evaluated. Thu et al. presented findings on TB symptom screening performed on adults in a private hospital, followed by CXR screening for those with symptoms. They added a mobile application to reduce dropouts in the cascade of care. This showed high rates of uptake in investigations by persons with possible symptoms of TB and of treatment by those diagnosed with TB [7]. In another study from Vietnam, Vo et al. showed an increase of 8.5% in all forms of TB notifications through subsidized CXR screening and Xpert MTB/RIF testing among private practitioners, with support of improved reporting to the national TB program [8]. In their study, they note that many people treated for TB at private facilities remain unreported, suggesting that further improvements in the intervention process can produce higher yields. Chry et al. reported on a comparison of individual sputum testing compared with a sputum pooling strategy, where both were tested using Xpert MTB/RIF Ultra. The pooling strategy detected 100% of bacteriologically positive people detected by the individual strategy, saving 27% of cartridges and processing time. The authors note that pooling sputum samples for use with Xpert will only have a significant impact on time and costs when programs test a large number of samples in a population with a low yield of TB [9].

HHCs of TB patients are at increased risk of developing TB, especially within the first year after exposure [10]. Four studies in this special issue report on findings from household investigations. Zayar et al. reported on an intervention in which HHCs are screened for diabetes mellitus and active TB. They observed that 14% of HHCs had diabetes mellitus and 5% had active TB, and there was no difference in TB prevalence among HHCs based on diabetes status of the index TB case [11]. Two studies reported on evaluations of HHCs among multi-drug resistant (MDR) TB index patients in Myanmar. Phyo et al. reported on the diagnostic cascade of care and noted significant disparities in reaching health care facilities and in investigations for persons with possible symptoms of TB. Kyaw et al. reported a yield of active TB of 3.9% among HHCs of MDR-TB index patients, with the highest yield of 10% among children under 5 years old. However, only a minority of TB patients diagnosed had rifampicin resistant (RR) TB [12,13]. Finally, Paryani et al. reported an incidence rate of TB of 2072/100,000 person years in the HHCs of index patients with pre-extensively drug resistant (pre-XDR) and XDR-TB following initial screening, which shows the importance of ongoing follow up and preventive treatment among HHCs [14].

Das et al. reported on a before and after intervention study in a conflict-affected area in India, with the introduction of Xpert MTB/RIF and patient follow-up supported by community health workers, implemented in mobile clinics [15]. This showed an increase in bacteriological confirmation and a reduction in pre-treatment loss to follow up. Anh et al. reported on high treatment success rates with levofloxacin and an injectable containing short treatment regimen for patients with RR-TB in Vietnam [16]. Lohiya et al. described the outcomes for patients with drug resistant (DR)-extrapulmonary TB in a retrospective analysis in three DR-TB treatment centers in Delhi, India, showing that one-third of patients had unfavorable treatment outcomes [17].

Finally, three perspective pieces describe some of the broader aspects required to improve TB care. Creswell et al. described the experience of the STOP TB Partnership's TB REACH initiative. This novel mechanism funds projects that develop, evaluate, and expand innovative approaches to improve TB case finding, treatment, biosocial approaches, and prevention [18]. Satyanarayana et al. described the opportunities to address the major socioeconomic determinants of TB through the lens of the Sustainable Development Goals [19]. Harries et al. examined the important role of TB preventive treatment in achieving TB elimination. They describe how research can improve the implementation of TB preventive treatment, highlighting the need for innovation, improved diagnostic tools, better biomarkers for the progression of TB infection to TB disease, and improved adherence monitoring tools [20].

While the challenges for TB elimination remain large, there is still cause for optimism, with new evidence on screening and ACF, improved all-oral MDR-TB treatment regimens, an increasing array of novel TB diagnostics, and shorter treatment regimens for TB preventive treatment. While progress has been made, the COVID-19 pandemic has highlighted how fragile progress on TB can be, with 1.4 million fewer TB patients diagnosed in 2020 [21]. With increased TB transmission and mortality due to TB predicted, the pandemic may set back progress by a decade [21]. Achieving TB elimination will require greater investments in screening, diagnosis, treatment, and prevention as well as major socioeconomic change.

It will also require increased research, innovation, and evaluation in order to find the most appropriate people-centered models of care for all countries and contexts.

Funding: This work received no external funding.

Conflicts of Interest: The authors declare no conflict of interest.

References

1. Uplekar, M.; Weil, D.; Lonnroth, K.; Jaramillo, E.; Lienhardt, C.; Dias, H.M.; Falzon, D.; Floyd, K.; Gargioni, G.; Getahun, H.; et al. WHO's new End TB Strategy. *Lancet* **2015**, *385*, 1799–1801. [CrossRef]
2. Keshavjee, S.; Dowdy, D.; Swaminathan, S. Stopping the body count: A comprehensive approach to move towards zero tuberculosis deaths. *Lancet* **2015**, *386*, e46–e47. [CrossRef]
3. Ortiz-Brizuela, E.; Menzies, D. Tuberculosis active case-finding: Looking for cases in all the right places? *Lancet Public Health* **2021**, *6*, e261–e262. [CrossRef]
4. Nguyen, L.H.; Codlin, A.J.; Vo, L.N.Q.; Dao, T.; Tran, D.; Forse, R.J.; Vu, T.N.; Le, G.T.; Luu, T.; Do, G.C.; et al. An Evaluation of Programmatic Community-Based Chest X-ray Screening for Tuberculosis in Ho Chi Minh City, Vietnam. *Trop. Med. Infect. Dis.* **2020**, *5*, 185. [CrossRef] [PubMed]
5. Mac, T.H.; Phan, T.H.; Nguyen, V.V.; Dong, T.T.T.; Le, H.V.; Nguyen, Q.D.; Nguyen, T.D.; Codlin, A.J.; Mai, T.D.T.; Forse, R.J.; et al. Optimizing Active Tuberculosis Case Finding: Evaluating the Impact of Community Referral for Chest X-ray Screening and Xpert Testing on Case Notifications in Two Cities in Viet Nam. *Trop. Med. Infect. Dis.* **2020**, *5*, 181. [CrossRef] [PubMed]
6. Siahaan, E.S.; Bakker, M.I.; Pasaribu, R.; Khan, A.; Pande, T.; Hasibuan, A.M.; Creswell, J. Islands of Tuberculosis Elimination: An Evaluation of Community-Based Active Case Finding in North Sumatra, Indonesia. *Trop. Med. Infect. Dis.* **2020**, *5*, 163. [CrossRef] [PubMed]
7. Do Thu, T.; Kumar, A.M.V.; Ramaswamy, G.; Htun, T.; Le Van, H.; Nguyen Quang Vo, L.; Thi Thu Dong, T.; Codlin, A.; Forse, R.; Crewsell, J.; et al. An Innovative Public–Private Mix Model for Improving Tuberculosis Care in Vietnam: How Well Are We Doing? *Trop. Med. Infect. Dis.* **2020**, *5*, 26. [CrossRef] [PubMed]
8. Vo, L.N.Q.; Codlin, A.J.; Huynh, H.B.; Mai, T.D.T.; Forse, R.J.; Truong, V.V.; Dang, H.M.T.; Nguyen, B.D.; Nguyen, L.H.; Nguyen, T.D.; et al. Enhanced Private Sector Engagement for Tuberculosis Diagnosis and Reporting through an Intermediary Agency in Ho Chi Minh City, Viet Nam. *Trop. Med. Infect. Dis.* **2020**, *5*, 143. [CrossRef] [PubMed]
9. Chry, M.; Smelyanskaya, M.; Ky, M.; Codlin, A.J.; Cazabon, D.; Tan Eang, M.; Creswell, J. Can the High Sensitivity of Xpert MTB/RIF Ultra Be Harnessed to Save Cartridge Costs? Results from a Pooled Sputum Evaluation in Cambodia. *Trop. Med. Infect. Dis.* **2020**, *5*, 27. [CrossRef] [PubMed]
10. Fox, G.J.; Barry, S.E.; Britton, W.J.; Marks, G.B. Contact investigation for tuberculosis: A systematic review and meta-analysis. *Eur. Respir. J.* **2013**, *41*, 140–156. [CrossRef] [PubMed]
11. Zayar, N.-N.; Sangthong, R.; Saw, S.; Aung, S.T.; Chongsuvivatwong, V. Combined Tuberculosis and Diabetes Mellitus Screening and Assessment of Glycaemic Control among Household Contacts of Tuberculosis Patients in Yangon, Myanmar. *Trop. Med. Infect. Dis.* **2020**, *5*, 107. [CrossRef] [PubMed]
12. Kyaw, N.T.T.; Sithu, A.; Satyanarayana, S.; Kumar, A.M.V.; Thein, S.; Thi, A.M.; Wai, P.P.; Lin, Y.N.; Kyaw, K.W.Y.; Tun, M.M.T.; et al. Outcomes of Community-Based Systematic Screening of Household Contacts of Patients with Multidrug-Resistant Tuberculosis in Myanmar. *Trop. Med. Infect. Dis.* **2020**, *5*, 2. [CrossRef] [PubMed]
13. Phyo, A.M.; Kumar, A.M.V.; Soe, K.T.; Kyaw, K.W.Y.; Thu, A.S.; Wai, P.P.; Aye, S.; Saw, S.; Win Maung, H.M.; Aung, S.T. Contact Investigation of Multidrug-Resistant Tuberculosis Patients: A Mixed-Methods Study from Myanmar. *Trop. Med. Infect. Dis.* **2020**, *5*, 3. [CrossRef] [PubMed]
14. Paryani, R.H.; Gupta, V.; Singh, P.; Verma, M.; Sheikh, S.; Yadav, R.; Mansoor, H.; Kalon, S.; Selvaraju, S.; Das, M.; et al. Yield of Systematic Longitudinal Screening of Household Contacts of Pre-Extensively Drug Resistant (PreXDR) and Extensively Drug Resistant (XDR) Tuberculosis Patients in Mumbai, India. *Trop. Med. Infect. Dis.* **2020**, *5*, 83. [CrossRef] [PubMed]
15. Das, M.; Pasupuleti, D.; Rao, S.; Sloan, S.; Mansoor, H.; Kalon, S.; Hossain, F.N.; Ferlazzo, G.; Isaakidis, P. GeneXpert and Community Health Workers Supported Patient Tracing for Tuberculosis Diagnosis in Conflict-Affected Border Areas in India. *Trop. Med. Infect. Dis.* **2020**, *5*, 1. [CrossRef] [PubMed]
16. Anh, L.T.N.; Kumar, A.M.V.; Ramaswamy, G.; Htun, T.; Thanh Hoang Thi, T.; Hoai Nguyen, G.; Quelapio, M.; Gebhard, A.; Nguyen, H.B.; Nguyen, N.V. High Levels of Treatment Success and Zero Relapse in Multidrug-Resistant Tuberculosis Patients Receiving a Levofloxacin-Based Shorter Treatment Regimen in Vietnam. *Trop. Med. Infect. Dis.* **2020**, *5*, 43. [CrossRef] [PubMed]
17. Lohiya, S.; Tripathy, J.P.; Sagili, K.; Khanna, V.; Kumar, R.; Ojha, A.; Bhatnagar, A.; Khanna, A. Does Drug-Resistant Extrapulmonary Tuberculosis Hinder TB Elimination Plans? A Case from Delhi, India. *Trop. Med. Infect. Dis.* **2020**, *5*, 109. [CrossRef] [PubMed]
18. Creswell, J.; Khan, A.; Bakker, M.I.; Brouwer, M.; Kamineni, V.V.; Mergenthaler, C.; Smelyanskaya, M.; Qin, Z.Z.; Ramis, O.; Stevens, R.; et al. The TB REACH Initiative: Supporting TB Elimination Efforts in the Asia-Pacific. *Trop. Med. Infect. Dis.* **2020**, *5*, 164. [CrossRef] [PubMed]

19. Satyanarayana, S.; Thekkur, P.; Kumar, A.M.V.; Lin, Y.; Dlodlo, R.A.; Khogali, M.; Zachariah, R.; Harries, A.D. An Opportunity to END TB: Using the Sustainable Development Goals for Action on Socio-Economic Determinants of TB in High Burden Countries in WHO South-East Asia and the Western Pacific Regions. *Trop. Med. Infect. Dis.* **2020**, *5*, 101. [CrossRef] [PubMed]
20. Harries, A.D.; Kumar, A.M.V.; Satyanarayana, S.; Thekkur, P.; Lin, Y.; Dlodlo, R.A.; Khogali, M.; Zachariah, R. The Growing Importance of Tuberculosis Preventive Therapy and How Research and Innovation Can Enhance Its Implementation on the Ground. *Trop. Med. Infect. Dis.* **2020**, *5*, 61. [CrossRef] [PubMed]
21. World Health Organization. *Impact of the COVID 19 Pandemic on TB Detection and Mortality in 2020*; World Health Organization: Geneva, Switzerland, 2021; Available online: https://cdn.who.int/media/docs/default-source/hq-tuberculosis/impact-of-the-covid-19-pandemic-on-tb-detection-and-mortality-in-2020.pdf?sfvrsn=3fdd251c_16&download=true (accessed on 14 June 2021).

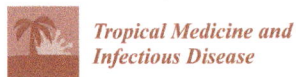 *Tropical Medicine and Infectious Disease*

Article

An Evaluation of Programmatic Community-Based Chest X-ray Screening for Tuberculosis in Ho Chi Minh City, Vietnam

Lan Huu Nguyen [1], Andrew J. Codlin [2,*], Luan Nguyen Quang Vo [2,3], Thang Dao [4], Duc Tran [2], Rachel J. Forse [2], Thanh Nguyen Vu [5], Giang Truong Le [5], Tuan Luu [6], Giang Chau Do [1], Vinh Van Truong [1], Ha Dang Thi Minh [1], Hung Huu Nguyen [7], Jacob Creswell [8], Maxine Caws [9,10], Hoa Binh Nguyen [11] and Nhung Viet Nguyen [11]

1. Pham Ngoc Thach Hospital, Ho Chi Minh City 700 000, Vietnam; nguyenhuulan1965@gmail.com (L.H.N.); do_giang68@yahoo.com (G.C.D.); drvinhpnt2020@gmail.com (V.V.T.); hadtm2018@gmail.com (H.D.T.M.)
2. Friends for International TB Relief, Ho Chi Minh City 700 000, Vietnam; luan.vo@tbhelp.org (L.N.Q.V.); tmduc93@gmail.com (D.T.); rachel.forse@tbhelp.org (R.J.F.)
3. Interactive Research and Development, Singapore 238884, Singapore
4. IRD VN, Ho Chi Minh City 700 000, Vietnam; thang.dao@tbhelp.org
5. Ho Chi Minh City Public Health Association, Ho Chi Minh City 700 000, Vietnam; thanhnguyen246@yahoo.com (T.N.V.); letruonggiang05@gmail.com (G.T.L.)
6. Clinton Health Access Initiative Vietnam, Ha Noi 100 000, Vietnam; tluu@clintonhealthaccess.org
7. Ho Chi Minh City Department of Health, Ho Chi Minh City 700 000, Vietnam; bsnguyenhuuhung102@gmail.com
8. Stop TB Partnership, 1218 Geneva, Switzerland; jacobc@stoptb.org
9. Department of Clinical Sciences, Liverpool School of Tropical Medicine, Liverpool L3 5QA, UK; maxine.caws@lstmed.ac.uk
10. Birat Nepal Medical Trust Nepal, Kathmandu 44600, Nepal
11. Viet Nam National Lung Hospital, Ha Noi 100 000, Vietnam; nguyenbinhhoatb@yahoo.com (H.B.N.); vietnhung@yahoo.com (N.V.N.)
* Correspondence: andrew.codlin@tbhelp.org; Tel.: +84-352512847

Received: 30 September 2020; Accepted: 12 November 2020; Published: 10 December 2020

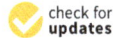

Abstract: Across Asia, a large proportion of people with tuberculosis (TB) do not report symptoms, have mild symptoms or only experience symptoms for a short duration. These individuals may not seek care at health facilities or may be missed by symptom screening, resulting in sustained TB transmission in the community. We evaluated the yields of TB from 114 days of community-based, mobile chest X-ray (CXR) screening. The yields at each step of the TB screening cascade were tabulated and we compared cohorts of participants who reported having a prolonged cough and those reporting no cough or one of short duration. We estimated the marginal yields of TB using different diagnostic algorithms and calculated the relative diagnostic costs and cost per case for each algorithm. A total of 34,529 participants were screened by CXR, detecting 256 people with Xpert-positive TB. Only 50% of those diagnosed with TB were detected among participants reporting a prolonged cough. The study's screening algorithm detected almost 4 times as much TB as the National TB Program's standard diagnostic algorithm. Community-based, mobile chest X-ray screening can be a high yielding strategy which is able to identify people with TB who would likely otherwise have been missed by existing health services.

Keywords: tuberculosis; TB; chest X-ray; active TB case-finding; diagnostic algorithm

1. Introduction

An estimated 170,000 people developed tuberculosis (TB) in Vietnam in 2019, resulting in 11,400 TB-related deaths [1]. Vietnam recently completed its second national TB prevalence survey [2], which documented a 59.9% reduction in smear-positive TB prevalence in the 11 years since the country's first TB prevalence survey was conducted [3]. However, the new prevalence survey results demonstrated that Vietnam's total estimated TB burden was higher than previously thought, due to improved survey methods and the use of more sensitive TB diagnostic tests. In light of these findings, the World Health Organization (WHO) revised Vietnam's official TB burden, and between 2018 [4] and 2019 [1], the National TB Program's (NTP) official estimated TB treatment coverage declined from 83% to 60%. Low TB treatment coverage presents an immense challenge to achieving the WHO's End TB Strategy's 90% TB incidence rate reduction target by 2035 [5], as people with untreated TB continue to transmit the disease.

One of the major barriers to improving TB treatment coverage is that a large proportion of people with TB either do not report symptoms (sub-clinical) or they have mild symptoms and/or have been experiencing symptoms for a short-duration of time (low-grade). These individuals often do not feel compelled to seek out screening and care services and, thus, are frequently missed by health programs. Across Asia, modern TB prevalence surveys have shown that 40–79% of adults with culture-confirmed, pulmonary TB do not report a prolonged cough (≥ 2 weeks) [6], and a recent meta-analysis indicates that the proportion of people with sub-clinical and low-grade TB may be significantly higher in Asia compared to Africa [7]. Vietnam's second TB prevalence survey results seem to affirm these findings; 42% of the people with TB detected by the survey did not report a prolonged cough [2]. These individuals were only indicated for diagnostic testing through the use of chest X-ray (CXR) screening. However, WHO guidelines on the use of CXR for TB screening indicate that access to high-quality radiography services can also form a barrier to health-seeking [8]. One root cause is the potentially limited availability of radiography equipment and radiologists. Even if high-quality radiography services are available, their facility-based nature and dependency on opening hours, travel time and associated costs further hinder the integration and use of CXR screening for TB in programmatic settings [9].

A second major barrier to improving TB treatment coverage in Vietnam is the continued reliance on acid fast bacilli (AFB) smear microscopy for diagnosis of TB and the need for smear-negative individuals to undergo a lengthy clinical evaluation process in accordance with NTP guidelines [10]. To address some of these barriers, Vietnam's NTP recently endorsed projects which pilot the use of CXR screening to both triage symptomatic individuals away from follow-on molecular diagnostic testing with the Xpert MTB/RIF assay (Xpert; Cepheid, Sunnyvale, CA, USA) and to indicate testing for people with mild or no TB symptoms [11]. This screening and testing approach is locally dubbed the 'Double-X' or '2X' diagnostic algorithm (X-ray to Xpert).

Several recent active case-finding campaigns across Asia have used CXRs to increase the detection of TB, particularly sub-clinical and low-grade TB. On Palawan island in the Philippines, mobile X-ray trucks were used to screen 25,000 people across various target populations [12]. Between 24.0% and 54.7% of those diagnosed with TB did not report a prolonged cough. In Cambodia, mobile X-rays were used to screen over 21,000 older people (aged ≥ 55 years) in the community [13]. If prolonged cough had been used as the only positive screening criterion, just 31.6% the people diagnosed with TB by the initiative would have been detected. In Pakistan, a fleet of mobile X-ray trucks were used to screen over 127,000 people in the community and also those visiting hospital outpatient departments [14]. Just 45.0% of the people screened by CXR reported a prolonged cough. This initiative did not report its case detection yields disaggregated by symptom status, as only computer-aided reading (CAR) software interpretations of CXR images were used to indicate follow-on diagnostic testing. Several other small-scale studies have also used CXR screening among key populations, including household contacts [15,16] and inmates [17,18], and have reported the detection of high proportions of sub-clinical and low-grade TB.

In Vietnam, due to the cost of human resource capacity-building, laboratory and equipment infrastructure and molecular assay kits, the Ministry of Health requires further evidence on the marginal yield and associated costs to formalize the scale up and transition to the X-ray to Xpert algorithm. We conducted an evaluation to quantify the benefit of using CXR screening and molecular testing in a programmatic, community-based active TB case finding initiative in Ho Chi Minh City, Vietnam.

2. Materials and Methods

2.1. Study Setting

Between 24 March 2018 and 13 October 2019, Friends for International TB Relief and its partners organized 114 days of CXR screening for TB at 235 unique locations (Figure 1) across seven intervention districts of Ho Chi Minh City, Vietnam (Districts 06, 08, 12, Binh Chanh, Go Vap, Hoc Mon and Tan Binh). These seven districts had a combined population of over 3.4 million people in 2017, the year before this intervention began, and their combined TB notification rate was 141 per 100,000 population. Each district contained one District TB Unit (DTU), which managed TB diagnosis and treatment in collaboration with a network of Commune Health Stations and under the technical supervision of the Provincial TB Program at Pham Ngoc Thach Hospital (PNTH).

These seven districts were selected for inclusion in a two-year, controlled evaluation study comparing the performance of different community healthcare worker (CHW) employment models on the yields, impact and cost of community-based active TB case-finding due to their low case detection and notification rates [19]. In this evaluation study, CHWs screened household contacts and other urban priority groups for symptoms of TB and made referrals for facility-based CXR screening services and follow-on diagnostic testing [20]. Community-based, mobile CXR screening was implemented as a secondary strategy to reduce some of the barriers study participants faced when trying to access facility-based radiography services.

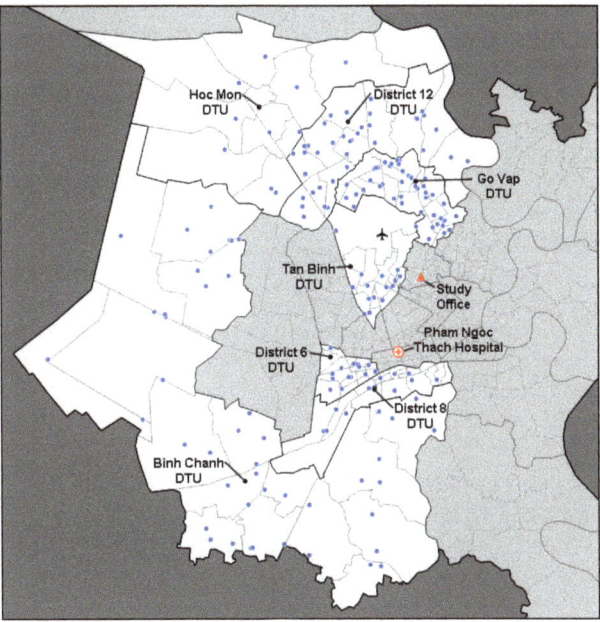

Figure 1. Map mobile chest X-ray (CXR) screening event locations (blue dots) in Ho Chi Minh City, Vietnam.

2.2. Participant Mobilization

The location for each CXR screening event was selected at least two weeks in advance of implementation. Commune Health Stations, local government offices, schools and churches/pagodas were the most commonly selected sites for screening due to their prominent placement in communities, open spaces for group congregation and availability of water, stable electricity and sanitary facilities. The project's X-ray truck was frequently moved to a second or third location during the day in an attempt to further reduce geographical access barriers to screening. Community members living in the catchment area of each screening location were sensitized about TB and the availability of upcoming CXR screening services with support from the District- and Commune-level government health staff, civil society organizations (e.g., Women's Union, Retirement Association, Red Cross, etc.) and the study's network of CHWs. Participant mobilization was enhanced through the distribution of individualized letters of invitation from each Commune's People's Committees, notices on community announcement boards and banners hung in highly visible areas. To maximize TB yields, we targeted urban priority populations for TB, including household contacts, older individuals ($\geq$55 years), people living with HIV or diabetes, people living in socioeconomically disadvantaged areas and others who had TB symptoms. CXR screening events were primarily hosted on Saturdays and Sundays, and occasionally on Fridays, in an attempt to improve access for people who were otherwise obligated during the work week. The events provided screening for additional diseases such as chronic obstructive pulmonary disorder (COPD), asthma, high blood pressure and diabetes to reduce any perceived stigma associated with hosting TB-focused events among the target populations. A VND 10,000 (approximately USD 0.44) cash incentive was provided to all study participants who completed CXR screening, to defray some of the costs of travel to the event.

2.3. Screening and Diagnosis of TB

At the screening events, medical student volunteers and CHWs administered a TB symptom questionnaire using a custom-built mHealth app loaded onto Android tablets (Clinton Health Access Initiative/TechUp, Ha Noi, Vietnam), but symptom-screening data were not used to indicate follow-on diagnostic testing. Instead, all participants were referred for CXR screening, whether or not they had symptoms of TB. Digital CXR images were immediately read and classified by a certified radiologist who was instructed to intentionally over-read the CXR images, in line with WHO's guidelines for CXR classification during TB prevalence surveys [21]. All individuals with an abnormal CXR were guided to provide a good-quality sputum specimen using an instructional aide. Sputum specimens were stored locally until the end of each screening day and were subsequently transported to a nearby laboratory for testing with Xpert.

If an individual was unable to provide a good-quality sputum specimen during the event, a CHW attempted another collection at their home to improve sputum submission rates. People diagnosed with drug-sensitive TB were initiated on treatment at the District TB Units, while people with rifampicin-resistant Xpert results were referred to PNTH for additional testing and drug-resistant TB treatment initiation.

2.4. Statistical Analyses

De-identified data were extracted from the study's mHealth database. The yields at each step of the TB screening cascade [22] were then tabulated, disaggregated by cough duration, age group and gender. Pearson's χ^2 test was used to measure the significance of differences between cohorts of participants who reported having a prolonged cough ($\geq$2 weeks) and those with a cough of short duration (<2 weeks) or no cough at all.

We estimated the marginal yields of bacteriologically-confirmed (Bac[+]) TB for various screening and diagnostic algorithms using a mix of study data (e.g., proportions of participants having a prolonged cough or a cough of any duration) and AFB smear microscopy testing performance characteristics from the literature. Actual Xpert yields were converted into estimated culture yields using an 85% sensitivity rate for Xpert [23] and then AFB smear microscopy yields were estimated using a 43% sensitivity rate [24]. We did not attempt to estimate the yields of TB for participants with symptoms and normal CXR results, as the TB prevalence in this cohort was estimated to be <10 per 100,000 in Vietnam's second TB prevalence survey [2]. The following six screening and diagnostic algorithms were investigated: (1) cough for ≥2 weeks followed by AFB smear microscopy testing, (2) cough for ≥2 weeks followed by Xpert testing, (3) any cough followed by AFB smear microscopy testing, (4) any cough followed by Xpert testing, (5) CXR abnormal followed by AFB smear microscopy testing and (6) CXR abnormal followed by Xpert testing.

Finally, we estimated the relative diagnostic costs and cost per Bac(+) TB case incurred by the health system for each of the aforementioned screening and diagnostic algorithms. Diagnostic costs were obtained from a Vietnamese health systems costing study [25], including USD 0.18 per AFB smear microscopy test performed and USD 11.12 per Xpert test performed (USD 0.83 for consumables, USD 9.98 for the Xpert cartridge [26] and USD 0.31 for shipping (obtained from the study's Cepheid shipping documents)). The cost of a provincial-level laboratory technician (USD 216 per month) was also included for the full 19-month project duration. When a diagnostic algorithm resulted in more than an average of 20 sputum tests being conducted per working day, the costs for additional laboratory technicians were included, in line with global TB laboratory standards [27]. We estimated the cost of each CXR image captured and read to be USD 1.53, based on the study's contract with the X-ray truck rental company (VND 35,000 per image) and used the average interbank exchange rate during the study period to convert into USD (VND 22,949 per 1 USD) [28]. We modeled the number of CXR screens and sputum tests for each algorithm and applied the aforementioned unit costs and added the laboratory technician costs. The cost per Bac(+) case was calculated by dividing the total diagnostic testing costs by each algorithm's estimated yield. We did not differentiate between the detection of drug-sensitive and -resistant TB; the incremental costs for confirming a drug-resistant TB diagnosis have been reported elsewhere [25].

2.5. Ethical Considerations

The Institutional Review Board of PNTH (155/NCKH-PNT) granted scientific and ethical approval for this study. The Provincial People's Committee of Ho Chi Minh City approved the implementation of the intervention (4699/QD-UBND).

3. Results

3.1. Yields of TB

Table 1 shows the yields of TB at defined points along the screening cascade. A total of 34,529 participants were screened by CXR, an average of 302 people per day. Over 4700 people had their CXR image classified as abnormal (13.7%) and 2670 people were tested on Xpert (56.5% of eligible). Screening resulted in the detection of 256 people with Xpert-positive TB (9.6% of those tested) translating to an overall TB detection/prevalence rate of 741 per 100,000. Furthermore, 84.4% of participants diagnosed with TB were male and 62.9% were aged 55 years and over.

Just 27.3% of all participants (n = 9430) reported having a cough lasting ≥2 weeks. This cohort of participants had a significantly higher CXR abnormality rate (16.1% vs. 12.8%, $p < 0.001$), sputum collection and testing rate (64.3% vs. 52.9%, $p < 0.001$) and Xpert test positivity (13.1% vs. 7.5%, $p < 0.001$) compared to participants with a cough of short duration or no cough at all. Participants with a prolonged cough had a TB detection/prevalence rate of 1357 per 100,000 screened, compared to 510 per 100,000 screened for participants with a cough of short duration or no cough at all. However, only 50% of the total number of people diagnosed with TB by the study (128/256) were detected among participants with a prolonged cough. Among those diagnosed with TB, a higher proportion of people with sub-clinical and low-grade TB was observed among older compared to younger people (52.8% vs. 45.3%) and men compared to women (51.9% vs. 40.0%).

Table 1. Yields of tuberculosis (TB) screening by cough status, age group and gender.

	All Participants	Cough ≥ 2 Weeks	Cough < 2 Weeks and No Cough
All Participants			
Screened by chest X-ray (CXR)	34,529	9430	25,099
CXR abnormal	4722 (13.7%)	1515 (16.1%)	3207 (12.8%)
Tested using the Xpert MTB/RIF assay (Xpert)	2670 (56.5%)	974 (64.3%)	1696 (52.9%)
Xpert(+) TB detected	256 (9.6%)	128 (13.1%)	128 (7.5%)
Xpert(+) TB prevalence rate	741	1357	510
Aged 15–54 Years			
Screened by CXR	12,896	3311	9585
CXR abnormal	1063 (8.2%)	337 (10.2%)	726 (7.6%)
Tested by Xpert	664 (62.5%)	253 (75.1%)	411 (56.6%)
Xpert(+) TB detected	95 (14.3%)	52 (20.6%)	43 (10.5%)
Xpert(+) TB prevalence rate	737	1571	449
Aged ≥ 55 Years			
Screened by CXR	21,633	6119	15,514
CXR abnormal	3659 (16.9%)	1178 (19.3%)	2481 (16.0%)
Tested by Xpert	2006 (54.8%)	721 (61.2%)	1285 (51.8%)
Xpert(+) TB detected	161 (8.0%)	76 (10.5%)	85 (6.6%)
Xpert(+) TB prevalence rate	744	1242	548
Males			
Screened by CXR	14,609	4409	10,200
CXR abnormal	2980 (20.4%)	1023 (23.2%)	1957 (19.2%)
Tested by Xpert	1950 (65.4%)	724 (70.8%)	1226 (62.6%)
Xpert(+) TB detected	216 (11.1%)	104 (14.4%)	112 (9.1%)
Xpert(+) TB prevalence rate	1479	2359	1098
Females			
Screened by CXR	19,920	5021	14,899
CXR abnormal	1742 (8.7%)	492 (9.8%)	1250 (8.4%)
Tested by Xpert	720 (41.3%)	250 (50.8%)	470 (37.6%)
Xpert(+) TB detected	40 (5.6%)	24 (9.6%)	16 (3.4%)
Xpert(+) TB prevalence rate	201	478	107

3.2. Marginal Yield Analysis and Relative Diagnostic Costing

Table 2 shows the results of the marginal yield analysis and relative diagnostic costing. If the NTP's standard diagnostic algorithm of testing people with a cough for ≥2 weeks with AFB smear microscopy had been followed, we estimate that just 65 would have been diagnosed with smear-positive TB. This algorithm has the lowest total diagnostic costs at USD 9915 and second lowest cost per Bac(+) case detected of USD 153.12. Identification of cough of any duration, followed by Xpert testing proved to the most expensive algorithm to implement overall at USD 176,131. Although this algorithm is estimated to detect 2.8× more people with TB than the NTP's standard diagnostic algorithm, it still had a cost per case of USD 978.51. CXR screening followed by Xpert testing detected the most people with TB-almost 4× as many as the NTP's standard diagnostic algorithm. Since CXRs were used to triage people with symptoms away from Xpert testing and the cost for a CXR is substantially lower than that of an Xpert test in Vietnam, the overall diagnostic costs were cheaper than direct Xpert testing for participants with either a cough of any duration or only those with a cough lasting ≥2 weeks. The X-ray to Xpert algorithm had an overall cost of USD 109,274 and a cost per TB case detected of

USD 426.85. This cost per case figure was substantially lower than any other diagnostic algorithm involving Xpert testing.

Table 2. Marginal yields of TB from various diagnostic algorithms and their relative diagnostic costs (USD).

	CXR Screens	AFB Tests	Xpert Tests	Estimated TB Yield	Marginal TB Yield	Total Diagnostic Costs	Cost per Bac(+) Case Detected
Cough ≥ 2 weeks followed by acid-fast bacilli smear microscopy (AFB)	0	9430	0	65	-	9915	153.12
Any cough followed by AFB	0	15,101	0	91	+40.6%	10,941	120.16
Cough ≥ 2 weeks followed by Xpert MTB/RIF assay (Xpert)	0	0	9430	128	+97.7%	113,070	883.36
Chest X-ray (CXR) abnormal followed by AFB	34,529	4722	0	130	+100.0%	57,620	444.92
Any cough followed by Xpert	0	0	15,101	180	+178.0%	176,131	978.51
CXR abnormal followed by Xpert	34,529	0	4722	256 *	+295.3%	109,274	426.85

* Actual total yield.

4. Discussion

This evaluation shows that programmatic community-based CXR screening followed by Xpert testing can result in high yields of TB among people who are likely to be missed by existing government health services. We recorded an Xpert-positive TB prevalence which is more than 2.5× the Xpert-positive TB prevalence in the Southern Region of Vietnam [2], indicating that our community sensitization efforts were effective at targeting and mobilizing higher risk individuals. In addition, half of the people diagnosed in this study had sub-clinical or low-grade TB and we estimate that only one quarter of our yield would have been detected if we had followed standard NTP screening and diagnostic guidelines. This finding is in line with a comparison of WHO's yield estimates for these two diagnostic algorithms during active case finding [29].

The relative diagnostic costing component of this evaluation shows that no matter what screening approach is used, the roll out of Xpert testing services will be significantly more costly than maintaining routine AFB smear microscopy testing. Despite the X-ray to Xpert algorithm having the lowest total costs and cost per TB case of any Xpert-based diagnostic algorithm, it still cost more than 10× the standard NTP diagnostic algorithm, although the cost per case detected was less than 3×. In order to end the TB epidemic, a surge of investment is needed in strategies such as this, so that they can be consistently implemented with enough population coverage and for a sufficient duration of time to impact TB incidence [30]. A recent trial from Vietnam showed that systematic mass diagnostic testing coverage over a 3-year period was associated with a 44% reduction in TB incidence [31]. This trial was able to test between 35–45% of the intervention area's adult population each year for three years. Due to funding constraints, our study was only able to reach roughly a total 1% of the population living in the intervention districts over a 19-month period.

Our intervention offers a blueprint for an economically viable model that can promote early and increased TB detection, which is essential for breaking the chain of TB transmission in communities and reducing TB incidence. The role which sub-clinical and low-grade TB plays in transmission dynamics is not well understood. However, the literature shows that people with paucibacillary disease, even those with negative nucleic acid amplification tests, can still transmit TB [32,33] and that transmission can occur in the absence of a cough [34]. People with sub-clinical TB may have only transient active infections which self-resolve, or they may be at risk for progression to more serious forms of TB disease [35]. A cohort study from South Africa involving untreated, laboratory-confirmed multidrug-resistant TB (MDR-TB) patients who reported minimal TB symptoms showed that patients with CXR abnormalities were four-times more likely to experience unfavorable outcomes, including death, loss to follow-up or second-line TB treatment initiation, during a 12 month follow-up period [36]. These findings suggest that the people with sub-clinical and low-grade TB who were diagnosed after an abnormal CXR screen by this study are at risk for progressing to more serious forms of TB.

This form of community-based active TB case finding was also a highly person-centered complement to the traditional facility-based referral system, as it directly addressed access barriers. This is evidenced by the higher proportion of women and girls participating in our screening events, even though they have traditionally faced greater access barriers to and longer delays with TB care in Vietnam [37,38]. In our study, for females in particular, it is possible that low sputum collection could explain the observed gender differences in sub-clinical and low-grade TB detection. Studies have shown that simple instructions are able to improve sputum collection among women [39]. We developed and used a visual aide to teach participants how to cough up a good specimen featuring an animated female character, but still recorded a lower sputum collection rate among women. Future community screening should consider additional ways to improve this metric, including by considering where sputum will be collected at the community events and providing a more private place that is shielded from view and inaudible to others for participants to cough up their specimens.

Meanwhile, the effectiveness in our targeting and community mobilization efforts were substantiated by the high case detection among men, particularly in the detection of sub-clinical and low-grade TB. As observed on both prevalence surveys, Vietnam ranks first globally in the male:female ratio (MFR) of people with TB at 5.1 [2,3]. However, the NTP reported an MFR of 2.6 among notified TB patients in 2018 [1], suggesting there are many missed males with TB. Our study has an MFR of 5.4, suggesting that community-based active TB case-finding is critical for reaching persons, especially men, with TB currently missed by the public health system.

There were many programmatic learnings from the implementation of this kind of active TB case-finding. Unlike a TB prevalence survey, participants did not have to be representative of the community in which they live. Thus, the targeting and mobilization of key populations for TB in advance of screening days helped to ensure that CXR throughput and TB yields were sufficiently high to justify this kind of human resource and financial investment. We relied heavily on the health infrastructure of the District TB program; TB Officers from the Commune Health Stations and District TB Units helped to supervise the events from a technical perspective but also helped to mobilize participants in advance of screening days. We also benefited from implementing in a highly structured government system where it was possible to send personalized invitations to all residents of a screening event's catchment area who were aged over 55 years.

The study used only one X-ray system per event location and we rarely implemented screening events in multiple locations in parallel. We did not purchase an X-ray system for this study as there is a vibrant occupational health screening market in urban Vietnam. There were no missed days due to the lack of X-ray truck rentals, or to damaged X-ray systems; when issues were encountered, a replacement X-ray truck was always available. Although for long-term ACF interventions, procurement of an X-ray system likely makes the most financial sense, this system of commoditized X-ray supply worked extremely well for our short-term study as we were able to rely on private companies that had the scale and technical capacity to meet our needs.

Certified radiologists immediately read and classified all of the CXR images before participants moved to the next station at the screening event. Although the radiologists were instructed to 'intentionally over-read' the CXR images, interpretation quality and reader fatigue were real concerns due to the high number of CXRs being read per day. The use of a CAR software to aide CXR interpretation would have been ideal in this high CXR throughput setting. Few CAR software platforms perform as well as experienced radiologists [40,41], and given the availability, quality and cost of radiologists in this setting, it is unlikely that a CAR software would be used to entirely replace human readers. However, a CAR software could be used to reduce workloads by triaging high-confidence normal CXR images, so that the radiologist can focus on providing clinical reports for abnormal images and interpreting the borderline abnormal images. In addition, a CAR software could be used as a live external quality assessment (EQA) tool, such that any abnormal CXR result, either from the radiologist or CAR software, could be used to indicate follow-on Xpert testing. Our study recorded a relatively low sputum collection rate after an abnormal CXR result (56.5%). We believe this was primarily driven by excessive over-reading of CXR images in the first third of our screening events. Using a CAR software as a live EQA tool could also help programs address this challenge by making evidence-based decisions to deprioritize some indicated sputum collection. Prospective feasibility and performance evaluations of CAR software should be conducted in settings where there are few access barriers to radiologists.

One of the most persistent challenges we faced during implementation was ensuring follow-on Xpert testing occurred in a timely fashion. Since a large number of people were screened each weekend, there were an average of 47 sputum specimens waiting every Monday morning to be tested when the laboratories re-opened. Each District TB Unit only has one four-module GeneXpert system, so we had to incentivize laboratory staff to perform tests past normal working hours to ensure a fast turnaround time and minimize sputum quality decay. In urban settings, it may make sense to set up a specialized high-volume Xpert testing facility that can handle the peaks of sputum testing which result from this type of active TB case-finding. Alternately, recent studies from other ACF initiatives in the region have shown that a pooled sputum testing approach could reduce workloads [42].

We estimated the performance of the different algorithms using published literature for the sensitivity of Xpert and AFB smear microscopy. However, these studies were primarily done in passive case-finding settings. Some literature has shown the sensitivity of Xpert during active case-finding to be just 50% [43]. The use of AFB smear microscopy during active case-finding is also highly discouraged due to its suboptimal specificity and common occurrence of false positive results [43]. Since the X-ray to Xpert algorithm is likely to detect people with paucibacillary disease, it is possible that our model over-estimated yields from other screening and diagnostic algorithms. Our study did not test symptomatic individuals with normal CXR results because prevalence survey results indicated that TB yields would be extremely low. We also did not estimate TB yields for this screening cohort when assessing the performance of different diagnostic algorithms for this same reason. However, it is possible that since our study mobilized higher risk populations, that TB yields in this screening cohort could possibly have been higher. We also were unable to assess how diagnosis would be impacted by systematic clinical evaluations, particularly for AFB smear microscopy-based algorithms.

5. Conclusions

Programmatic community-based CXR screening can be implemented in urban Vietnam and can achieve high overall yields of TB while detecting a large proportion of people who would likely otherwise have been missed by existing health services. Enhanced case-finding activities such as this are needed in order to improve the coverage of TB testing and treatment so that we can reach the End TB strategy goal of eliminating TB by 2035. However, this strategy is technically more complex and significantly more costly than using routine AFB smear microscopy testing. Thus, additional resources are required in order to scale up and sustain the types of strategies which are necessary to end TB.

Author Contributions: Conceptualization, A.J.C., L.N.Q.V., M.C., R.J.F. and T.N.V.; methodology, A.J.C., L.N.Q.V., M.C. and R.J.F.; formal analysis, A.J.C., L.N.Q.V. and R.J.F.; investigation, A.J.C., D.T., L.N.Q.V., R.J.F., T.D. and T.N.V.; resources A.J.C., L.N.Q.V., M.C. and R.J.F.; data curation A.J.C., D.T., L.N.Q.V., R.J.F., T.D., T.L. and T.N.V.; writing—original draft preparation, A.J.C., L.N.Q.V. and R.J.F.; writing—review and editing A.J.C., D.T., G.C.D., G.T.L., H.B.N., H.D.T.M., L.H.N., L.N.Q.V., M.C., N.V.N., R.J.F., T.D., T.L., H.H.N., T.N.V and V.V.T.; supervision, A.J.C., G.C.D., G.T.L., H.B.N., H.D.T.M., J.C., L.H.N., L.N.Q.V., M.C., N.V.N., R.J.F., T.L., H.H.N., T.N.V., V.V.T.; funding acquisition, A.J.C., L.N.Q.V., M.C. and R.J.F. All authors have read and agreed to the published version of the manuscript.

Funding: The IMPACT-TB study and A.J.C., L.N.Q.V., R.J.F., D.T. and M.C. were supported by the European Commission's Horizon 2020 Programme under grant agreement number 733174. We received additional support from the Stop TB Partnership's TB REACH initiative, with funding from Global Affairs Canada, to implement community activities.

Acknowledgments: The authors would like to thank Vietnam's NTP, Pham Ngoc Thach Hospital in Ho Chi Minh City and the District People's Committee, District General Hospital and District TB Unit in Districts 06, 08, 12, Binh Chanh, Go Vap, Hoc Mon and Tan Binh of Ho Chi Minh City. We would also like to thank the field staff of the Ho Chi Minh City Public Health Association, community health workers and student volunteers who worked to support the study, their communities and their patients.

Conflicts of Interest: The authors declare that there is no conflict of interest. A.J.C. works for the Stop TB Partnership's TB REACH initiative but was not involved in the decision to fund the grant which supported this work.

References

1. *Global Tuberculosis Report 2020*; World Health Organization: Geneva, Switzerland, 2020.
2. Nguyen, H.V.; Tiemersma, E.W.; Nguyen, H.B.; Cobelens, F.G.J.; Finlay, A.; Glaziou, P.; Dao, C.H.; Mirtskhulava, V.; Nguyen, H.V.; Pham, H.T.T.; et al. The second national tuberculosis prevalence survey in Vietnam. *PLoS ONE* **2020**, *15*, e0232142. [CrossRef]
3. Hoa, N.B.; Sy, D.N.; Nhung, N.V.; Tiemersma, E.W.; Borgdorff, M.W.; Cobelens, F.G. National survey of tuberculosis prevalence in Viet Nam. *Bull. World Health Organ.* **2010**, *88*, 273–280. [CrossRef]
4. *Global Tuberculosis Report 2018*; World Health Organization: Geneva, Switzerland, 2018.
5. *The End TB Strategy*; World Health Organization: Geneva, Switzerland, 2015.
6. Onozaki, I.; Law, I.; Sismanidis, C.; Zignol, M.; Glaziou, P.; Floyd, K. National tuberculosis prevalence surveys in Asia, 1990–2012: An overview of results and lessons learned. *Trop. Med. Int. Health* **2015**, *20*, 1128–1145. [CrossRef]
7. Frascella, B.; Richards, A.S.; Sossen, B.; Emery, J.C.; Odone, A.; Law, I.; Onozaki, I.; Esmail, H.; Houben, R.M.G.J. Subclinical tuberculosis disease—A review and analysis of prevalence surveys to inform definitions, burden, associations and screening methodology. *Clin. Infect. Dis.* **2020**. [CrossRef]
8. *Chest Radiography in Tuberculosis Detection: Summary of Current WHO Recommendations and Guidance on Programmatic Approaches*; World Health Organization: Geneva, Switzerland, 2016.
9. Biermann, O.; Lönnroth, K.; Caws, M.; Viney, K. Factors influencing active tuberculosis case-finding policy development and implementation: A scoping review. *BMJ Open* **2019**, *9*, e031284. [CrossRef]
10. *Guidelines on TB Diagnosis, Treatment and Prevention (1314/QĐ-BYT)*; Viet Nam Ministry of Health: Ha Noi, Viet Nam, 2020.
11. *2019 Final Report: Activities of the National TB Program*; National TB Program: Ha Noi, Viet Nam, 2020.
12. Morishita, F.; Garfin, A.M.C.G.; Lew, W.; Oh, K.H.; Yadav, R.-P.; Reston, J.C.; Infante, L.L.; Acala, M.R.C.; Palanca, D.L.; Kim, H.J.; et al. Bringing state-of-the-art diagnostics to vulnerable populations: The use of a mobile screening unit in active case finding for tuberculosis in Palawan, the Philippines. *PLoS ONE* **2017**, *12*, e0171310. [CrossRef]
13. Camelique, O.; Scholtissen, S.; Dousset, J.-P.; Bonnet, M.; Bastard, M.; Hewison, C. Mobile community-based active case-finding for tuberculosis among older populations in rural Cambodia. *Int. J. Tuberc. Lung Dis.* **2019**, *23*, 1107–1114. [CrossRef]
14. Madhani, F.; Maniar, R.A.; Burfat, A.; Ahmed, M.; Farooq, S.; Sabir, A.; Domki, A.K.; Page-Shipp, L.; Khowaja, S.; Safdar, N.; et al. Automated chest radiography and mass systematic screening for tuberculosis. *Int. J. Tuberc. Lung Dis.* **2020**, *24*, 665–673. [CrossRef]
15. Muyoyeta, M.; Maduskar, P.; Moyo, M.; Kasese, N.; Milimo, D.; Spooner, R.; Kapata, N.; Hogeweg, L.; van Ginneken, B.; Ayles, H. The Sensitivity and Specificity of Using a Computer Aided Diagnosis Program for Automatically Scoring Chest X-Rays of Presumptive TB Patients Compared with Xpert MTB/RIF in Lusaka Zambia. *PLoS ONE* **2014**, *9*, e93757. [CrossRef]
16. Ananthakrishnan, R.; Thiagesan, R.; Auguesteen, S.; Karunakaran, N.; Jayabal, L.; Stevens, R.; Codlin, A.; Creswell, J. The impact of chest radiography and Xpert MTB/RIF testing among household contacts in Chennai, India. *PLoS ONE* **2020**, *15*, e0241203. [CrossRef]
17. Kim, H.-Y.; Zishiri, V.; Page-Shipp, L.; Makgopa, S.; Churchyard, G.J.; Dowdy, D.; Charalambous, S.; Hoffmann, C.J. Symptom and digital chest X-ray TB screening in South African prisons: Yield and cost-effectiveness. *Int. J. Tuberc. Lung Dis.* **2020**, *24*, 295–302. [CrossRef] [PubMed]

18. Pelissari, D.M.; Kuhleis, D.C.; Bartholomay, P.; Barreira, D.; Oliveira, C.L.P.; de Jesus, R.S.; Possa, L.A.; Jarczewski, C.A.; Nemeth, L.T.; de Araujo, N.D.; et al. Prevalence and screening of active tuberculosis in a prison in the South of Brazil. *Int. J. Tuberc. Lung Dis.* **2018**, *22*, 1166–1171. [CrossRef] [PubMed]
19. Vo, L.N.Q.; Forse, R.J.; Codlin, A.J.; Vu, T.N.; Le, G.T.; Do, G.C.; Van Truong, V.; Dang, H.M.; Nguyen, L.H.; Nguyen, H.B.; et al. A comparative impact evaluation of two human resource models for community-based active tuberculosis case finding in Ho Chi Minh City, Viet Nam. *BMC Public Health* **2020**, *20*, 934. [CrossRef] [PubMed]
20. Vo, L.N.Q.; Forse, R.J.; Codlin, A.J.; Nguyen, N.T.; Vu, T.N.; Le, G.T.; Do, G.C.; Truong, V.V.; Dang, H.M.; Nguyen, L.H.; et al. Evaluating the yield of systematic screening for tuberculosis among three priority groups in Ho Chi Minh City, Viet Nam. *Infect. Dis. Poverty* **2020**, *20*, 1–12.
21. *Tuberculosis Prevalence Surveys: A Handbook*; World Health Organization: Geneva, Switzerland, 2011.
22. MacPherson, P.; Houben, R.M.G.J.; Glynn, J.R.; Corbett, E.L.; Kranzer, K. Pre-treatment loss to follow-up in tuberculosis patients in low- and lower-middle-income countries and high-burden countries: A systematic review and meta-analysis. *Bull. World Health Organ.* **2014**, *92*, 126–138. [CrossRef]
23. Steingart, K.R.; Schiller, I.; Horne, D.J.; Pai, M.; Boehme, C.C.; Dendukuri, N. Xpert® MTB/RIF assay for pulmonary tuberculosis and rifampicin resistance in adults. *Cochrane Database Syst. Rev.* **2014**, CD009593. [CrossRef]
24. *Toman's Tuberculosis: Case Detection, Treatment and Monitoring: Questions and Answers*, 2nd ed.; World Health Organization: Geneva, Switzerland, 2004.
25. Minh, H.V.; Mai, V.Q.; Nhung, N.V.; Hoi, L.V.; Giang, K.B.; Chung, L.H.; Kien, V.D.; Duyen, N.T.; Ngoc, N.B.; Anh, T.T.; et al. Costs of providing tuberculosis diagnosis and treatment services in Viet Nam. *Int. J. Tuberc. Lung Dis.* **2017**, *21*, 1035–1040. [CrossRef]
26. *Global Drug Facility (GDF) Diagnostics Catalog*; Stop TB Partnership: Geneva, Switzerland, 2020.
27. *External Quality Assessment for AFB Smear Microscopy*; Association of Public Health Laboratories (U.S.): Silver Spring, MD, USA; Centers for Disease Control and Prevention (U.S.): Atlanta, GA, USA; International Union against Tuberculosis and Lung Disease: Paris, France; World Health Organization: Geneva, Switzerland, 2002.
28. *Systematic Screening for Active Tuberculosis: An Operational Guide*; World Health Organization: Geneva, Switzerland, 2015.
29. *The Global Plan to End TB 2016–2020*; Stop TB Partnership: Geneva, Switzerland, 2015.
30. Marks, G.B.; Nguyen, N.V.; Nguyen, P.T.B.; Nguyen, T.-A.; Nguyen, H.B.; Tran, K.H.; Nguyen, S.V.; Luu, K.B.; Tran, D.T.T.; Vo, Q.T.N.; et al. Community-wide Screening for Tuberculosis in a High-Prevalence Setting. *N. Engl. J. Med.* **2019**, *381*, 1347–1357. [CrossRef]
31. Behr, M.A.; Warren, S.A.; Salamon, H.; Hopewell, P.C.; Ponce de Leon, A.; Daley, C.L.; Small, P.M. Transmission of Mycobacterium tuberculosis from patients smear-negative for acid-fast bacilli. *Lancet* **1999**, *353*, 444–449. [CrossRef]
32. Xie, Y.L.; Cronin, W.A.; Proschan, M.; Oatis, R.; Cohn, S.; Curry, S.R.; Golub, J.E.; Barry, C.E.; Dorman, S.E. Transmission of Mycobacterium tuberculosis From Patients Who Are Nucleic Acid Amplification Test Negative. *Clin. Infect. Dis.* **2018**, *67*, 1653–1659. [CrossRef]
33. Patterson, B.; Wood, R. Is cough really necessary for TB transmission? *Tuberculosis* **2019**, *117*, 31–35. [CrossRef] [PubMed]
34. Cadena, A.M.; Fortune, S.M.; Flynn, J.L. Heterogeneity in tuberculosis. *Nat. Rev. Immunol.* **2017**, *17*, 691–702. [CrossRef] [PubMed]
35. Loveday, M.; Ramjee, A.; Osburn, G.; Master, I.; Kabera, G.; Brust, J.C.M.; Padayatchi, N.; Warren, R.; Theron, G. Drug-resistant tuberculosis in patients with minimal symptoms: Favourable outcomes in the absence of treatment. *Int. J. Tuberc. Lung Dis.* **2017**, *21*, 556–563. [CrossRef] [PubMed]
36. Huong, N.T.; Vree, M.; Duong, B.D.; Khanh, V.T.; Loan, V.T.; Co, N.V.; Borgdorff, M.W.; Cobelens, F.G. Delays in the diagnosis and treatment of tuberculosis patients in Vietnam: A cross-sectional study. *BMC Public Health* **2007**, *7*, 110. [CrossRef] [PubMed]
37. Johansson, E.; Long, N.H.; Diwan, V.K.; Winkvist, A. Gender and tuberculosis control: Perspectives on health seeking behaviour among men and women in Vietnam. *Health Policy* **2000**, *52*, 33–51. [CrossRef]

38. Khan, M.S.; Dar, O.; Sismanidis, C.; Shah, K.; Godfrey-Faussett, P. Improvement of tuberculosis case detection and reduction of discrepancies between men and women by simple sputum-submission instructions: A pragmatic randomised controlled trial. *Lancet* **2007**, *369*, 1955–1960. [CrossRef]
39. Qin, Z.Z.; Ahmed, S.; Sarker, M.S.; Paul, K.; Adel, A.S.S.; Naheyan, T.; Banu, S.; Creswell, J. Can artificial intelligence (AI) be used to accurately detect tuberculosis (TB) from chest x-ray? A multiplatform evaluation of five AI products used for TB screening in a high TB-burden setting. *arXiv* **2020**, arXiv:200605509.
40. Qin, Z.Z.; Sander, M.S.; Rai, B.; Titahong, C.N.; Sudrungrot, S.; Laah, S.N.; Adhikari, L.M.; Carter, E.J.; Puri, L.; Codlin, A.J.; et al. Using artificial intelligence to read chest radiographs for tuberculosis detection: A multi-site evaluation of the diagnostic accuracy of three deep learning systems. *Sci. Rep.* **2019**, *9*, 15000. [CrossRef]
41. Chry, M.; Smelyanskaya, M.; Ky, M.; Codlin, A.J.; Cazabon, D.; Tan Eang, M.; Creswell, J. Can the High Sensitivity of Xpert MTB/RIF Ultra Be Harnessed to Save Cartridge Costs? Results from a Pooled Sputum Evaluation in Cambodia. *Trop. Med. Infect. Dis.* **2020**, *5*, 27. [CrossRef]
42. Sander, M.; Laah, S.; Titahong, C.; Lele, C.; Kinge, T.; de Jong, B.; Abena, J.-L.; Codlin, A.; Creswell, J. Systematic screening for tuberculosis among hospital outpatients in Cameroon: The role of screening and testing algorithms to improve case detection. *J. Clin. Tuberc. Other Mycobact. Dis.* **2019**, *15*, 100095. [CrossRef]
43. *Systematic Screening for Active Tuberculosis: Principles and Recommendations*; World Health Organization: Geneva, Switzerland, 2013.

Publisher's Note: MDPI stays neutral with regard to jurisdictional claims in published maps and institutional affiliations.

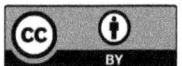

© 2020 by the authors. Licensee MDPI, Basel, Switzerland. This article is an open access article distributed under the terms and conditions of the Creative Commons Attribution (CC BY) license (http://creativecommons.org/licenses/by/4.0/).

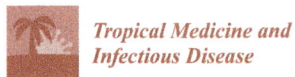

Article

Optimizing Active Tuberculosis Case Finding: Evaluating the Impact of Community Referral for Chest X-ray Screening and Xpert Testing on Case Notifications in Two Cities in Viet Nam

Tuan Huy Mac [1], Thuc Huy Phan [2], Van Van Nguyen [3], Thuy Thu Thi Dong [4], Hoi Van Le [5], Quan Duc Nguyen [2], Tho Duc Nguyen [1], Andrew James Codlin [4], Thuy Doan To Mai [4], Rachel Jeanette Forse [4], Lan Phuong Nguyen [4], Tuan Ho Thanh Luu [6], Hoa Binh Nguyen [5], Nhung Viet Nguyen [5], Xanh Thu Pham [2], Phap Ngoc Tran [7], Amera Khan [8], Luan Nguyen Quang Vo [4,9,*] and Jacob Creswell [8]

1 Hai Phong Lung Hospital, Hai Phong 180000, Vietnam; drtuanhpl@gmail.com (T.H.M.); tholaohp@gmail.com (T.D.N.)
2 Provincial Department of Health, Hai Phong 180000, Vietnam; thucphanhuy@gmail.com (T.H.P.); nguyenyquanhp@gmail.com (Q.D.N.); phamthuxanh@gmail.com (X.T.P.)
3 Provincial Department of Health, Quang Nam 560000, Vietnam; nhivan6@gmail.com
4 Friends for International TB Relief, Ha Noi 100000, Vietnam; thuy.dong@tbhelp.org (T.T.T.D.); andrew.codlin@tbhelp.org (A.J.C.); thuy.mai@tbhelp.org (T.D.T.M.); rachel.forse@tbhelp.org (R.J.F.); lan.nguyen@tbhelp.org (L.P.N.)
5 Viet Nam National Lung Hospital, Ha Noi 100000, Vietnam; hoilv@yahoo.com (H.V.L.); nguyenbinhhoatb@yahoo.com (H.B.N.); vietnhung@yahoo.com (N.V.N.)
6 Clinton Health Access Initiative, Ha Noi 100000, Vietnam; tluu@clintonhealthaccess.org
7 Pham Ngoc Thach Quang Nam Hospital, Quang Nam 560000, Vietnam; phapqnam@gmail.com
8 Stop TB Partnership, 1218 Geneva, Switzerland; amerak@stoptb.org (A.K.); jacobc@stoptb.org (J.C.)
9 Interactive Research and Development, Singapore 189677, Singapore
* Correspondence: luan.vo@tbhelp.org; Tel.: +84-902-908004

Received: 30 September 2020; Accepted: 7 November 2020; Published: 30 November 2020

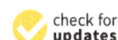

Abstract: To accelerate the reduction in tuberculosis (TB) incidence, it is necessary to optimize the use of innovative tools and approaches available within a local context. This study evaluated the use of an existing network of community health workers (CHW) for active case finding, in combination with mobile chest X-ray (CXR) screening events and the expansion of Xpert MTB/RIF testing eligibility, in order to reach people with TB who had been missed by the current system. A controlled intervention study was conducted from January 2018 to March 2019 in five intervention and four control districts of two low to medium TB burden cities in Viet Nam. CHWs screened and referred eligible persons for CXR to TB care facilities or mobile screening events in the community. The initial diagnostic test was Xpert MTB/RIF for persons with parenchymal abnormalities suggestive of TB on CXR or otherwise on smear microscopy. We analyzed the TB care cascade by calculating the yield and number needed to screen (NNS), estimated the impact on TB notifications and conducted a pre-/postintervention comparison of TB notification rates using controlled, interrupted time series (ITS) analyses. We screened 30,336 individuals in both cities to detect and treat 243 individuals with TB, 88.9% of whom completed treatment successfully. All forms of TB notifications rose by +18.3% (95% CI: +15.8%, +20.8%). The ITS detected a significant postintervention step-increase in the intervention area for all-form TB notification rates (IRR(β6) = 1.221 (95% CI: 1.011, 1.475); p = 0.038). The combined use of CHWs for active case findings and mobile CXR screening expanded the access to and uptake of Xpert MTB/RIF testing and resulted in a significant increase in TB notifications. This model could serve as a blueprint for expansion throughout Vietnam. Moreover, the results demonstrate the need to optimize the use of the best available tools and approaches in order to end TB.

Keywords: tuberculosis; active case finding; community health workers; mobile X-ray screening

---

1. Introduction

In 2014, the Government of Viet Nam passed legislation with the vision of ending tuberculosis (TB) by 2030 [1]. This goal seemed within reach, with a reported treatment coverage of 87% in 2018 [2]. However, the second national prevalence survey revealed that a large detection gap remained as treatment coverage estimates were revised downwards to 57% in 2019 [3]. This gap, in human terms, means that approximately 74,000 people with TB are unreached by the National TB Control Program (NTP), and this is a formidable barrier to the nation's ambitions to end TB.

The prevalence survey results also demonstrated that a "business-as-usual" approach was insufficient to end TB and evinced the need for active case finding (ACF), as many people with TB identified in the survey were previously undiagnosed. To generate the evidence in support of an ACF scale-up, Viet Nam conducted a randomized controlled trial that featured population-wide outreach with dedicated teams conducting door-to-door visits to offer unrestricted testing on the Xpert MTB/RIF (Xpert) assay as the initial diagnostic test on any obtainable expectorate [4]. While the trial demonstrated the possibility of drastic reductions in TB prevalence through ACF, the approach was extremely resource-intensive.

The programmatic implementation of resource-intensive strategies, even if strongly evidenced, has traditionally faced challenges [5–7]. Common barriers are unsustainable human, financial and technical resource requirements [8]. In Viet Nam, these barriers are exacerbated by the resource needs to compensate for lower-than-expected treatment coverage following the second prevalence survey as well as delays in the transition of TB program financing to national social health insurance [9]. Hence, the NTP is keen to optimize its resource utilization by providing Xpert testing mainly to persons with the highest risk of suffering from active TB disease.

There is extensive evidence that parenchymal abnormalities suggestive of TB on chest radiography (CXR) represent a critical risk factor of active TB disease [10,11]. Based on this evidence, CXR has been recommended as a screening and triage tool placed early in TB diagnostic algorithms [12]. The NTP has committed to expand the use of CXR as a triage tool for the indication of Xpert testing as part of its national diagnostic roadmap [9]. This diagnostic algorithm, locally dubbed the "Double-X" or "2X" algorithm, is cited to have the potential to significantly reduce laboratory burdens, costs per true case detected and false-positive bacteriological test results [13,14]. Previous studies have also found that this algorithm offers a good balance between sensitivity and costs [15,16].

There is a growing consensus that a comprehensive, intensified approach is needed to progress towards ending TB [17]. Critical components of such a comprehensive approach include ACF and prompt treatment initiation as a means to stop transmission, treating subclinical TB infection for persons most likely to progress to active TB disease and addressing the social determinants of TB treatment [18–20]. In 2017, the NTP launched the Zero TB Viet Nam (ZTV) project as a pilot for such an approach in Viet Nam. As part of its ACF activities, the project tested an intensified TB case finding approach with a targeted case detection through the engagement of community health workers (CHW) as well as an early diagnosis and initiation of appropriate treatment via the 2X diagnostic algorithm [21].

2. Materials and Methods

2.1. Study Design

This study was a prospective controlled cohort intervention study that aimed to measure the yield, treatment outcomes and additional impact on case notifications of an intensified community-based active case finding intervention.

2.2. Study Setting

The study was conducted from January 2018 until March 2019 in nine districts in Viet Nam. These included five intervention and four control districts (Figure 1).

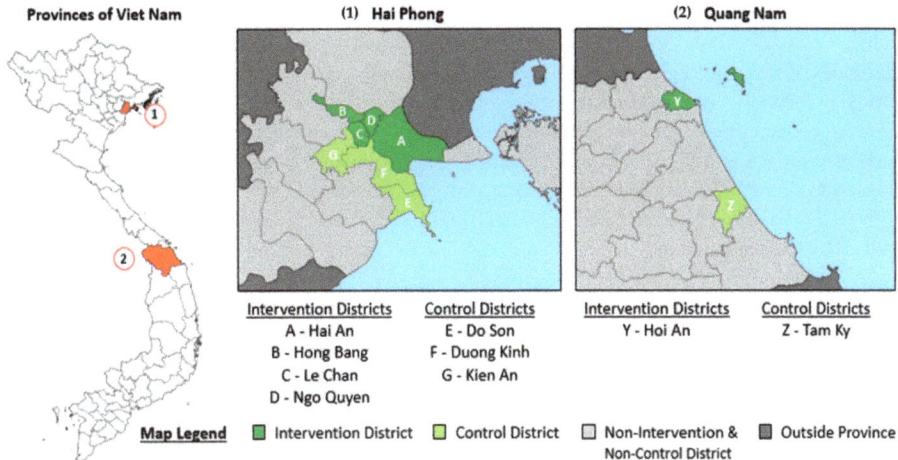

Figure 1. Map of intervention and control provinces and districts. Hai Phong and Quang Nam, Viet Nam. January 2018 to March 2019.

The intervention area included four districts in Hai Phong provincial city and the district-level city of Hoi An in the Quang Nam province. The five intervention districts had a population of 717,343 and notified 376 people with all forms TB in 2017 for a case notification rate (CNR) of 52/100,000. The control area was selected based on recommendations from the provincial TB programs to match the intervention areas in approximate size and TB burden as well as the absence of any case finding interventions. The control area included three districts in Hai Phong and the district-level city of Tam Ky in Quang Nam. The cumulative control district population was 377,130 and notified 150 people with all forms TB in 2017 for a CNR of 40/100,000. The District TB Unit (DTU) and other NTP-affiliated TB clinics managed diagnosis, treatment and notification according to national guidelines under the technical supervision of the Hai Phong and Quang Nam provincial lung hospitals.

2.3. Community Health Workers

The study recruited a cadre of 60 CHWs in both cities to carry out ACF activities. The community network engaged in Hai Phong and Hoi An was provided by the General Department of Population and Family Planning (GDPFP) under the Ministry of Health. The GDPFP employs a network of over 11,000 commune coordinators, who are full-time government staff responsible for coordinating a government network of community volunteers at the subcommune level. Their primary duties consist of population surveillance as well as advocacy and care in the fields of sexual and reproductive health, and maternal and child health [22]. Most coordinators hold intermediate college degrees in the fields of midwifery and nursing. The 60 individuals selected by the study to be CHWs received a two-day training focused on a basic level of TB literacy, core study objectives and responsibilities, and associated recording and reporting requirements on the study's Android-based, mobile health (mHealth) application. Each CHW received a remuneration package that included a stipend of USD 22.70 per month as well as performance-based incentives of USD 0.45 per successful CXR referral and USD 2.27 per successful linkage to treatment of a person diagnosed with TB.

2.4. Target Populations

The target groups consisted of contacts of a TB index case and urban priority groups, including people aged 55 years and over, individuals with a history of TB treatment during the prior two years (2016–2017) and urban poor households based on national poverty definitions. These groups were prioritized at the discretion of the Provincial TB control programs based on the historically observed higher incidence in these groups.

Index cases were defined as anyone prospectively notified with drug-susceptible TB regardless of bacteriological status or disease site (all forms). Anyone who shared a kitchen with the index case or close contacts who had interacted with the index case at least once per week met the inclusion criteria for contact investigation. CHWs obtained index patient details from NTP patient registers. Household contacts (HHC) were enumerated and screened during home visits. Index patients were requested to identify other close contacts and provide relevant phone numbers and/or addresses. Elderly individuals were identified through the GDPFP's local census. Low income households were identified by local authorities.

2.5. ACF Activities

The study's process flow of the ACF activities is depicted in Figure 2. CHWs systematically screened target populations though home visits and mobile screening events using a bespoke mHealth application (TechUp/Clinton Health Access Initiative; Ha Noi, Viet Nam). Screening activities were promoted and enhanced through the distribution of educational pamphlets to encourage awareness and participation. During home visits, CHWs verbally screened all individuals for clinical symptoms and a history of TB. Clinical symptoms included (productive) cough, hemoptysis, fever, weight loss, night sweats, dyspnea, chest pain and fatigue, as per national guidelines. Any household contact was eligible for CXR referral, irrespective of symptomatic presentation. All other individuals targeted for screening were eligible for CXR if they reported at least one symptom or had a history of TB. Eligible individuals received a voucher for a free CXR at NTP-designated facilities. In addition to the home visits, the provincial TB programs organized 46 community CXR screening events in Hai Phong and four in Hoi An using mobile CXR vans to improve uptake. CXR images were read by a NTP-trained radiologist, and persons with abnormalities suggestive of TB provided a sputum sample for testing on the Xpert MTB/RIF assay (Cepheid; Sunnyvale, CA, USA). Any symptomatic individual without CXR results or with chest radiograph findings not associated with TB was referred for smear microscopy. Persons with a positive Xpert result and a history of TB were further tested on smear and culture, if needed, as per NTP guidelines. Symptomatic persons with negative sputum test results were evaluated for a clinical diagnosis according to NTP guidelines. Children with presumptive TB were referred to the Provincial Lung Hospital for further evaluation. Persons diagnosed with active TB were linked to care at their provider of choice and followed up until treatment completion.

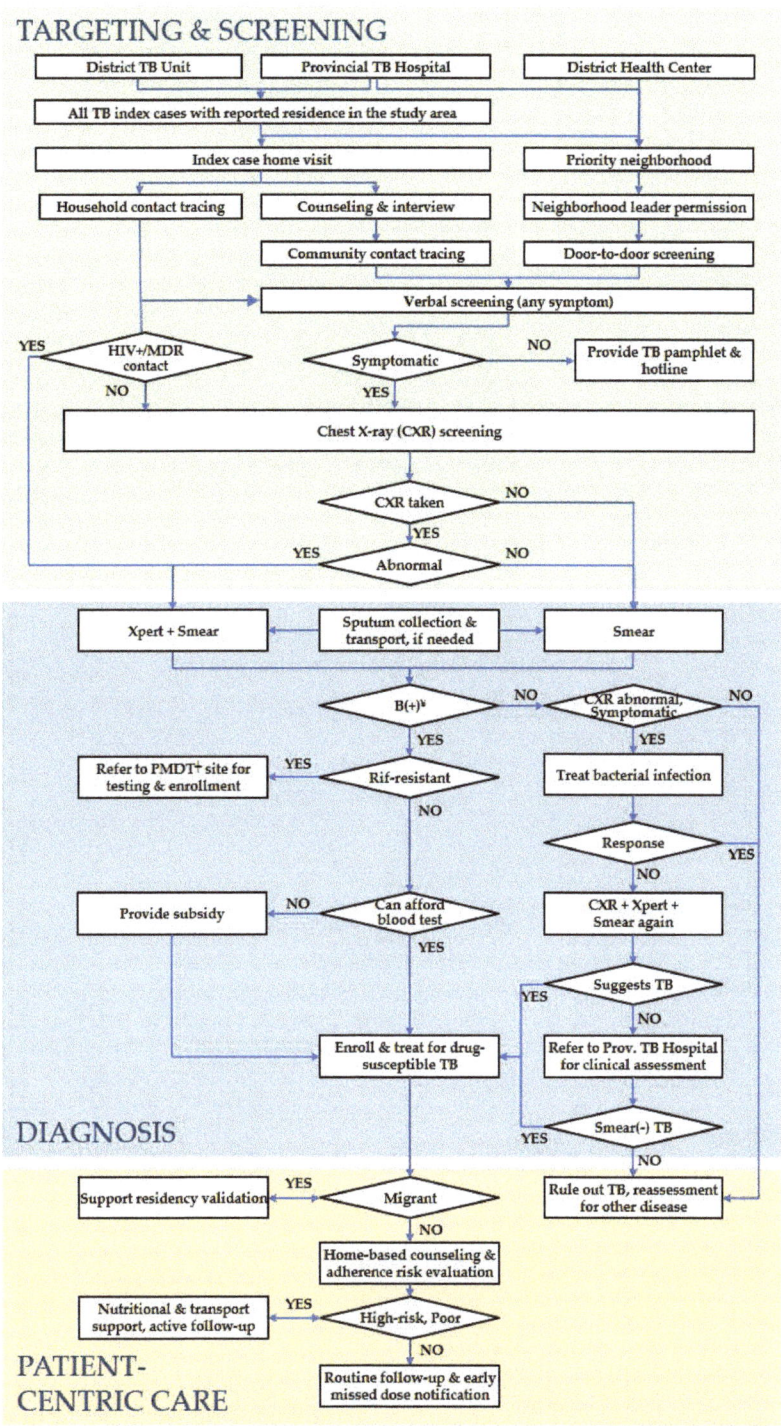

Figure 2. Process flow of the ACF activities. Hai Phong and Quang Nam, Viet Nam. January 2018 to March 2019. ¥ Bacteriologically-confirmed; ‡ Programmatic Management of Drug-Resistant TB.

2.6. Data Analysis

We calculated the number and proportion of persons in each step in the TB care cascade starting with those verbally screened and eligible for CXR until treatment completion [23] by city and further bifurcated the cascade by CXR screening site, i.e., facility vs. mobile van. We calculated the cumulative and city-disaggregated changes in all forms and bacteriologically confirmed TB notifications applying historical and contemporaneous controls [24]. To verify these results in light of secular trends, we conducted comparative interrupted time series (ITS) analyses of population-standardized aggregated quarterly all-form and bacteriologically confirmed TB notification rates. The ITS analyses employed segmented methods to model a postintervention step-change (β_6) and subsequent trend differences (β_6). The time series data consisted of 21 observations of quarterly TB notification rates in intervention and control areas. This included 16 preintervention quarters and five quarters of implementation of ACF interventions [25]. These methods were applied to marginal log-linear Poisson regression models using the generalized estimating equation (GEE) approach. We tested for serial autocorrelation using the Cumby–Huizinga test with a threshold of $p < 0.05$, and specified lag parameters of the model based on the lowest quasi-likelihood information criterion values. Statistical analyses were performed on Stata 13 (StataCorp; College Station, TX, USA). Hypothesis tests were two-sided, and point estimates included 95% confidence intervals.

2.7. Ethical Considerations

The study protocol was approved by the Scientific and Ethics Committee of the Hai Phong University of Medicine and Pharmacy (82/QD-YDHP) and the Ethics Committee for Biomedical Research & Committee for Science and Technology of Pham Ngoc Thach Hospital (430/HDDD-PNT). The NTP (909/QD-BVPTW) and the Ministry of Health (3651/QD-BYT) granted technical and administrative approval for the study's implementation. We obtained written informed consent from participants during each screening encounter and de-identified all personal data. Persons who did not consent still received testing and treatment per the study protocol and NTP guidelines, but were excluded from all analyses.

3. Results

3.1. ACF Outputs

The aggregate TB care cascade is shown in Figure 3. Over 15 months, the CHWs verbally screened 30,336 individuals. CXR results were recorded for 67.2% (20,389/30,336), among whom the abnormality rate was 18.4% (3749/20,389). We tested the sputum of 2249 individuals, including 1655 with Xpert tests (44.1% of those eligible) and 594 smear tests. We diagnosed 268 people with TB. Of these individuals with TB, 90.7% (243/268) initiated treatment. This represents a yield of 801/100,000 and an NNS of 125. Of these people with TB, 88.9% (216/243) completed treatment successfully, 7.8% (19/243) were lost to follow-up, 1.6% (4/243) were not evaluated due to a transfer to an MDR-TB treatment regimen and 1.6% (4/243) died.

Table 1 shows the disaggregated TB care cascade and treatment outcomes by the three urban priority groups. Of the 30,336 individuals screened, 14.0% (4259/30,336) were HHCs, among whom 41 were initiated on TB treatment for a prevalence of 963/100,000 and an NNS of 104. Close contacts comprised just 4.3% (1313/30,336) of the sample. Eight close contacts were initiated on treatment for a prevalence of 609/100,000 or an NNS of 164. The proportion of urban priority area residents among screened individuals was 82.1% (24,764/30,336), of whom 194 individuals were initiated on treatment for a prevalence of 783/100,000 and an NNS of 128. Overall, 88.9% (216/243) of those enrolled successfully completed treatment (Table 2). The treatment success rates among household contacts, social and close contacts, and urban priority area residents were 87.8% (36/41), 100.0% (8/8) and 88.7% (172/194), respectively.

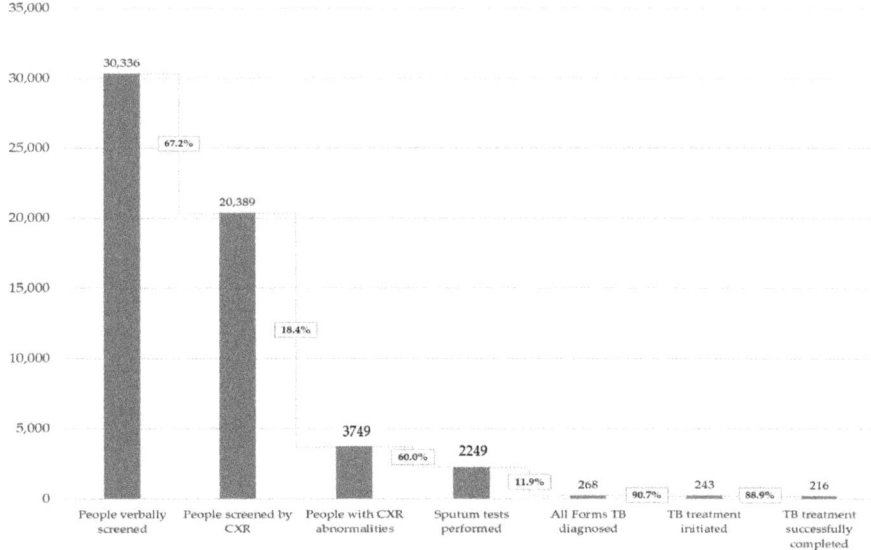

Figure 3. Aggregate TB care cascade. Hai Phong and Quang Nam, Viet Nam. January 2018 to March 2019.

Table 1. TB care cascade disaggregated by urban priority group. Hai Phong and Quang Nam, Viet Nam. January 2018 to March 2019.

	Total N (%)	Household Contacts N (%)	Social & Close Contacts N (%)	Urban Priority Area Residents N (%)
Individuals verbally screened	30,336 (100.0%)	4259 (100.0%)	1313 (100.0%)	24,764 (100.0%)
Individuals screened by CXR	20,389 (67.2%)	2087 (49.0%)	563 (42.9%)	17,739 (71.6%)
–Individuals with abnormal CXR screen	3749 (12.4%)	266 (6.2%)	101 (7.7%)	3382 (13.7%)
Individuals tested for TB (any sputum test)	2249 (7.4%)	184 (4.3%)	65 (5.0%)	2000 (8.1%)
–Individuals tested for TB with Xpert	1655 (5.5%)	120 (2.8%)	45 (3.4%)	1490 (6.0%)
Individuals diagnosed with All Forms TB	268 (0.9%)	44 (1.0%)	9 (0.7%)	215 (0.9%)
–Individuals diagnosed Xpert(+)	149 (0.5%)	14 (0.3%)	8 (0.6%)	127 (0.5%)
All Forms TB patients started on treatment	243 (0.8%)	41 (1.0%)	8 (0.6%)	194 (0.8%)
–NNS	125	104	164	128

Table 2. TB treatment outcomes by urban priority group. Hai Phong and Quang Nam, Viet Nam. January 2018 to March 2019.

	Total N (%)	Household Contacts N (%)	Social & Close Contacts N (%)	Urban Priority Area Residents N (%)
Treated successfully	216 (88.9%)	36 (87.8%)	8 (100.0%)	172 (88.7%)
Lost to follow-up	19 (7.8%)	5 (12.2%)	0 (0.0%)	14 (7.2%)
Died	4 (1.6%)	0 (0.0%)	0 (0.0%)	4 (2.1%)
Not evaluated/failure	4 (1.6%)	0 (0.0%)	0 (0.0%)	4 (2.1%)

Figure 4 shows the TB care cascade disaggregated by city and by facility-based or community-based CXR screening location. There were notable differences between the two cities. In Hai Phong, CHWs engaged and verbally screened 23,967 persons from the target populations, of whom 71.7% (17,191/23,967) presented for a CXR. In comparison, only 50.2% (3198/6369) of the individuals screened in Hoi An had a recorded CXR result. Of the total number of CXRs taken in Hai Phong, only 19.9% (3428/17,191) were facility-based, while 80.1% (13,763/17,191) of CXRs originated from mobile CXR screening events. In comparison, 71.2% (2278/3198) of CXRs in Hoi An were taken at a facility, and only

28.8% (920/3198) of CXRs were recorded from mobile screening events. Similarly, the aggregate proportion of Xpert testing among all sputum tests in Hai Phong was 85.0% (1516/1783) compared to 29.8% (139/466) in Hoi An. ACF activities in Hai Phong yielded 223 persons diagnosed with TB, of whom 88.8% (198/223) were initiated on treatment, corresponding to a yield of 826/100,000 and an NNS of 121. In Hoi An, ACF activities resulted in 45 persons diagnosed with TB and initiated on treatment, corresponding to a yield of 707/100,000 and an NNS of 142.

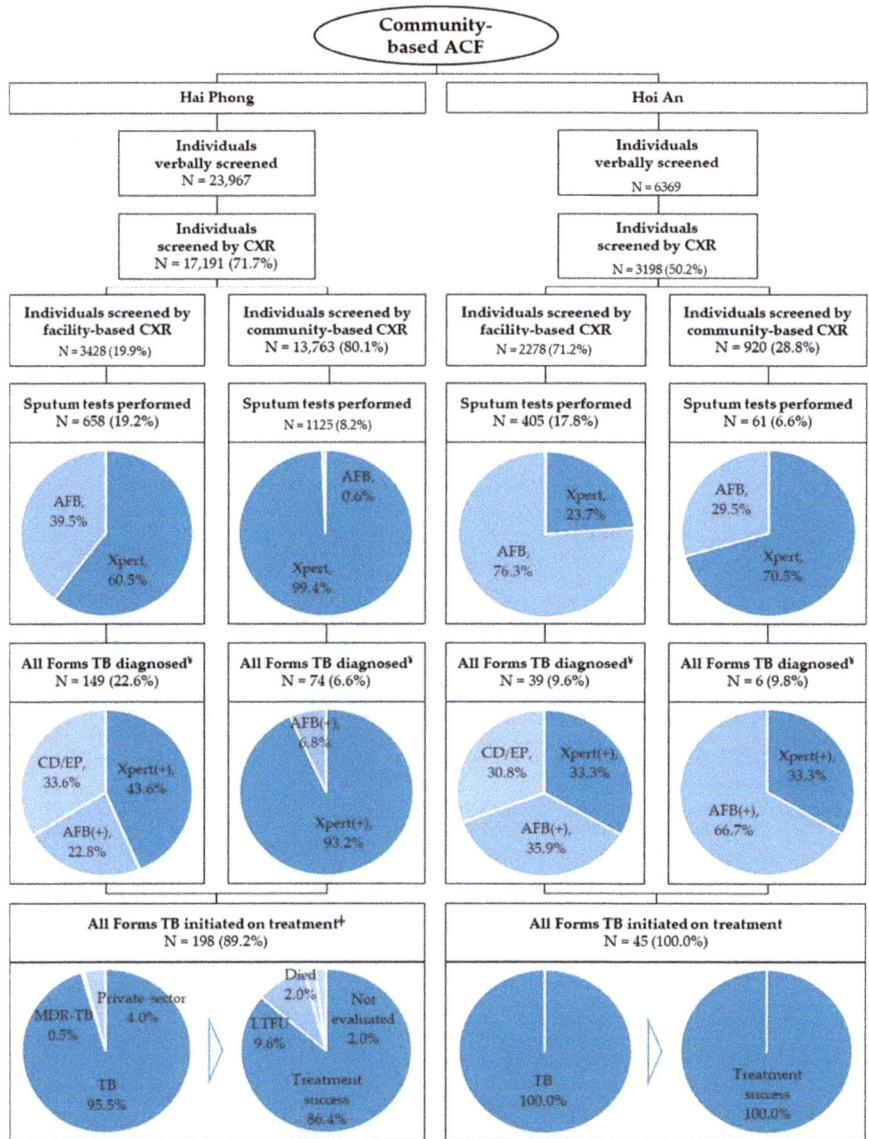

Figure 4. TB care cascade by city and CXR screening site. Hai Phong and Quang Nam, Viet Nam. January 2018 to March 2019. ¥ In the event that a positive AFB and Xpert result was recorded, the patient was categorized as an AFB(+) case. ‡ All private sector patients had rifampicin-susceptible TB.

3.2. Impact on Notifications

All forms TB notifications across both intervention cities (Table 3) increased by +18.3% (+15.8%, +20.8%), corresponding to 165 (142, 188) additional TB notifications. All-form TB notifications by city rose by +11.0% (+9.2%, +12.9%) in Hai Phong compared to +35.4% (+26.8%, +44.1%) in Hoi An. These rates corresponded to 123 (102, 144) additional all-form TB notifications in Hai Phong and 42 (32, 52) in Hoi An. Bacteriologically-confirmed TB notifications increased by +32.9% (+27.8%, +37.9%), corresponding to 108 (91, 125) additional TB cases over the baseline. In Hai Phong, the estimated impact on notifications was +30.6% (+24.9%, +36.3%), corresponding to 76 (62, 90) additional cases. In Hoi An, the increase in notifications was +36.5% (+26.4%, +46.5%), corresponding to 32 (23, 41) additional people with bacteriologically confirmed TB.

Table 3. Impact analysis [24] of all forms and bacteriologically confirmed TB notifications by city. Hai Phong and Quang Nam, Viet Nam. January 2018 to March 2019.

	Cumulative Notifications		Trend Differences			
	Baseline Period [†]	Intervention Period	# Cases	95% CI	% Change [§]	95% CI
All forms TB						
Cumulative additional notifications			165	(142,188)	18.3%	(15.8%, 20.8%)
Hai Phong			123	(102,144)	11.0%	(9.2%, 12.9%)
Intervention area	706	850	144	(123,165)	20.4%	(17.4%, 23.4%)
Control area	224	245	21	(12,30)	9.4%	(5.6%, 13.2%)
Hoi An			42	(32,52)	35.4%	(26.8%, 44.1%)
Intervention area	112	148	36	(26,46)	32.1%	(23.5%, 40.8%)
Control area	182	176	−6	(−11,−1)	−3.3%	(−5.9%, −0.7%)
Bacteriologically confirmed TB						
Cumulative additional notifications			108	(91,125)	32.9%	(27.8%, 37.9%)
Hai Phong			76	(62,90)	30.6%	(24.9%, 36.3%)
Intervention area	354	419	65	(51,79)	18.4%	(14.3%, 22.4%)
Control area	90	79	−11	(−17,−5)	−12.2%	(−19.0%, −5.5%)
Hoi An			32	(23,41)	36.5%	(26.4%, 46.5%)
Intervention area	77	93	16	(9,23)	20.8%	(11.7%, 29.8%)
Control area	102	86	−16	(−23,−9)	−15.7%	(−22.7%, −8.6%)

[†] The baseline period consists of the January 2017–December 2017 timeframe; the cumulative baseline notifications are the sum of notifications matched by quarter to the intervention period of January 2018–March 2019 to account for seasonality, i.e., Q1 2018 matched with Q1 2017, Q2 2018 matched with Q2 2017, Q3 2018 matched with Q3 2017, Q4 2018 matched with Q4 2017 and Q1 2019 matched with Q1 2017. [§] The sums of the percentage point estimates include rounding effects; The number of cases denotes the double difference between pre- and postimplementation and between intervention and control areas.

The ITS analyses results are in Table 4 and Figure 5. The baseline median quarterly all-form TB notification rate was 24.7 (IQR: 21.9–27.1) per 100,000 in the intervention area and 22.0 (IQR: 19.1–23.6) in the control area. In the post-implementation period, there was a significant step-change in all-form TB notification rates (IRR(β_6) = 1.221 (1.011, 1.475); p = 0.038) and bacteriologically confirmed TB notification rates (IRR(β_6) = 1.535 (1.067, 2.210); p = 0.021).

Table 4. Comparative ITS analysis model parameters of population-standardized quarterly notification rates of all-form and bacteriologically confirmed TB cases for intervention vs. control districts ¥. Hai Phong and Quang Nam, Viet Nam. January 2018 to March 2019.

Comparative ITS Analysis Model Parameters	Intervention vs. Control Districts		
	IRR ‡	95% CI	p-Value ⌐
All Forms TB			
Baseline rate (β_0)	21.563	(20.108, 23.124)	<0.001
Preintervention trend, control (β_1)	0.998	(0.990, 1.006)	0.590
Postintervention step change, control (β_2)	1.116	(0.952, 1.308)	0.178
Postintervention trend, control (β_3)	0.977	(0.923, 1.034)	0.427
Difference in baseline (β_4)	1.378	(1.270, 1.495)	<0.001
Difference in preintervention trends (β_5)	0.977	(0.967, 0.986)	<0.001
Difference in postintervention step change (β_6)	1.221	(1.011, 1.475)	0.038
Difference in postintervention trends (β_7)	1.015	(0.948, 1.086)	0.676
Bacteriologically confirmed TB			
Baseline rate (β_0)	11.107	(9.562, 12.901)	<0.001
Preintervention trend, control (β_1)	0.992	(0.975, 1.009)	0.361
Postintervention step change, control (β_2)	0.807	(0.587, 1.109)	0.186
Postintervention trend, control (β_3)	1.043	(0.935, 1.163)	0.448
Difference in baseline (β_4)	1.141	(0.956, 1.362)	0.144
Difference in preintervention trends (β_5)	1.001	(0.981, 1.021)	0.928
Difference in postintervention step change (β_6)	1.535	(1.067, 2.210)	0.021
Difference in postintervention trends (β_7)	0.902	(0.796, 1.023)	0.108

¥ The parameters were obtained for a segmented regression model with the following structure: $Y_t = \beta_0 + \beta_1 T_t + \beta_2 X_t + \beta_3 X_t T_t + \beta_4 Z + \beta_5 ZT_t + \beta_6 ZX_t + \beta_6 ZX_t T_t + \epsilon_t$. Here, Y_t is the outcome measure along time t; T_t is the monthly time counter; X_t indicates pre- and postintervention periods, Z denotes the intervention cohort, and ZT_t, ZX_t, and $ZX_t T_t$ are interaction terms. β_0 to β_3 relate to the control group as follows: β_0, intercept; β_1, preintervention trend; β_2, postintervention step change; β_3, postintervention trend. β_4 to β_7 represent differences between the control and intervention districts: β_4, difference in baseline intercepts; β_5, difference in preintervention trends; β_6, difference in postintervention step changes; β_7, difference in postintervention trend. ‡ IRR is based on a log-linear GEE Poisson regression with correlation structures, as determined by the Cumby–Huizinga test and Quasi-Information Criteria; ⌐, Wald test.

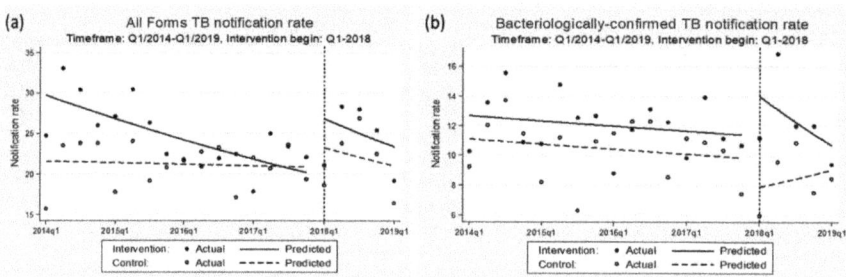

Figure 5. Comparative ITS analysis model graphs of population-standardized quarterly notification rates of (**a**) all-form TB case notification rates and (**b**) bacteriologically confirmed TB case notification rates for intervention vs. control areas. Hai Phong and Quang Nam, Viet Nam. January 2018 to March 2019. Notes: In the baseline period, the predicted line indicates the fitted model based on historical actual notification rates.

4. Discussion

The results of our study demonstrate that CHWs were effective in mobilizing and verbally screening a large number of people and in ultimately detecting persons suffering from TB. The analysis of notification data showed that a substantial portion of this yield translated to additional TB notifications over the baseline. Adjusting for demographic changes and other secular confounders showed that the additional TB notifications comprised a significant change from the status quo. Our results add to a growing literature documenting the impact of community-based ACF on increasing TB case notifications [26,27].

The yield achieved on this project underlines the high number of people in the community who have TB yet remain unreached and were underestimated prior to Viet Nam's second prevalence survey. In this study, this was particularly evident among urban priority area residents without documented exposure to an index patient. A key catalyst for the high yield was the use of the 2X diagnostic algorithm and the use of Xpert as the initial diagnostic tool. Prior to this project, Hai Phong and Hoi An used smear as the primary diagnostic tool, while Xpert was reserved for drug-susceptibility testing. The impact of using Xpert for TB diagnosis on the yield was evidenced by the intercity differences in the number of people tested and bacteriologically confirmed on Xpert. Specifically, the Hai Phong provincial TB program was able to avail Xpert to a larger proportion of people screened and as such achieved a higher yield. This elevated yield from the introduction of Xpert as the initial diagnostic test has been previously documented in many other settings [28–30].

However, studies have shown that a high yield and low NNS from more sensitive diagnostic tools and algorithms in isolation does not necessarily translate to additional notifications [31,32]. As vulnerable groups with low NNS are often also small in numbers, it has been noted that the use of more sensitive diagnostic tools and algorithms must be complemented by efforts to increase the number of people referred for screening and testing [33]. This particularly applies to individuals who may otherwise not have sought care [34] due to the lack of symptomatic presentation or recognition, challenging socioeconomic conditions or indomitable sociocultural barriers [35–38]. One way of reaching more people with TB is effective community engagement.

In this study, community engagement was facilitated by the GDPFP network of CHWs. These CHWs were able to seamlessly integrate the study's ACF activities into their daily responsibilities. As Viet Nam's population growth and demographics have stabilized, the GDPFP is looking to repurpose its community network to address other public health concerns. This type of repurposing of existing health worker networks has also been successfully implemented in other settings [39]. As such, the study raised notifications without creating new or redundant community structures and thereby offers a potential avenue for a national scale-up. Accessing the existing GDPFP network played an important role in the fidelity of this study [40]. Coordination with the provincial branches of the GDPFP generated operational efficiencies by simplifying the recruitment process, given that GDPFP coordinator rosters were readily available. Since these coordinators were experienced in the delivery of public health services, it was possible to impart TB literacy in a relatively short amount of time at a high level of quality [40]. As these coordinators were full-time employees, attrition was also lower than what was typically observed in community health worker and volunteer networks [41,42].

The synergies of combining responsibilities likely also contributed to the high efficiency in our study. Both cities exhibited a similar NNS that was relatively low in comparison to reported values from systematic screening in other target groups [43]. Similarly, our study recorded a high rate of CXR screening among persons that were verbally engaged. According to field staff, the CHWs leveraged their existing relationships with community leaders to establish a personal referral system. Through this system, symptomatic persons could confide in a trusted community member before presenting at a health facility. This trust in CHWs is a key reason why their services are often considered more person-centric than that of formal healthcare providers [44]. A critical question consists in the ability of repurposed CHWs to multitask without making concessions on the quality of care. While we did not systematically measure the level of multitasking and performance across all of the individual CHWs' duties or the CHWs' contribution to the measured treatment outcomes on this study, the ability of CHWs to effectively manage multiple responsibilities for TB and other public health indications has been documented elsewhere [45–47]. For example, Ethiopian health workers reported receiving positive feedback from their communities on the provision of multiple tasks and noticed the impact that their work made, which was motivating for them [48].

Nevertheless, we still faced challenges in community mobilization efforts despite the support from the CHWs. Specifically, we found that CXR triaging could work as an access barrier to care as health-seeking persons had to present at an X-ray facility. This risk is noted in the WHO guidelines on the role of chest radiography in TB [13]. Studies have also linked facility-based health-seeking to higher directly incurred expenses and lost time [49]. To reduce these diagnostic access barriers, the project implemented weekend community screening events using mobile CXR vans. These vans are abundant in the Vietnamese context for statutory occupational health screening in formal workplace settings and have been used in the past for TB screening in closed settings and on prevalence surveys [50]. The benefit of this strategy was evident in Hai Phong, where the participation rate in CXR screening was substantially higher than in Hoi An. The consequence of the higher CXR participation rate was that more health-seeking persons were able to access Xpert testing. The utility of mobile CXR events and their ability to reduce TB care access barriers, particularly for vulnerable populations such as the urban priority area residents, has also been demonstrated in other settings [51,52]. Another limitation of the approach consisted in the potential heterogeneity in CXR interpretations across different human readers. Future studies should further explore this limitation and the utility of computer-aided reading solutions in active case finding settings such as the one implemented in this project [53].

Our study was limited by confounding effects in the control districts of Hai Phong from a concurrent scale-up of public-private mix (PPM) activities in the city [54]. This resulted in a positive notification trend in the control districts, which affected the additionality results. This PPM scale-up was also evident in the proportion of TB patients detected by our intervention who chose private sector treatment. The ITS analysis detected a significant step-change but did not detect a change in long-term trends, suggesting diminishing returns from our ACF activities. This lack of sustained impact may have been a result of the short timeframe of the project and should be further investigated through appropriately powered cluster randomized trials. Moreover, the additional notifications constituted only half of the estimated case detection gap, suggesting that a more comprehensive evaluation, inclusive of ACF and PPM activities, is required to close the TB treatment coverage gap.

Last, the study focused mainly on active tuberculosis, and future studies should investigate the possibility of integrated screening, testing and treatment of TB and latent TB infection. Similarly, as high-burden countries begin to expand Xpert coverage through strategies such as the 2X diagnostic algorithm in Viet Nam, the cost-effectiveness of these strategies need further investigation to complement their potential epidemiologic benefits.

5. Conclusions

Our study evidenced that ACF, through a combination of community engagement through CHWs and the reduction of access barriers to CXR screening and subsequent Xpert testing, can locate previously unreached persons with TB. These findings may serve as further evidence in favor of the scale-up of intensified case finding activities for TB in Viet Nam and other high-burden settings.

Author Contributions: Conceptualization, T.H.M., P.N.T., V.V.N., T.T.T.D., H.V.L., L.N.Q.V., R.J.F., L.P.N., T.H.T.L., H.B.N., N.V.N. and J.C.; methodology, H.V.L., L.N.Q.V., R.J.F., L.P.N., A.J.C., H.B.N., N.V.N., A.K. and J.C.; software, L.N.Q.V., R.J.F., A.J.C. and T.H.T.L.; formal analysis, L.N.Q.V., A.J.C. and T.D.T.M.; investigation, T.H.M., P.N.T., T.H.P., V.V.N., Q.D.N., T.D.N., T.T.T.D., L.P.N., L.N.Q.V., R.J.F. and A.J.C.; data curation, T.T.T.D., A.J.C., T.D.T.M., T.H.T.L. and L.N.Q.V.; writing—original draft preparation, L.N.Q.V., A.J.C.; writing—review and editing, L.N.Q.V., A.J.C., A.K. and J.C.; visualization, A.J.C. and L.N.Q.V.; supervision, T.H.M., P.N.T., V.V.N., H.V.L., T.H.P., X.T.P., L.N.Q.V., H.B.N., N.V.N. and J.C.; project administration, T.T.T.D., L.P.N., L.N.Q.V., R.J.F., A.J.C., T.H.T.L., Q.D.N. and A.K.; funding acquisition, L.N.Q.V., L.P.N., R.J.F., T.H.T.L. and H.V.L. All authors have read and agreed to the published version of the manuscript.

Funding: This research was supported by the TB REACH initiative of the Stop TB Partnership through a Project Cooperation Agreement with the Government of Viet Nam with funding from the Global Affairs Canada.

Acknowledgments: We acknowledge the contributions of Dong Thi Huong, Nguyen Thi Thanh Thuy, Nguyen Thi Thanh Thao and Tran Minh Duc in preparing, anonymizing and cleaning the data. We further acknowledge the contribution of the Clinton Health Access Initiative and TechUp. We thank the staff of the District health centers and DTUs in the intervention districts for the provision of routine program surveillance data. We are deeply grateful for the tireless efforts and dedication of the Community Health Workers to the wellbeing of their patients.

Conflicts of Interest: The authors declare no conflict of interest. The funders had no role in the design of the study; in the collection, analyses, or interpretation of data; in the writing of the manuscript, or in the decision to publish the results.

References

1. Office of the Prime Minister. *Approval of the National Strategy for TB Prevention and Control Until 2020 with Vision to 2030 [Vietnamese]*; Government of Viet Nam: Ha Noi, Vietnam, 2014.
2. World Health Organization. *Global Tuberculosis Report 2018*; World Health Organization: Geneva, Switzerland, 2018.
3. World Health Organization. *Global Tuberculosis Report 2019*; World Health Organization: Geneva, Switzerland, 2019.
4. Marks, G.B.; Nguyen, N.V.; Nguyen, P.T.B.; Nguyen, T.A.; Nguyen, H.B.; Tran, K.H.; Nguyen, S.V.; Luu, K.B.; Tran, D.T.T.; Vo, Q.T.N.; et al. Community-wide screening for tuberculosis in a high-prevalence setting. *N. Engl. J. Med.* **2019**, *381*, 1347–1357. [CrossRef] [PubMed]
5. Fajans, P.; Simmons, R.; Ghiron, L. Helping public sector health systems innovate: The strategic approach to strengthening reproductive health policies and programs. *Am. J. Public Health* **2006**, *96*, 435–440. [CrossRef] [PubMed]
6. World Health Organization. *Guidelines for Intensified Tuberculosis Case-Finding and Isoniazid Preventive Therapy for People Living with HIV in Resource-Constrained Settings*; World Health Organization: Geneva, Switzerland, 2011.
7. Thanh, T.H.T.; Ngoc, S.D.; Viet, N.N.; Van, H.N.; Horby, P.; Cobelens, F.G.; Wertheim, H.F. A household survey on screening practices of household contacts of smear positive tuberculosis patients in Vietnam. *BMC Public Health* **2014**, *14*, 713. [CrossRef] [PubMed]
8. ExpandNet. *Beginning with the End in Mind: Planning Pilot Projects and Other Programmatic Research for Successful Scaling Up*; World Health Organization: Geneva, Switzerland, 2011.
9. Viet Nam National TB Control Programme. *NTP Year-End Report 2019 [Vietnamese]*; National Lung Hospital: Ha Noi, Vietnam, 2020.
10. World Health Organization. *Systematic Screening for Active Tuberculosis: Principles and Recommendations*; World Health Organization: Geneva, Switzerland, 2013.
11. World Health Organization. *Tuberculosis Prevalence Surveys: A Handbook*; World Health Organization: Geneva, Switzerland, 2007; ISBN 978 92 4 154816 8.
12. World Health Organization. *Chest Radiography in Tuberculosis Detection—Summary of Current WHO Recommendations and Guidance on Programmatic Approaches*; World Health Organization: Geneva, Switzerland, 2016.
13. World Health Organisation. *Chest Radiography in Tuberculosis*; WHO Libr. Cat. Data: Geneva, Switzerland, 2016.
14. Van't Hoog, A.H.; Cobelens, F.; Vassall, A.; Van Kampen, S.; Dorman, S.E.; Alland, D.; Ellner, J. Optimal triage test characteristics to improve the cost-effectiveness of the Xpert MTB/RIF assay for TB diagnosis: A decision analysis. *PLoS ONE* **2013**, *8*, e82786. [CrossRef] [PubMed]
15. Shazzadur Rahman, A.A.M.; Langley, I.; Galliez, R.; Kritski, A.; Tomeny, E.; Squire, S.B. Modelling the impact of chest X-ray and alternative triage approaches prior to seeking a tuberculosis diagnosis. *BMC Infect. Dis.* **2019**, *19*, 93. [CrossRef]
16. Creswell, J.; Qin, Z.Z.; Gurung, R.; Lamichhane, B.; Yadav, D.K.; Prasai, M.K.; Bista, N.; Adhikari, L.M.; Rai, B.; Sudrungrot, S. The performance and yield of tuberculosis testing algorithms using microscopy, chest x-ray, and Xpert MTB/RIF. *J. Clin. Tuberc. Other Mycobact. Dis.* **2019**, *14*, 1–6. [CrossRef]
17. Keshavjee, S.; Dowdy, D.; Swaminathan, S. Stopping the body count: A comprehensive approach to move towards zero tuberculosis deaths. *Lancet* **2015**, *386*, e46–e47. [CrossRef]
18. Yuen, C.M.; Amanullah, F.; Dharmadhikari, A.; Nardell, E.A.; Seddon, J.A.; Vasilyeva, I.; Zhao, Y.; Keshavjee, S.; Becerra, M.C. Turning off the tap: Stopping tuberculosis transmission through active case-finding and prompt effective treatment. *Lancet* **2015**, *386*, 2334–2343. [CrossRef]
19. Rangaka, M.X.; Cavalcante, S.C.; Marais, B.J.; Thim, S.; Martinson, N.A.; Swaminathan, S.; Chaisson, R.E. Controlling the seedbeds of tuberculosis: Diagnosis and treatment of tuberculosis infection. *Lancet* **2015**, *386*, 2344–2353. [CrossRef]

20. Ortblad, K.F.; Salomon, J.A.; Bärnighausen, T.; Atun, R. Stopping tuberculosis: A biosocial model for sustainable development. *Lancet* **2015**, *386*, 2354–2362. [CrossRef]
21. Nguyen, T.H.; Vo Nguyen Quang, L.; Le, T.G.; Vu, N.T.; Nguyen, H.D. Results of the community—Based intervention for the prevention and control of TB in Go Vap district, Ho Chi Minh city, 2014 [vietnamese]. *Viet Nam J. Public Heal.* **2015**, *38*, 6–12.
22. General Department of Population and Family Planning. *End-Year Report 2019*; Ministry of Health: Ha Noi, Vietnam, 2019.
23. MacPherson, P.; Houben, R.M.; Glynn, J.R.; Corbett, E.L.; Kranzer, K. Pre-treatment loss to follow-up in tuberculosis patients in low- and lower-middle-income countries and high-burden countries: A systematic review and meta-analysis. *Bull. World Health Organ.* **2014**, *92*, 126–138. [CrossRef]
24. Blok, L.; Creswell, J.; Stevens, R.; Brouwer, M.; Ramis, O.; Weil, O.; Klatser, P.; Sahu, S.; Bakker, M.I. A pragmatic approach to measuring monitoring and evaluating interventions for improved tuberculosis case detection. *Int. Health* **2014**, *6*, 181–188. [CrossRef]
25. Bernal, J.L.; Cummins, S.; Gasparrini, A. Interrupted time series regression for the evaluation of public health interventions: A tutorial. *Int. J. Epidemiol.* **2017**, *46*, 348–355. [CrossRef]
26. Mhimbira, F.A.; Cuevas, L.E.; Dacombe, R.; Mkopi, A.; Sinclair, D. Interventions to increase tuberculosis case detection at primary healthcare or community-level services. *Cochrane Database Syst. Rev.* **2017**. [CrossRef]
27. Shewade, H.D.; Gupta, V.; Ghule, V.H.; Nayak, S.; Satyanarayana, S.; Dayal, R.; Mohanty, S.; Singh, S.; Biswas, M.; Kumar Reddy, K.; et al. Impact of advocacy, communication, social mobilization and active case finding on TB notification in Jharkhand, India. *J. Epidemiol. Glob. Health* **2019**, *9*, 233–242. [CrossRef]
28. Calligaro, G.L.; Zijenah, L.S.; Peter, J.G.; Theron, G.; Buser, V.; Mcnerney, R.; Bara, W.; Bandason, T.; Govender, U.; Tomasicchio, M.; et al. Effect of new tuberculosis diagnostic technologies on community-based intensified case finding: A multicentre randomised controlled trial. *Lancet* **2017**, *3099*, 441–450. [CrossRef]
29. Ho, J.; Nguyen, P.T.B.; Nguyen, T.A.; Tran, K.H.; Van Nguyen, S.; Nguyen, N.V.; Nguyen, H.B.; Luu, K.B.; Fox, G.J.; Marks, G.B. Reassessment of the positive predictive value and specificity of Xpert MTB/RIF: A diagnostic accuracy study in the context of community-wide screening for tuberculosis. *Lancet Infect. Dis.* **2016**, *16*, 1045–1051. [CrossRef]
30. Creswell, J.; Codlin, A.J.; Andre, E.; Micek, M.A.; Bedru, A.; Carter, E.J.; Yadav, R.P.; Mosneaga, A.; Rai, B.; Banu, S.; et al. Results from early programmatic implementation of Xpert MTB/RIF testing in nine countries. *BMC Infect. Dis.* **2014**, *14*. [CrossRef]
31. Theron, G.; Peter, J.; Dowdy, D.; Langley, I.; Squire, S.B.; Dheda, K. Do high rates of empirical treatment undermine the potential effect of new diagnostic tests for tuberculosis in high-burden settings? *Lancet Infect. Dis.* **2014**, *14*, 527–532. [CrossRef]
32. Theron, G.; Zijenah, L.; Chanda, D.; Clowes, P.; Rachow, A.; Lesosky, M.; Bara, W.; Mungofa, S.; Pai, M.; Hoelscher, M.; et al. Feasibility, accuracy, and clinical effect of point-of-care Xpert MTB/RIF testing for tuberculosis in primary-care settings in Africa: A multicentre, randomised, controlled trial. *Lancet* **2014**, *383*, 424–435. [CrossRef]
33. Creswell, J.; Rai, B.; Wali, R.; Sudrungrot, S.; Adhikari, L.M.; Pant, R.; Pyakurel, S.; Uranw, D.; Codlin, A.J. Introducing new tuberculosis diagnostics: The impact of Xpert MTB/RIF testing on case notifications in Nepal. *Int. J. Tuberc. Lung Dis.* **2015**, *19*, 545–551. [CrossRef]
34. Wells, W.A. Onions and prevalence surveys: How to analyze and quantify tuberculosis case-finding gaps. *Int. J. Tuberc. Lung Dis.* **2017**, *21*, 1101–1113. [CrossRef]
35. Mason, P.H.; Roy, A.; Spillane, J.; Singh, P. Social, historical and cultural dimensions of tuberculosis. *J. Biosoc. Sci.* **2015**, *48*, 206–232. [CrossRef]
36. Stop TB Partnership. *Stop TB Field Guide 3: Finding Missing People with TB in Communities*; Stop TB Partnership: Geneva, Switzerland, 2018.
37. Long, N.H.; Johansson, E.; Lönnroth, K.; Eriksson, B.; Winkvist, A.; Diwan, V.K. Longer delays in tuberculosis diagnosis among women in Vietnam. *Int. J. Tuberc. Lung Dis.* **1999**, *3*, 388–393.
38. Lönnroth, K.; Jaramillo, E.; Williams, B.G.; Dye, C.; Raviglione, M. Drivers of tuberculosis epidemics: The role of risk factors and social determinants. *Soc. Sci. Med.* **2009**, *68*, 2240–2246. [CrossRef]
39. Datiko, D.G.; Yassin, M.A.; Theobald, S.J.; Blok, L.; Suvanand, S.; Creswell, J.; Cuevas, L.E. Health extension workers improve tuberculosis case finding and treatment outcome in Ethiopia: A large-scale implementation study. *BMJ Glob. Heal.* **2017**, *2*, e000390. [CrossRef]

40. World Health Organization. *ENGAGE-TB: Integrating Community-Based Tuberculosis Activities into the Work of Nongovernmental and Other Civil Society Organizations: Training of Community Health Workers and Community Volunteers: Facilitators' Guide*; World Health Organization: Geneva, Switzerland, 2015.
41. Agarwal, S.; Kirk, K.; Sripad, P.; Bellows, B.; Abuya, T.; Warren, C. Setting the global research agenda for community health systems: Literature and consultative review. *Hum. Resour. Health* **2019**, *17*, 22. [CrossRef] [PubMed]
42. Scott, K.; Beckham, S.W.; Gross, M.; Pariyo, G.; Rao, K.D.; Cometto, G.; Perry, H.B. What do we know about community-based health worker programs? A systematic review of existing reviews on community health workers. *Hum. Resour. Health* **2018**, *16*, 39. [CrossRef]
43. Shapiro, A.; Akande, T.; Lonnroth, K.; Golub, J.; Chakravorty, R. *A Systematic Review of the Number Needed to Screen to Detect a Case of Active Tuberculosis in Different Risk Groups*; World Health Organization: Geneva, Switzerland, 2013.
44. Getahun, H.; Raviglione, M. Transforming the global tuberculosis response through effective engagement of civil society organizations: The role of the World Health Organization. *Bull. World Health Organ.* **2011**, *89*, 616–618. [CrossRef] [PubMed]
45. Shelley, K.D.; Frumence, G.; Mpembeni, R.; George, A.S.; Stuart, E.A.; Killewo, J.; Baqui, A.H.; Peters, D.H. Can volunteer community health workers manage multiple roles? An interrupted time-series analysis of combined HIV and maternal and child health promotion in Iringa, Tanzania. *Health Policy Plan.* **2018**, *33*, 1096–1106. [CrossRef]
46. Datiko, D.G.; Lindtjørn, B. Health extension workers improve tuberculosis case detection and treatment success in southern Ethiopia: A community randomized trial. *PLoS ONE* **2009**, *4*, e5443. [CrossRef]
47. Sinha, P.; Shenoi, S.V.; Friedland, G.H. Opportunities for community health workers to contribute to global efforts to end tuberculosis. *Glob. Public Health* **2019**, 474–484. [CrossRef]
48. Datiko, D.G.; Yassin, M.A.; Tulloch, O.; Asnake, G.; Tesema, T.; Jamal, H.; Markos, P.; Cuevas, L.E.; Theobald, S. Exploring providers' perspectives of a community based TB approach in Southern Ethiopia: Implication for community based approaches. *BMC Health Serv. Res.* **2015**, *15*, 501. [CrossRef]
49. Nhung, N.V.; Hoa, N.B.; Anh, N.T.; Anh, L.T.N.; Siroka, A.; Lönnroth, K.; Garcia Baena, I. Measuring catastrophic costs due to tuberculosis in Viet Nam. *Int. J. Tuberc. Lung Dis.* **2018**, *22*, 983–990. [CrossRef] [PubMed]
50. Viet Nam National TB Control Programme. *Viet Nam Global Fund Funding Request 2018–2020*; National Lung Hospital: Ha Noi, Vietnam, 2016.
51. Morishita, F.; Eang, M.T.; Nishikiori, N.; Yadav, R.P. Increased case notification through active case finding of tuberculosis among household and neighbourhood contacts in Cambodia. *PLoS ONE* **2016**, *11*, e150405. [CrossRef]
52. Morishita, F.; Garfin, A.M.C.G.; Lew, W.; Oh, K.H.; Yadav, R.P.; Reston, J.C.; Infante, L.L.; Acala, M.R.C.; Palanca, D.L.; Kim, H.J.; et al. Bringing state-of-the-art diagnostics to vulnerable populations: The use of a mobile screening unit in active case finding for tuberculosis in Palawan, the Philippines. *PLoS ONE* **2017**, *12*, e171310. [CrossRef]
53. Khan, F.A.; Pande, T.; Tessema, B.; Song, R.; Benedetti, A.; Pai, M.; Lönnroth, K.; Denkinger, C.M. Computer-aided reading of tuberculosis chest radiography: Moving the research agenda forward to inform policy. *Eur. Respir. J.* **2017**, *50*. [CrossRef]
54. Do, T.T.; Kumar, A.M.; Ramaswamy, G.; Htun, T.; Le, V.H.; Vo, L.N.Q.; Dong, T.T.T.; Codlin, A.; Forse, R.; Crewsell, J.; et al. An innovative public—Private mix model for improving tuberculosis care in vietnam: How well are we doing? *Trop. Med. Infect. Dis.* **2020**, *5*, 26. [CrossRef]

Publisher's Note: MDPI stays neutral with regard to jurisdictional claims in published maps and institutional affiliations.

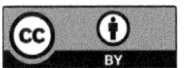

© 2020 by the authors. Licensee MDPI, Basel, Switzerland. This article is an open access article distributed under the terms and conditions of the Creative Commons Attribution (CC BY) license (http://creativecommons.org/licenses/by/4.0/).

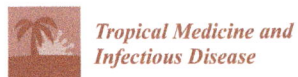 *Tropical Medicine and Infectious Disease*

Article

Islands of Tuberculosis Elimination: An Evaluation of Community-Based Active Case Finding in North Sumatra, Indonesia

Elvi S. Siahaan [1], Mirjam I. Bakker [2], Ratna Pasaribu [1], Amera Khan [3], Tripti Pande [4], Alwi Mujahit Hasibuan [5] and Jacob Creswell [3,*]

1. Yayasan Menara Agung Pengharapan Internasional, Medan Johor 20211, Indonesia; elvi.siahaan@gmail.com (E.S.S.); ratnapasaribu@gmail.com (R.P.)
2. KIT Royal Tropical Institute, 1092 Amsterdam, The Netherlands; M.Bakker@kit.nl
3. Stop TB Partnership, 1218 Geneva, Switzerland; amerak@stoptb.org
4. McGill International Tuberculosis Center, Montreal, QC H4A 3J1, Canada; tripti.pande@mail.mcgill.ca
5. Kepala Dinas Kesehatan Provinsi Sumatera Utara, Medan 20028, Indonesia; alwi.mujahit@gmail.com
* Correspondence: jacobc@stoptb.org

Received: 25 September 2020; Accepted: 23 October 2020; Published: 26 October 2020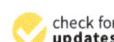

Abstract: Community-based active case finding (ACF) is needed to reach key/vulnerable populations with limited access to tuberculosis (TB) care. Published reports of ACF interventions in Indonesia are scarce. We conducted an evaluation of a multicomponent community-based ACF intervention as it scaled from one district to nine in Nias and mainland North Sumatra. Community and health system support measures including laboratory strengthening, political advocacy, sputum transport, and community awareness were instituted. ACF was conducted in three phases: pilot (18 months, 1 district), intervention (12 months, 4 districts) and scale-up (9 months, 9 districts). The pilot phase identified 215 individuals with bacteriologically positive (B+) TB, representing 42% of B+ TB notifications. The intervention phase yielded 509, representing 54% of B+ notifications and the scale-up phase identified 1345 individuals with B+ TB (56% of notifications). We observed large increases in B+ notifications on Nias, but no overall change on the mainland despite district variation. Overall, community health workers screened 377,304 individuals of whom 1547 tested positive, and 95% were initiated on treatment. Our evaluation shows that multicomponent community-based ACF can reduce the number of people missed by TB programs. Community-based organizations are best placed for accessing and engaging hard to reach populations and providing integrated support which can have a large positive effect on TB notifications.

Keywords: tuberculosis; active case finding; community outreach; Indonesia; key population

1. Introduction

Tuberculosis (TB) has existed for millennia yet is the leading infectious disease killer worldwide [1]. In 2018, a United Nations (UN) High-Level Meeting reaffirmed the global commitment to meeting previously established ambitious targets and strategies to end TB by 2030 and set out interim targets for 2022 on the numbers of people treated for TB [2]. Every year, it is estimated that 3 million people with TB are undetected and/or remain unnotified to National TB Programs (NTPs) globally [1]. Lack of accessibility and availability of TB services are major drivers for this [3]. Those who are missed are often members of key/vulnerable populations (i.e., miners, prisoners, elderly, people living with human immunodeficiency virus (HIV), or people in hard to reach areas) [4,5]. Various global initiatives have been launched in an attempt to reach all people with TB including the Global Fund's Strategic Initiative on TB and the Find.Treat.All initiative which focus attention on reaching people with TB who are missed by routine services [6,7]. To reach more people with TB, active case finding (ACF) strategies focused outside traditional health facilities are needed [8–10].

Previous literature indicates that numerous approaches have been explored to identify and diagnose people with TB through ACF. A study in Ethiopia documented the high impact on TB case notifications by using existing health extension workers to perform numerous tasks, such as community-based screening, sputum collection and laboratory techniques (i.e., community-based slide fixing) [11,12]. In Cambodia and Myanmar there have been multiple efforts to reach people with TB using mobile chest X-ray units. [13–16]. In India, ACF encompassing the use of mobile vans as well as house-to-house screening by community workers on a massive scale has been conducted through Global Fund projects and more recently by the government's ambitious initiatives [17,18]. Initiatives conducted outside of health facilities to reach individuals who are either not seeking care or are seeking care in the informal sector require a critical component of community mobilization and acceptance [19]. The inclusion of communities in such interventions to ensure access and local acceptance is crucial and, therefore, many ACF interventions are supported by community-based organizations. The Global Plan to End TB highlights the importance of increased involvement by the communities and civil society in the fight to end TB [4] and it is a critical part of the development of national strategic plans for TB [20].

Indonesia contributes to 8% of the global TB incidence, making it the third highest burden country after India and China [1]. In 2018, an estimated 845,000 people developed TB and only 563,879 (67%) were notified, meaning that 275,000 (33%) people with TB were missed [1]. Indonesia's health system is decentralized, and district health offices have the responsibility of organizing public health services through local facilities at the sub-district level called *Puskesmas* [21]. Encouraging ACF and community engagement in the TB response is one of the main strategies in Indonesia's National Strategic Plan [22].

TB patient-pathway analyses from Indonesia documented that more than 67% of symptomatic TB patients initially sought care in the private sector. The analyses highlighted the importance of 'community referrals' within the pathway [21]. However, there is limited published literature on ACF interventions in Indonesia. One study compared contact investigation and door-to-door screening by community health workers (CHWs) in Bandung City. The authors concluded that CHWs can be used to improve acceptance by the community, however no people with TB were detected in the study [23]. A modeling study comparing three case finding strategies concluded that if ACF is used to lower the proportion of people not accessing care, it can reduce mortality [24]. Due to the paucity of literature on ACF in Indonesia and the need to improve case detection, we report on the results of an evaluation of an ACF intervention in Nias archipelago and mainland North Sumatra, Indonesia funded by Stop TB partnership's TB REACH initiative [25].

2. Materials and Methods

2.1. Setting

We conducted an evaluation of scaled ACF interventions implemented in North Sumatra province. North Sumatra is the fourth most populous province in Indonesia consisting of 419 islands. The ACF intervention was conducted on Nias archipelago and mainland North Sumatra. Nias is an archipelago off the western coast of Northern Sumatra consisting of 32 inhabited islands. Many of the islands are difficult to reach and are only accessible by boat. The total population of the archipelago is approximately 800,000 people [26]. Nias is one of the poorest areas in Sumatra, and many of the indigenous residents are illiterate and do not speak Bahasa, limiting their access to official health information. Additionally, access to healthcare in Nias is often limited due to distances, high staff turnover, and lack of funding and training for healthcare staff in these remote areas. For much of the project period, Nias had only one GeneXpert machine which was mostly non-functional. Mainland North Sumatra is more developed than Nias. The total population is approximately 3 million people. Despite better access to health services compared to Nias, North Sumatra has a medium ranking for its health development index indicators (education, life expectancy and per capita income) in most districts [27]. The districts on the mainland each had a single GeneXpert machine which was used primarily to test for drug resistance rather than diagnosis. Yayasan Menara Agung Pengharapan Internasional (YMAPI), a local non-governmental organization based in North Sumatra has provided access to health services and medicine for more than 15 years. YMAPI was the main implementer of this intervention, working in collaboration with the local District Health Offices and the NTP.

2.2. Timeline and Coverage

This community-based ACF intervention was conducted in three phases. Figure 1 presents a map of the area and timeline for the intervention and control districts. A pilot phase began in October 2014 in Nias Selatan District (population approximately 182,000) to test the intervention and help train project staff, lasting through March 2016. The ACF intervention phase (hereafter intervention phase) took place in four of the five districts within Nias (population approximately 450,000) between July 2017 and June 2018. Between April and December 2019, the ACF scale-up phase (hereafter scale-up phase) was implemented in all five districts on Nias as well as four additional districts in the mainland North Sumatra (population approximately 740,000). Two purposefully selected districts in North Sumatra with stable notifications rates and lacking other case detection interventions were used as control districts as part of TB REACH's standard monitoring and evaluation methodology [28]. Throughout the different areas and across the phases, the ACF interventions were similar but lessons learned from earlier phases were incorporated during implementation of subsequent phases.

2.3. Community-Based Outreach Intervention

A multicomponent community based ACF intervention was developed in coordination with the NTP and was conducted as part of the TB programme operations (see Figure 2). Predominantly female community-based volunteers (health promoters) who lived and worked in the communities were the core of this intervention. There were 1505 health promoters engaged in the pilot phase; 3730 in the intervention phase; and 7835 during the scale-up phase. In the pilot and intervention phase, health promoters were selected by the head of the different villages and other community leaders, while during the scale-up phase existing CHW (*posyandu kader*) were selected. The health promoters did not receive a salary but were provided small in-kind support such as transport reimbursements, T-shirts, caps, notebooks, and an official inauguration ceremony with a certificate. Health promoters were trained and supervised by project staff (health facilitators) to raise TB awareness, to sensitize community members on the importance of TB diagnosis and treatment and to screen community members for signs and symptoms of TB. The health promoters also advocated for health-seeking behaviors and provided information on nutrition, sanitation, and the harmful effects of tobacco use. The health facilitators, who received a small salary, travelled to hard-to-reach areas and villages by foot, bicycle, motorbike, and/or boat to support the screening and referral of people with presumptive TB to link them to testing, diagnosis and treatment.

The intervention targeted people at the village level. The health promoters and facilitators disseminated their health awareness messages and conducted TB screening during house to house visits and informal meetings where people congregated such as town meetings and events. A primary focus of their work was to promote the value of the local *Puskesmas* in providing high-quality medicine and care for TB as confidence in the health system was perceived as low.

Individuals were screened verbally for seven symptoms. The symptoms included: cough for more than 2 weeks, weight loss, loss of appetite, difficulty breathing, prolonged fever, night sweats and coughing blood. Anyone reporting two or more symptoms was considered to have presumptive TB and was eligible for diagnostic testing. All individuals with presumptive TB were asked to provide two sputum samples. In most situations, a health promoter or health facilitator accompanied them to the nearest *Puskesmas* for testing. A small enabler was provided to support the travel. For individuals living far from the *Puskesmas*, a health facilitator collected samples in the village and transported them to the nearest laboratory using a cold box by motorcycle and/or boat. In some instances, in very remote islands, laboratory technicians visited the communities, collected sputum and fixed slides on site. All diagnostic testing was done with sputum microscopy and individuals were eligible to initiate treatment if one of the smear results was positive/scanty in accordance with NTP guidelines. All individuals with TB were provided treatment support through the health facilitators and were also offered nutritional support consisting of food packages.

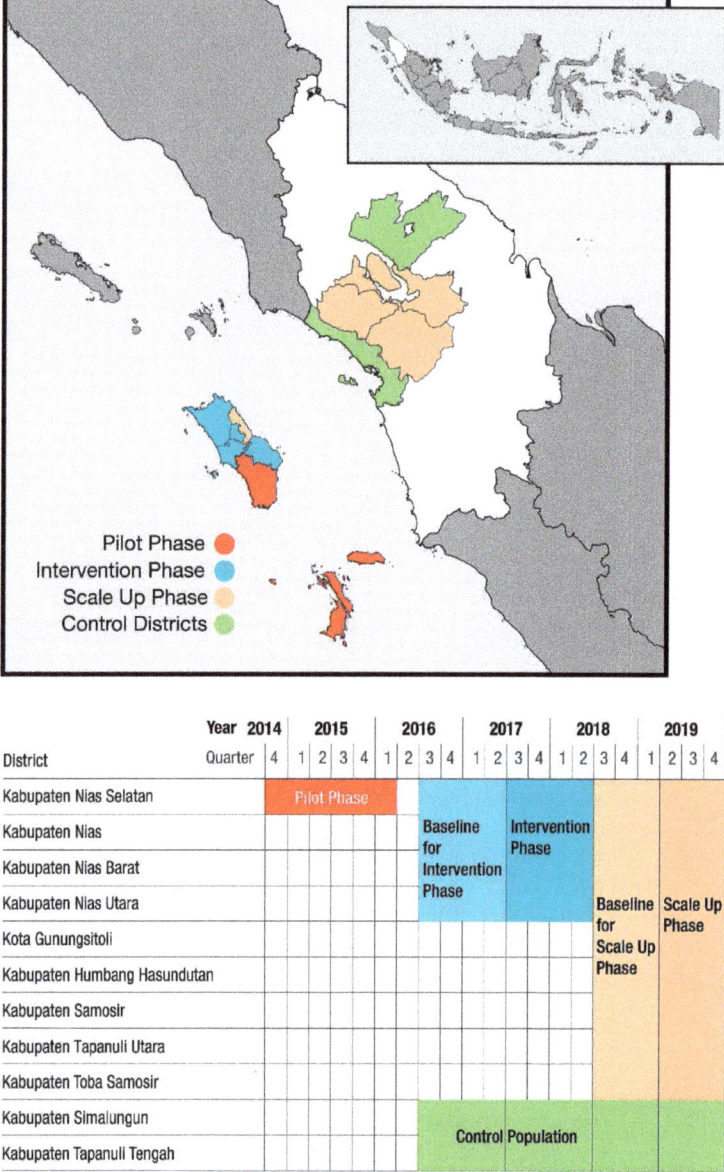

Figure 1. Active case finding in North Sumatra—timelines and geographic areas.

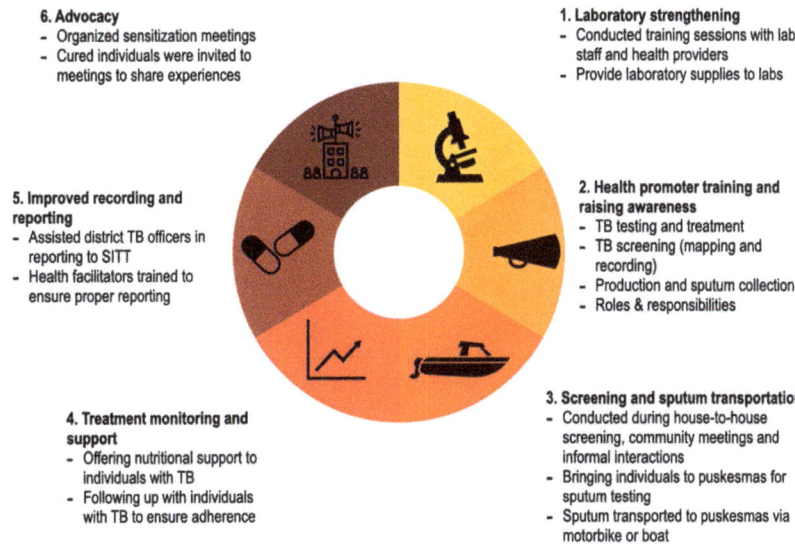

Figure 2. Multicomponent community-based active case-finding intervention in North Sumatra, Indonesia.

To ensure the ACF activities did not overwhelm the health system's ability to provide care, YMAPI procured laboratory equipment including 17 microscopes and supplies for 85 diagnostic facilities in the intervention areas. Training sessions for laboratory and facility staff on screening, diagnostics and laboratory procedures, and treatment were also provided. People initiating TB treatment were notified through the TB registers as per standard NTP practice. YMAPI also worked with district TB officers to ensure timely and accurate reporting in the SITT (*Sistem Informasi Terpadu TB*), the national TB reporting system.

Finally, the project organized sensitization and results sharing meetings for village leaders, district heads and government staff. In these meetings people with TB currently on treatment or those who had completed their treatment were invited to participate to share their stories and advocate for more local funding for the TB program (see Figure 2).

2.4. Data Collection

Quarterly notification data from the SITT from the district and provincial offices from October 2013 to December 2019 were extracted. If online reporting data were incomplete, we complemented the reports with facility level data directly from the *Puskesmas*. The numbers of people screened and identified as having presumptive TB were collected by the health facilitators directly from the health promoters and then tracked into the facility laboratory registers to determine yield.

2.5. Data Analysis

Evaluation of the ACF intervention followed the standard monitoring and evaluation framework of TB REACH to determine the impact of case finding in a given area [28]. For all three phases, official NTP notification data were analyzed using a pre-post evaluation methodology of bacteriologically positive (B+) TB notifications in intervention areas. In addition, a control area was used for the intervention and scale-up phases. We compared the notifications in a baseline period to the notifications during the ACF intervention and did the same in control districts. Since the pilot phase lasted 6 quarters, for the baseline data we multiplied the four previous quarters of notifications by 1.5 to get a comparable result. Other periods all used actual notification numbers. We calculated the percentage change in TB notifications between baseline and intervention periods, as well as the absolute number of additional people notified. In addition, project data were used to track indicators relating to the number of presumptive cases among screened and the yield of testing during the ACF intervention to complement the results of the change in TB notifications.

2.6. Ethics Statement

This intervention was approved by the District Administration as part of programmatic services thus no additional ethical approval was required. All patient information was anonymized, and only aggregate data were used in the analyses.

3. Results

During the 18-month pilot phase (Q4 2014–Q1 2016), ACF in one district (Nias Selatan) was conducted. This involved five of the 11 Puskesmas with TB testing facilities and three Satellite Puskesmas. As shown in Table 1, during the pilot phase, health facilitators identified 3261 people who had presumptive TB, and were able to ensure 2983 (91.5%) were tested by linking them to laboratory services. Data on numbers of people screened were not collected in a systematic manner during the pilot phase. The ACF yielded 215 people with B+ TB (7.2% positivity rate), all of whom initiated treatment. Overall, there were 509 people with B+ TB notified in Nias Selatan during this phase, meaning community outreach efforts were responsible for 42% of the total B+ notifications during the pilot period. The computed 18-month B+ TB notifications prior to the pilot phase in Nias Selatan were 444, signifying a 15% increase using a pre/post analysis (Table 2).

Table 1. Active case finding intervention data from all phases, North Sumatra.

	Pilot Phase [#]	Intervention Phase [+]	Scale-up Phase [&]			Overall Total
			Nias	Mainland	Total	
People Screened	N/A	124,430	126,384	126,390	252,774	377,204
People Referred for Testing	3261	6084	5464	4280	9744	19,089
People Tested	2983	5807	5287	3675	8962	17,752
People with B+ TB	215	509	429	394	823	1547
People Initiated on Treatment	215	492	388	370	758	1465
Presumptive Rate (Presumptive/Screened)		4.9%	4.3%	3.4%	3.9%	4.2% [**]
% of presumptive people tested	91.5%	95.4%	96.8%	85.9%	92.0%	93.0%
% yield of TB testing	7.2%	8.8%	8.1%	13.1%	9.2%	8.7%
% B+ linked to treatment	100.0%	96.7%	90.4%	91.7%	92.1%	94.7%

TB: tuberculosis; N/A: data unavailable, B+: bacteriologically positive. [#] Pilot Phase included 1 district (Q4 2014–Q1 2016). [+] Intervention Phase included 4 districts on Nias Island (Q3 2017–Q2 2018). [&] Scale up Phase included 9 districts total (5 districts on Nias Island and 4 districts on mainland North Sumatra; Q2 2019–Q4 2019). Diagnosis was through sputum smear microscopy. [**] Includes only data from active case finding (ACF) Intervention phase and Scale-up phase since pilot phase did not track screening numbers.

Table 2. Active case finding yield and impact on bacteriologically positive TB notifications, North Sumatra.

	B+ TB Notifications Intervention Districts	B+ TB Notifications Control Districts
Pilot phase Nias [*]		
Baseline ^	444	NA
Intervention	509	NA
ACF direct yield	215	NA
% notifications identified by ACF	42%	NA
Number and (%) change from baseline	65 (+15%)	NA
Intervention phase Nias [+]		
Baseline	495	1424
Intervention	916	1653
ACF direct yield	492	NA
% notifications identified by ACF	54%	NA
Number and (%) change from baseline	421 (+85%)	229 (+16%)

Table 2. Cont.

	B+ TB Notifications Intervention Districts	B+ TB Notifications Control Districts
Scale-up phase Nias &		
Baseline	551	1176
Intervention	673	1184
ACF direct yield	388	NA
% notifications identified by ACF	58%	NA
Number and (%) change from baseline	122 (+22%)	8 (+1%)
Scale-up phase Mainland North Sumatra &		
Baseline	686	1176
Intervention	672	1184
ACF direct yield	370	NA
% notifications identified by ACF	55%	NA
Number and (%) change from baseline	−14 (−2%)	8 (+1%)

Notifications only include people who initiated anti-TB treatment. * Pilot Phase included 1 district (Q4 2014–Q1 2016). ˆ Baseline in pilot phase includes 4 quarters of notification numbers prior to pilot phase ($n = 296$) multiplied by 1.5 (for 6 quarters, $n = 444$) since the intervention in the pilot phase lasted 6 quarters. + ACF Intervention Phase included 4 districts on Nias Island (Q3 2017–Q2 2018). & Scale up Phase included 9 districts total (5 districts on Nias Island and 4 districts on mainland. North Sumatra; Q2 2019–Q4 2019). ACF = active case finding. B+ = bacteriologically positive.

During the 12-month intervention phase (Q3 2017–Q2 2018) outreach was conducted in four districts in Nias. Health facilitators verbally screened 124,430 individuals. There were 6084 individuals who screened positive and were referred for testing (4.9% of those screened). The vast majority of individuals with presumptive TB, were tested (5807 or 95.4%). Of those tested, 509 (8.8%) had B+ results and 492 (96.7%) of them initiated anti-TB treatment (Table 1). Total B+ notifications during the intervention phase in the evaluation area, including passive case finding, was 916, indicating that community based ACF contributed 54% of B+ notifications. In the four quarters prior to the intervention phase, there were 495 B+ notifications in the same districts meaning that B+ TB notifications increased 85% in the four intervention districts. At the same time, we observed a modest increase in B+ TB notifications in the control population during the intervention phase, moving from 1424 to 1653, (+16%) (Table 2).

The scale-up phase included an additional district on Nias and four districts on mainland North Sumatra meaning that a total of nine districts were covered. During the scale-up phase the number of people screened was 252,774 and the numbers were similar between Nias and the mainland. Of those screened, 9744 (3.9%) were referred for testing and 8962 symptomatic individuals (92.0%) were tested. Higher rates of presumptive TB were found on Nias compared to the mainland (4.3% vs. 3.4%), and the proportion tested among those referred was also higher on Nias (96.8% vs. 85.9%). Among people identified by the ACF who were tested, 823 (9.2%) had B+ results and 758 (92.1%) initiated treatment. Pretreatment loss to follow-up was slightly higher on Nias (9.6% vs. 8.3%). Across all the nine districts, there were 1345 B+ TB notifications during the scale-up phase meaning that the ACF activities identified 56% of the total B+ cases notified. ACF in districts on Nias contributed slightly more than the yield on the mainland (58% vs. 55%). B+ notifications on Nias island continued to rise compared to the baseline period (+22%), while on the mainland there was almost no change (−2%). When the change by district on the mainland was evaluated, we noted a wide range from an increase of 130% in Kabupaten Humbang Hasundutan, to a decrease of 41% in Kabupaten Tapanuli Utara, but the overall change was minimal. The control population had B+ notifications that also remained almost unchanged (+1%) with no variation between the control districts. Overall, the outreach activities screened 377,204 people, and tested 17,752 for TB, identifying 1547 people with B+ TB, and linking 94.7% of them to treatment.

4. Discussion

To our knowledge, our results are the first published account of large-scale ACF for TB in Indonesia. Our results show that combining health system strengthening, community mobilization, and ACF activities reached 1547 people with B+ TB and linked 95% of them to treatment. Despite a longstanding focus on bringing basic services to people with TB, our evaluation suggests many people in Indonesia with TB need additional measures to reach them. Previously, ACF has been used in numerous settings with different outreach models [11–18,29–32]. While Indonesia has a strong private sector where many people with TB seek care [22], evidently there are places, especially in remote rural areas, where community-based approaches are needed to reach people with TB.

ACF is often effective in situations where there is poor access to care due to stigma, travel times, distances, and/or cost barriers [15,31,32]. Although we did not measure the impact of this intervention on out-of-pocket costs for people with TB, ACF has been shown to reduce catastrophic costs for people with TB [33]. In addition, ACF reaches people earlier in their disease progression, although this has not translated into improved treatment outcomes, it may lessen individual suffering [34].

We believe our intervention was successful, not only because of the outreach efforts for screening of villagers, but because of the multifaceted approach that was taken including supporting public health facilities with laboratory supplies and political advocacy. While ACF found more than 50% of the total TB notifications during the intervention, the numbers of diagnostic tests undertaken were also very large. Identifying individuals with presumptive TB and getting their samples to laboratories through the provision of enablers and a transport system for sputum was critical [35]. To identify more people with TB, large numbers of people must be tested. In Nigeria and India, ACF studies demonstrated these increases in testing were necessary to generate gains in notifications [36,37]. ACF efforts can place an enormous burden on the laboratory system and this was one of the main reasons to also strengthen the infrastructure and the capacity of laboratories to diagnose TB.

In addition to the community-based screening, the intervention focused on improving health information and the promotion of health-seeking behavior in the communities. It also supported the district TB officers to improve recording and reporting and provided political advocacy for local government to provide more support for the health services in the area. These comprehensive actions were aimed at strengthening the overall health services and promoting the accessibility to the services within the community for longer-term sustainability [38].

While the ACF intervention increased the numbers of people detected with TB, national disease estimates suggest people with TB are still being missed. In our evaluation, the rates of bacteriologically negative TB (clinically diagnosed) overall were low (~24%), and in the first two phases it was only 10% of all forms (AF) notifications. On North Sumatra there were higher proportions, up to 55% (data not shown). On Nias and its surrounding islands it remains difficult to make a clinical diagnosis of TB at the *Puskesmas* level as there is only one X-ray machine available on the island. Presumptive individuals must be referred and bear the cost of the X-ray which is a disincentive. Additionally, we only used symptom screening to identify presumptive TB. Multiple prevalence surveys across Asia have shown that confining testing to only symptomatic people will miss a large proportion (40–79%) of people with TB [39]. Since we did not have access to X-ray services, people with TB were probably missed. Finally, it is well known that the sensitivity of smear microscopy is poor [40,41]. Ideally Xpert MTB/RIF testing would be used in ACF situations. However, despite large investments in Xpert in Indonesia with more than 500 machines procured as of 2017 [42] and efforts to expand testing, access to diagnostic Xpert testing on Nias Island and Sumatra was very low. Ensuring testing for all people with presumptive TB is a challenge globally; while it is recommended in many national guidelines, only a few countries are able to provide access to rapid molecular tests for initial diagnosis [21]. Expanding access to testing should be strongly considered to conform to World Health Organization (WHO) recommendations [43] and to identify more people with bacteriologically confirmed TB [44,45].

While the ACF contributed to large increases in B+ notifications on Nias, the same activities had a variable impact on mainland North Sumatra. We are not sure why these results were different but have some hypotheses. The interventions were implemented on the mainland for a short period of time, which did not permit the same level of collaboration with local authorities, a factor that is hard to measure, but we feel is important to community-based work. Mainland North Sumatra is also more developed and access to diagnostic and treatment facilities is better than on Nias. We did see variation between the districts on the mainland with the most developed districts showing a decrease in notifications while the less-developed districts had an increase. ACF will not perform the same in all areas and for all populations and thus tailoring the outreach to address local barriers is critical.

Limitations of this intervention include the fact that neither the intervention nor control areas were randomly selected, and by using as baseline for the scale-up phase in Nias the three quarters directly following the intervention phase, we may have slightly underestimated the effect, as some of the sensitization activities can be expected to have a lasting effect beyond the intervention itself. In addition, we were not able to use molecular diagnostic tests, culture, nor X-ray due to the resources available in the project areas. These tools would have likely helped identify more people with TB, however the reality in many countries is that access to modern tools of TB diagnosis are often limited to well-equipped urban areas [46]. Since smear microscopy and Xpert are not 100% specific there is a possibility that a proportion of the sputum smear positive individuals may have false positive results, a risk that all ACF interventions where positivity rates are low must consider [47]. The laboratory positivity rate in our interventions was close to 9%, which is actually higher than documented yields in some TB programs and similar to passive case finding [48,49]. As we describe the results of an evaluation of a specific programmatic intervention, the impact of a similar approach in other parts of Indonesia or other countries may not be generalizable. However, with the growing body of evidence around the impact of ACF interventions [50] we believe there are likely many areas where remote rural populations could benefit from similar activities. Our results are from a programmatic implementation, not a controlled research experiment, limiting the data we can collect and conclusions we can draw, but also providing a better understanding of what is feasible in a 'real world' situation.

5. Conclusions

Despite a well-established TB program, there are many poor and remote communities where access to health services is lacking in Indonesia. By combining community-based education and outreach with training and infrastructure support to health services and political advocacy, large numbers of people with TB can be reached. These comprehensive types of intervention should be considered in other areas with deficient access to care. Expanding the screening approach to include both X-ray and Xpert to identify asymptomatic cases through better screening and enhance diagnostic sensitivity would likely improve results even more.

Author Contributions: Conceptualization, E.S.S. and R.P.; methodology, E.S.S., R.P., M.I.B. and J.C.; validation, E.S.S., R.P., M.I.B., A.K., A.M.H. and T.P.; formal analysis, M.I.B., A.K., T.P. and J.C.; investigation, E.S.S., R.P., and A.M.H.; data curation, E.S.S., M.I.B. and R.P.; writing—original draft preparation, J.C.; writing—review and editing, E.S.S., R.P., M.I.B., A.K., T.P. and J.C.; visualization, T.P. and J.C.; supervision, E.S.S., R.P. and A.M.H.; funding acquisition, E.S.S. and R.P. All authors have read and agreed to the published version of the manuscript.

Funding: The intervention and the evaluation was supported by Stop TB Partnership's TB REACH initiative. TB REACH is funded by Global Affairs Canada.

Acknowledgments: We would like to acknowledge and thank the thousands of health volunteers and facilitators who worked to conduct the community outreach for this project. We also want to recognize and thank the district TB officers in Nias and North Sumatra, the National TB Program, and Ministry of Health of Indonesia for supporting the intervention over the years.

Conflicts of Interest: A.K. and J.C. are members of Stop TB Partnership and TB REACH. They do not make any funding decisions but provide technical assistance to selected projects. TP is a member of the Research Institute of McGill University Health Center which has a knowledge management grant from the Stop TB Partnership, TB REACH initiative.

References

1. World Health Organization. Global Tuberculosis Report 2019. Available online: https://www.who.int/teams/global-tuberculosis-programme/global-report-2019 (accessed on 18 September 2020).
2. Stop TB Partnership. UN High Level Meeting on TB: Key Targets & Commitments for 2022. 2018. Available online: http://stoptb.org/assets/documents/global/advocacy/unhlm/UNHLM_Targets&Commitments.pdf (accessed on 18 September 2020).

3. Creswell, J.; Sahu, S.; Blok, L.; Bakker, M.I.; Stevens, R.; Ditiu, L. A multi-site evaluation of innovative approaches to increase tuberculosis case notification: Summary results. *PLoS ONE* **2014**, *9*, e94465. [CrossRef]
4. Stop TB Partnership. *Partnership: The Paradigm Shift. 2016–2020. Global Plan to End TB*; United Nations Office for Project Services: Geneva, Switzerland, 2015.
5. De Vries, S.G.; Cremers, A.L.; Heuvelings, C.C.; Greve, P.F.; Visser, B.J.; Bélard, S.; Janssen, S.; Spijker, R.; Shaw, B.; Hill, R.A.; et al. Barriers and facilitators to the uptake of tuberculosis diagnostic and treatment services by hard-to-reach populations in countries of low and medium tuberculosis incidence: A systematic review of qualitative literature. *Lancet Infect. Dis.* **2017**, *17*, e128–e143. [CrossRef]
6. World Health Organization. Joint Initiative "FIND. TREAT. All. #ENDTB". 2018. Available online: https://www.who.int/tb/joint-initiative/en/ (accessed on 18 September 2020).
7. Stop TB Partnership. The Strategic Initiative to Find the Missing People with TB. Available online: https://stoptb-strategicinitiative.org/ (accessed on 20 August 2020).
8. Dowdy, D.W.; Basu, S.; Andrews, J.R. Is passive diagnosis enough? The impact of subclinical disease on diagnostic strategies for tuberculosis. *Am. J. Respir. Crit. Care Med.* **2013**, *187*, 543–551. [CrossRef]
9. Ho, J.; Fox, G.J.; Marais, B.J. Passive case finding for tuberculosis is not enough. *Int. J. Mycobacteriol.* **2016**, *5*, 374–378. [CrossRef]
10. Yuen, C.M.; Amanullah, F.; Dharmadhikari, A.; Nardell, E.A.; Seddon, J.A.; Vasilyeva, I.; Zhao, Y.; Keshavjee, S.; Becerra, M.C. Turning off the tap: Stopping tuberculosis transmission through active case-finding and prompt effective treatment. *Lancet* **2015**, *386*, 2334–2343. [CrossRef]
11. Datiko, D.G.; Yassin, M.A.; Theobald, S.J.; Blok, L.; Suvanand, S.; Creswell, J.; Cuevas, L.E. Health extension workers improve tuberculosis case finding and treatment outcome in Ethiopia: A large-scale implementation study. *BMJ Glob. Health* **2017**, *2*, e000390. [CrossRef]
12. Yassin, M.A.; Datiko, D.G.; Tulloch, O.; Markos, P.; Aschalew, M.; Shargie, E.B.; Dangisso, M.H.; Komatsu, R.; Sahu, S.; Blok, L.; et al. Innovative community-based approaches doubled tuberculosis case notification and improve treatment outcome in Southern Ethiopia. *PLoS ONE* **2013**, *8*, e63174. [CrossRef]
13. Codlin, A.J.; Monyrath, C.; Ky, M.; Gerstel, L.; Creswell, J.; Eang, M.T. Results from a roving, active case finding initiative to improve tuberculosis detection among older people in rural Cambodia using the Xpert MTB/RIF assay and chest X-ray. *J. Clin. Tuberc. Other Mycobact. Dis.* **2018**, *13*, 22–27. [CrossRef]
14. Eang, M.T.; Satha, P.; Yadav, R.P.; Morishita, F.; Nishikiori, N.; van-Maaren, P.; Lambregts-van Weezenbeek, C. Early detection of tuberculosis through community-based active case finding in Cambodia. *BMC Public Health* **2012**, *12*, 469. [CrossRef]
15. Morishita, F.; Eang, M.T.; Nishikiori, N.; Yadav, R.P. Increased case notification through active case finding of tuberculosis among household and neighbourhood contacts in Cambodia. *PLoS ONE* **2016**, *11*, e0150405. [CrossRef]
16. Myint, O.; Saw, S.; Isaakidis, P.; Khogali, M.; Reid, A.; Hoa, N.B.; Kyaw, T.T.; Zaw, K.K.; Khaing, T.M.; Aung, S.T. Active case-finding for tuberculosis by mobile teams in Myanmar: Yield and treatment outcomes. *Infect. Dis. Poverty* **2017**, *6*, 77. [CrossRef]
17. Prasad, B.; Satyanarayana, S.; Chadha, S.S.; Das, A.; Thapa, B.; Mohanty, S.; Pandurangan, S.; Babu, E.R.; Tonsing, J.; Sachdeva, K.S. Experience of active tuberculosis case finding in nearly 5 million households in India. *Public Health Action* **2016**, *6*, 15–18. [CrossRef]
18. Shewade, H.D.; Gupta, V.; Satyanarayana, S.; Kharate, A.; Sahai, K.N.; Murali, L.; Kamble, S.; Deshpande, M.; Kumar, N.; Kumar, S.; et al. Active case finding among marginalised and vulnerable populations reduces catastrophic costs due to tuberculosis diagnosis. *Glob. Health Action* **2018**, *11*, 1494897. [CrossRef]
19. Mitchell, E.M.; Golub, J.; Portocarrero, A. *Acceptability of TB Screening among at-Risk and Vulnerable Groups*; World Health Organization: Geneva, Switzerland, 2011.
20. World Health Organization. Toolkit to Develop a National Strategic Plan for TB Prevention, Care and Control. 2015. Available online: https://apps.who.int/iris/bitstream/handle/10665/153811/9789241507974_eng.pdf (accessed on 4 August 2020).
21. Surya, A.; Setyaningsih, B.; Suryani Nasution, H.; Gita Parwati, C.; Yuzwar, Y.E.; Osberg, M.; Hanson, C.L.; Hymoff, A.; Mingkwan, P.; Makayova, J.; et al. Quality tuberculosis Care in Indonesia: Using patient pathway analysis to optimize public–private collaboration. *J. Infect. Dis.* **2017**, *216* (Suppl. 7), S724–S732. [CrossRef]

22. Indonesia National TB Program. Current Status of Integrated Community Based TB Service Delivery and the Global Fund Work Plan to Find Missing TB Cases. 2018. Available online: https://www.who.int/tb/features_archive/indonesia_11apr18.pdf?ua=1 (accessed on 25 September 2020).
23. McAllister, S.; Wiem Lestari, B.; Sujatmiko, B.; Siregar, A.; Sihaloho, E.D.; Fathania, D.; Dewi, N.F.; Koesoemadinata, R.C.; Hill, P.C.; Alisjahbana, B. Feasibility of two active case finding approaches for detection of tuberculosis in Bandung City, Indonesia. *Public Health Action* **2017**, *7*, 206–211. [CrossRef]
24. Ahmad, R.A.; Mahendradhata, Y.; Cunningham, J.; Utarini, A.; de Vlas, S.J. How to optimize tuberculosis case finding: Explorations for Indonesia with a health system model. *BMC Infect. Dis.* **2009**, *9*, 87. [CrossRef]
25. Stop TB Partnership. The TB REACH Initiative. Available online: http://www.stoptb.org/global/awards/tbreach/ (accessed on 24 September 2020).
26. Kementerian Kesehatan Republik Indonesia. Estimasi Penduduk Menurut Umur Tunggal Dal Jenis Kelamin Menurut Kabupaten/Kota Tahun 2014. Available online: https://web.archive.org/web/20140208021950/http:/depkes.go.id/downloads/Penduduk%20Kab%20Kota%20Umur%20Tunggal%202014.pdf (accessed on 25 September 2020).
27. Wikipedia. North Sumatra. 2020. Available online: https://en.wikipedia.org/wiki/North_Sumatra (accessed on 25 September 2020).
28. Blok, L.; Creswell, J.; Stevens, R.; Brouwer, M.; Ramis, O.; Weil, O.; Klatser, P.; Sahu, S.; Bakker, M.I. A pragmatic approach to measuring, monitoring and evaluating interventions for improved tuberculosis case detection. *Int. Health* **2014**, *6*, 181–188. [CrossRef]
29. Corbett, E.L.; Bandason, T.; Duong, T.; Dauya, E.; Makamure, B.; Churchyard, G.J.; Williams, B.G.; Munyati, S.S.; Butterworth, A.E.; Mason, P.R.; et al. Comparison of two active case-finding strategies for community-based diagnosis of symptomatic smear-positive tuberculosis and control of infectious tuberculosis in Harare, Zimbabwe (DETECTB): A cluster-randomised trial. *Lancet* **2010**, *376*, 1244–1253. [CrossRef]
30. Miller, A.C.; Golub, J.E.; Cavalcante, S.C.; Durovni, B.; Moulton, L.H.; Fonseca, Z.; Arduini, D.; Chaisson, R.E.; Soares, E.C. Controlled trial of active tuberculosis case finding in a Brazilian favela. *Int. J. Tuberc. Lung Dis.* **2010**, *14*, 720–726.
31. Marks, G.B.; Nguyen, N.V.; Nguyen, P.T.; Nguyen, T.A.; Nguyen, H.B.; Tran, K.H.; Nguyen, S.V.; Luu, K.B.; Tran, D.T.; Vo, Q.T.; et al. Community-wide screening for tuberculosis in a high-prevalence setting. *N. Engl. J. Med.* **2019**, *381*, 1347–1357. [CrossRef]
32. Ayles, H.; Muyoyeta, M.; Du Toit, E.; Schaap, A.; Floyd, S.; Simwinga, M.; Shanaube, K.; Chishinga, N.; Bond, V.; Dunbar, R.; et al. Effect of household and community interventions on the burden of tuberculosis in southern Africa: The ZAMSTAR community-randomised trial. *Lancet* **2013**, *382*, 1183–1194. [CrossRef]
33. Gurung, S.C.; Dixit, K.; Rai, B.; Caws, M.; Paudel, P.R.; Dhital, R.; Acharya, S.; Budhathoki, G.; Malla, D.; Levy, J.W.; et al. The role of active case finding in reducing patient incurred catastrophic costs for tuberculosis in Nepal. *Infect. Dis. Poverty* **2019**, *8*, 99. [CrossRef]
34. Kranzer, K.; Afnan-Holmes, H.; Tomlin, K.; Golub, J.E.; Shapiro, A.E.; Schaap, A.; Corbett, E.L.; Lönnroth, K.; Glynn, J.R. The benefits to communities and individuals of screening for active tuberculosis disease: A systematic review [State of the art series. *Case finding/screening. Number 2 in the series]. Int. J. Tuberc. Lung Dis.* **2013**, *17*, 432–446. [CrossRef]
35. Albert, H.; Purcell, R.; Wang, Y.Y.; Kao, K.; Mareka, M.; Katz, Z.; Maama, B.L. Mots' oane T Designing an optimized diagnostic network to improve access to TB diagnosis and treatment in Lesotho. *PLoS ONE* **2020**, *15*, e0233620. [CrossRef]
36. John, S.; Gidado, M.; Dahiru, T.; Fanning, A.; Codlin, A.J.; Creswell, J. Tuberculosis among nomads in Adamawa, Nigeria: Outcomes from two years of active case finding. *Int. J. Tuberc. Lung Dis.* **2015**, *19*, 463–468. [CrossRef]
37. Vyas, A.; Creswell, J.; Codlin, A.J.; Stevens, R.; Rao, V.G.; Kumar, B.; Khaparde, S.; Sahu, S. Community-based active case-finding to reach the most vulnerable: Tuberculosis in tribal areas of India. *Int. J. Tuberc. Lung Dis.* **2019**, *23*, 750–755. [CrossRef]
38. Abdullahi, S.A.; Smelyanskaya, M.; John, S.; Adamu, H.I.; Ubochioma, E.; Kennedy, I.; Abubakar, F.A.; Ago, H.A.; Stevens, R.; Creswell, J. Providing TB and HIV outreach services to internally displaced populations in Northeast Nigeria: Results of a controlled intervention study. *PLoS Med.* **2020**, *17*, e1003218. [CrossRef]

39. Onozaki, I.; Law, I.; Sismanidis, C.; Zignol, M.; Glaziou, P.; Floyd, K. National tuberculosis prevalence surveys in Asia, 1990–2012: An overview of results and lessons learned. *Trop. Med. Int. Health* **2015**, *20*, 1128–1145. [CrossRef]
40. World Health Organization. Approaches to Improve Sputum Smear Microscopy for Tuberculosis Diagnosis: Expert Group Meeting Report. 2009. Available online: https://www.who.int/tb/laboratory/egmreport_microscopymethods_nov09.pdf (accessed on 4 July 2020).
41. World Health Organization. *Systematic Screening for Active Tuberculosis: Principles and Recommendations*; World Health Organization: Geneva, Switzerland, 2013.
42. rGLC Country Support Mission Report. 2017. Available online: https://www.who.int/docs/default-source/searo/tuberculosis/pmdt-indonesia-2017.pdf?sfvrsn=b07db6e9_2 (accessed on 20 August 2020).
43. World Health Organization. *Molecular Assays Intended as Initial Tests for the Diagnosis of Pulmonary and Extrapulmonary TB and Rifampicin Resistance in Adults and Children: Rapid Communication*; World Health Organization: Geneva, Switzerland, 2020.
44. Creswell, J.; Rai, B.; Wali, R.; Sudrungrot, S.; Adhikari, L.M.; Pant, R.; Pyakurel, S.; Uranw, D.; Codlin, A.J. Introducing new tuberculosis diagnostics: The impact of Xpert® MTB/RIF testing on case notifications in Nepal. *Int. J. Tuberc. Lung Dis.* **2015**, *19*, 545–551. [CrossRef]
45. Theron, G.; Zijenah, L.; Chanda, D.; Clowes, P.; Rachow, A.; Lesosky, M.; Bara, W.; Mungofa, S.; Pai, M.; Hoelscher, M.; et al. Feasibility, accuracy, and clinical effect of point-of-care Xpert MTB/RIF testing for tuberculosis in primary-care settings in Africa: A multicentre, randomised, controlled trial. *Lancet* **2014**, *383*, 424–435. [CrossRef]
46. TB CARE I Core Project: Intensified Implementation of GeneXpert MTB/RIF in 3 Countries. KNCV Tuberculosis Foundation to Eliminate TB 2013. Available online: https://www.kncvtbc.org/uploaded/2015/09/TB_CARE_I_GeneXpert_Core_Project_Final_Report.pdf (accessed on 20 August 2020).
47. Van't Hoog, A.H.; Onozaki, I.; Lonnroth, K. Choosing algorithms for TB screening: A modelling study to compare yield, predictive value and diagnostic burden. *BMC Infect. Dis.* **2014**, *14*, 532. [CrossRef] [PubMed]
48. Suárez, P.G.; Watt, C.J.; Alarcón, E.; Portocarrero, J.; Zavala, D.; Canales, R.; Luelmo, F.; Espinal, M.A.; Dye, C. The dynamics of tuberculosis in response to 10 years of intensive control effort in Peru. *J. Infect. Dis.* **2001**, *184*, 473–478. [CrossRef] [PubMed]
49. Creswell, J.; Codlin, A.J.; Oliva Flores, S.; Samayoa, M.; Ramis, O.; Guardado, M.E. Will more sensitive diagnostics identify tuberculosis missed by clinicians? Evaluating Xpert MTB/RIF testing in Guatemala. *Gac. Sanit.* **2020**, *34*, 127–132. [CrossRef]
50. Mhimbira, F.A.; Cuevas, L.E.; Dacombe, R.; Mkopi, A.; Sinclair, D. Interventions to increase tuberculosis case detection at primary healthcare or community-level services. *Cochrane Database Syst. Rev.* **2017**. [CrossRef]

Publisher's Note: MDPI stays neutral with regard to jurisdictional claims in published maps and institutional affiliations.

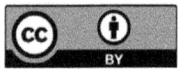

© 2020 by the authors. Licensee MDPI, Basel, Switzerland. This article is an open access article distributed under the terms and conditions of the Creative Commons Attribution (CC BY) license (http://creativecommons.org/licenses/by/4.0/).

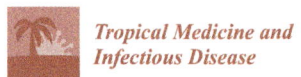

Perspective

The TB REACH Initiative: Supporting TB Elimination Efforts in the Asia-Pacific

Jacob Creswell [1,*], Amera Khan [1], Mirjam I Bakker [2], Miranda Brouwer [3], Vishnu Vardhan Kamineni [4], Christina Mergenthaler [2], Marina Smelyanskaya [1], Zhi Zhen Qin [1], Oriol Ramis [5], Robert Stevens [6], K Srikanth Reddy [7] and Lucie Blok [2]

1. Stop TB Partnership, 1218 Geneva, Switzerland; amerak@stoptb.org (A.K.); m.smelyanskaya@gmail.com (M.S.); zhizhenq@stoptb.org (Z.Z.Q.)
2. KIT Royal Tropical Institute, 1092 Amsterdam, The Netherlands; M.Bakker@kit.nl (M.I.B.); C.Mergenthaler@kit.nl (C.M.); L.Blok@kit.nl (L.B.)
3. PHTB Consult, 5014 DN Tilburg, The Netherlands; phtbconsult@gmail.com
4. Independent Consultant, Bangalore 560094, India; vvkamineni@gmail.com
5. Epirus, 08034 Barcelona, Spain; oriolramis@gmail.com
6. Independent Consultant, Manchester HX7 6AL, UK; robert.hartley.stevens@gmail.com
7. Global Affairs Canada, Global Health and Nutrition Bureau, Ottawa K1A 0G2, ON, Canada; SKondreddy@bruyere.org
* Correspondence: jacobc@stoptb.org

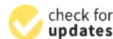

Received: 26 September 2020; Accepted: 16 October 2020; Published: 26 October 2020

Abstract: After many years of TB 'control' and incremental progress, the TB community is talking about ending the disease, yet this will only be possible with a shift in the way we approach the TB response. While the Asia-Pacific region has the highest TB burden worldwide, it also has the opportunity to lead the quest to end TB by embracing the four areas laid out in this series: using data to target hotspots, initiating active case finding, provisioning preventive TB treatment, and employing a biosocial approach. The Stop TB Partnership's TB REACH initiative provides a platform to support partners in the development, evaluation and scale-up of new and innovative technologies and approaches to advance TB programs. We present several approaches TB REACH is taking to support its partners in the Asia-Pacific and globally to advance our collective response to end TB.

Keywords: tuberculosis; active case finding; TB preventive therapy; innovation; End TB; TB REACH

1. Introduction

Since the tuberculosis (TB) epidemic was declared an emergency by the World Health Organization (WHO) in the 1990s, different global TB strategies, each growing more comprehensive and ambitious in their plans and goals, have been developed and deployed. Moving from a focus on adults with TB seeking care in the public sector, strategies have evolved to provide more emphasis on children, people living with HIV, engaging the private sector, involving communities, pro-actively reaching out to people with limited access to care and addressing catastrophic costs incurred by people who have TB [1–3]. Once aiming to identify 70% of incident TB cases, we now understand this will not suffice to end TB and new targets call for universal access to TB care and prevention [4–6]. In 2018, the TB community came together at a UN High Level Meeting (UNHLM) to agree on ambitious global targets and called for an end to the epidemic in the next decade [3,7,8]. Business as usual approaches will not be sufficient to reach these targets, and this is what drives Stop TB Partnership's Global Plan: The Paradigm Shift [7].

The TB community has been criticized for lacking ambition and being timid in its approach to combatting the disease [9,10]. The current series of this journal, Innovation and Evidence for

Achieving TB Elimination in the Asia–Pacific Region, brings together several important topics for the TB community. The Asia-Pacific region accounts for more than two thirds of incident TB globally (using generally accepted countries rather than WHO's grouping) [11,12]. However, the region has also been a leader in innovation and research in the TB field. Recent large increases in case notification primarily came from this region and bold new research is highlighting the path towards ending TB [11,13,14]. Strongly correlated with reductions in TB incidence, is socio-economic development and the Asia-Pacific region is also leading the world in GDP growth [15]. Below, we present how the Stop TB Partnership's TB REACH initiative has addressed the different areas outlined in the Lancet Series "How to Eliminate Tuberculosis" [16] with particular attention paid to the Asia-Pacific.

2. The TB REACH Initiative

The Stop TB Partnership's TB REACH initiative [17] was established in 2009 to bring new ideas and thinking to promote bold action in the fight against TB. With foundational support from Global Affairs Canada, and additional support from USAID and The Bill and Melinda Gates Foundation, TB REACH provides rapid funding to partners to quickly implement case finding and treatment support interventions whilst conducting continuous monitoring and evaluation. Despite a focus on service delivery, each TB REACH project is given strong independent monitoring and evaluation support to track historical and prospective TB notification data as well as intervention specific indicators, so results are rigorously documented. TB REACH works with innovators and grassroots organizations, testing new approaches and technologies that many traditional donors, are less inclined to support. With eight waves of funding, TB REACH has provided USD 63.4 million to countries in the Asia-Pacific region through 134 grants (Figure 1).

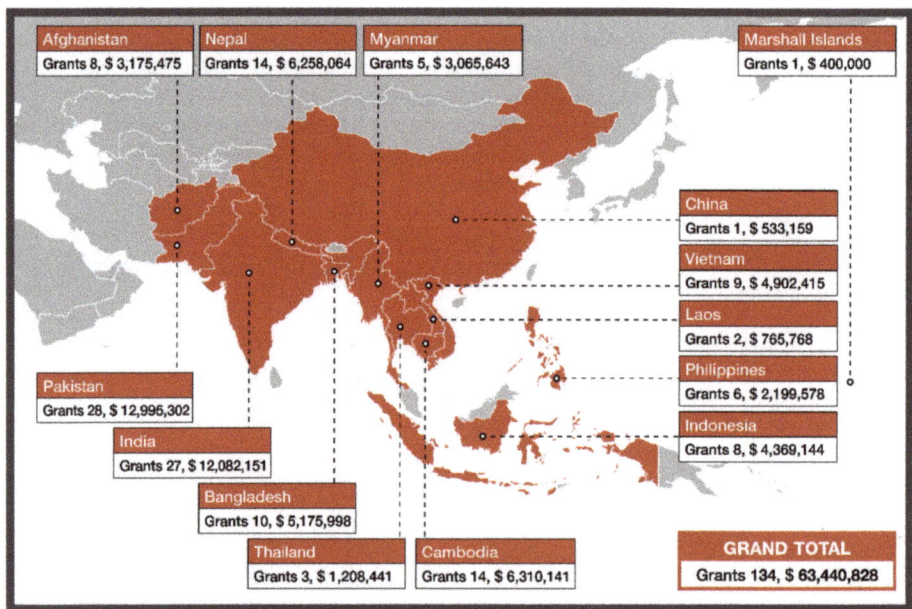

Figure 1. Map of TB REACH grants in the Asia-Pacific region.

Unlike other funding mechanisms, TB REACH is not constrained by WHO guidelines as to what it can fund, which allows implementers to take risks and test new approaches or technologies. For example, TB REACH supported Xpert testing in Tanzania in mobile vans before WHO guidance was issued on the assay in 2011. The assay was used by other TB REACH projects as a front-line diagnostic while most countries were still using it only as a drug sensitivity test [18,19]. Additionally, TB REACH efforts in Nigeria and Cambodia presented interesting results from a novel pooled sputum strategy to save Xpert cartridge costs and time [20,21]. While the use of artificial intelligence (AI) in health has gained interest recently, TB REACH has been supporting AI to read chest x-rays (CXR) well before this approach was reviewed by WHO [22–24]. Current projects are testing new handheld X-ray machines that can be brought into communities for screening.

TB REACH projects are limited in both time and scope. Projects generally last between 12–18 months and their funding cannot exceed USD 1 million. These limitations create the need for longer term support from governments and other donors to scale-up and sustain successful interventions. As such, TB REACH has worked with partners and donors to stimulate the adoption of new and innovative approaches by national TB programs, the Global Fund [25], and Unitaid among others [26].

Much of the data and examples included in this article come from experiences and results of TB REACH projects. Where possible, data has been referenced, but in some instances, results have not been published yet and been abstracted from project reports.

3. Data and Hotspots

The 3 million people with TB who are missed every year by routine health programs, "the missing millions", are at the center of global discussions. At the national level, treatment coverage quantifies how well TB programs are reaching all people with TB [11]. However, these numbers fail to capture the substantial heterogeneity in treatment coverage at regional or district levels. This heterogeneity exists because of geographic features, demographics, key populations and other factors such as access to health care [27,28]. Furthermore, because people with TB are not homogenously distributed across geographical areas, mapping hotspots to help identify where best to focus active case finding (ACF) efforts is critical [29]. Often, TB REACH projects are specifically designed to focus on these hotspot areas and key populations, such as sex workers, transgender populations, people who inject drugs, prisoners, migrants, miners, ethnic minorities and indigenous populations, and other poor and/or remote communities, who have poor access to care and high burdens of TB [30]. These projects use intervention data to improve case finding as part of a rigorous monitoring and evaluation process. The continued monitoring and evaluation of TB REACH interventions ensures an understanding of the target populations demographics and specifically, how many people are reached, screened, tested and diagnosed, and where people drop out of the care cascade. A number of mobile screening applications to track people through the care cascade as well as systems to track Xpert testing have been developed [31,32].

4. Active Case Finding

Passive case finding (PCF) is the standard approach for TB programs globally. PCF relies on people who have chest symptoms to visit diagnostic facilities and be tested, generally with smear microscopy. While the approach is inexpensive, and can reach large parts of the population, it often misses many groups such as children, people with HIV, and many of the key populations mentioned above who have difficulties accessing care because of stigma, financial, structural, cultural and/or socio-economic barriers [5,6]. Ten years ago, TB REACH began to support innovative approaches to improve case detection including ACF programs which involve moving outside the health facility to reach people who are ill [33]. ACF often uses community members to conduct activities, and increasingly has employed CXR to identify people with TB who do not complain about symptoms. ACF is a complement to routine PCF and usually is measured by how many undiagnosed people with TB are identified and how this impacts the total notifications in a population [34]. Some differences between ACF and PCF are presented in Table 1. ACF is now an integral part of many national strategic plans for TB [34–36]. Here, and in this Series, we document numerous examples demonstrating the power of ACF in the Asia-Pacific region. In Indonesia, a community-based organization (CBO) increased TB notification numbers significantly through ACF initiatives aimed at remote island populations [37]. Similar increases have been attributed to ACF initiatives in Pakistan [38,39] and Cambodia [40].

Table 1. Characteristics of Passive and Active Case Finding for Tuberculosis.

Passive Case Finding	Active Case Finding
• Sick individuals seek care at a health facility	• Health services expanded into the community
• Care is provided to those who present to the facility	• Targets specific groups/populations at elevated risk of TB or with limited access to services
• Presumptive TB usually defined as a prolonged cough	• Presumptive TB definition often more inclusive, such as any TB symptom (no duration indication) or chest X-ray abnormal
• Traditionally uses smear microscopy, and increasingly molecular assays for diagnosis	• Molecular assay recommended for diagnosis to reduce risk of false-positive results
• Likely to identify people with TB later in their disease progression	• Likely to identify people with TB earlier in their disease progression
• Low health system costs, and often high patient costs	• Higher health system costs, and lower patient costs
• Higher TB prevalence among those screened and tested	• Usually finds lower TB prevalence among those screened and tested
• Often (but not always) relies on clinical staff (e.g. doctors and nurses) to carry out diagnostic evaluations	• Often (but not always) relies on lay workers or community health workers to carry out diagnostic evaluations
• Contributes to routine surveillance and notification data	• Often measured by number needed to screen and test, and additional TB notifications
• Part of the routine care provision and seeks primarily to identify people who need TB care and treatment	• Focuses on reaching people with limited access to care, interrupting transmission, and decreasing TB disease incidence

Contact investigation is a core component of ACF. Although contact investigation has not lead to large increases in case notifications, it does focus on a high risk group, assists in early identification, and is the main entry point for TB preventive treatment (TPT). Furthermore, when done comprehensively, people with TB identified through contact investigation can contribute more than 10% of the total case notifications in a given population [41,42]. Despite being part of WHO and country guidelines, contact investigation is not always regularly conducted in many countries in the region.

While a systematic review has shown that ACF alone does not impact treatment outcomes [43], the outreach associated with ACF presents better opportunities to support people with TB and ensure they successfully complete treatment, often through community health workers. In India, a CBO developed a highly successful outreach effort employing local lay workers on motorcycles to visit, screen and provide treatment support to tribal communities. The results were impressive, with a first-year pilot improving case notifications by 84% and a scale-up intervention producing similar results [44]. Moreover, pre-treatment loss to follow-up and treatment outcomes improved even with the added testing and treatment burden as the lay workers supported people with TB by visiting them consistently throughout treatment. Cambodia has been one of the earliest adopters of ACF by repurposing prevalence survey equipment to reach communities with poor access to care with both CXR and modern diagnostics such as Xpert [20,40,45,46]. While it is clear that ACF reaches people with TB earlier and can greatly improve the numbers of people treated [47,48], it is also clear that ACF alone will not be enough to end TB.

5. Treating TB Infection

In this series, Harries et al. presents a strong argument for the importance of including treating TB infection as we move to end TB [49]. We note that while ACF has found a strong following in the last ten years, the scale up of TPT has seen many obstacles. Harries et al. describe several challenges for TPT scale up including imperfect and expensive diagnostic tests for TB infection, long regimens, high pill burden, expensive shorter regimens, and limited recommendations on risk groups to receive treatment. However, there are a few initiatives trying to address these issues. In many cases, ACF in the form of contact investigation will be a necessary precursor to successful TPT. Numerous early adopters, such as the Zero TB Cities Initiative [50], are combining ACF and TPT to move more quickly towards the goal of ending TB. On the islands of Cu Lao Cham and Cat Ba in Viet Nam, community screening campaigns called SWEEP-TB integrated ACF and TB infection testing and treatment to create islands of elimination. These campaigns consisted of community mobilization and TB infection testing, using either the tuberculin skin test (TST) or the QuantiFERON-TB Gold Plus (QFT), in public places of congregation and subsequent door-to-door campaigns. Two days later, participants presented for evaluation of the TST or QFT results and CXR screening for active TB disease and were placed on either TB treatment or TPT as appropriate. These efforts achieved an estimated 72% population coverage with a cumulative TB infection testing of 4782 people and screening over 3100 people by CXR for the detection and treatment of 20 TB patients, two individuals with multidrug-resistant TB, and 1494 persons with TB infection. Repeat visits will attempt to document the impact of the campaigns. In the Marshall Islands, similar work was conducted combining ACF and TPT to eliminate TB from the islands. In the process, the intervention treated 4237 people with TPT and 305 for active disease [51]. Projects in other countries in the region have also shown great promise including large increases in childhood TPT enrolment in Mymensingh, Bangladesh working with both public and private providers as well as the introduction of new shorter regimens. In Indonesia, large scale Zero TB efforts are getting underway as part of a TB REACH Wave 7 project in Yogyakarta which seeks to massively scale up new shorter TPT regimens by combining ACF, and integration with community-based Maternal Child Health and Sexual Reproductive Health activities. These initiatives on TPT will identify program bottlenecks and allow TB programs to address issues during the impending scale-up of prevention efforts to meet the ambitious targets set out at the UNHLM [8].

6. Biosocial Approaches

TB is linked to poverty; its epidemiology and biology are highly dependent on social and economic factors impacting the communities where it spreads [52]. TB also aggravates poverty due to the costs of seeking care even though diagnosis and treatment itself may be free [53]. Ending TB thus means tackling the root causes of poverty, and the causes of stigma and marginalization which includes gender inequality, discrimination, racial and ethnic biases, and others. The difficulty of navigating the health care sector can add additional costs and result in people to drop out of the care cascade [54]. TB REACH supported projects in India using Accredited Social Health Activists (commonly known as ASHAs), an existing cadre working in the community as outreach workers, to guide patients through the diagnostic and treatment process, have led to substantially increased notifications [55,56]. A study in Nepal demonstrated how ACF can reduce catastrophic costs for people with TB as well as bringing health services to the community [57]. Traditional facility-based directly observed therapy requires persons with TB to regularly travel to health facilities, which can result in the incurring of travel and time costs as well as the loss of autonomy and privacy [58]. TB REACH has supported novel ways to improve treatment outcomes and enhance TB care including a portfolio of projects exploring the use of digital adherence technologies (DAT) as treatment support. The use of DAT is part of a shift towards people-centred care, empowering people with TB to take charge of their treatment and enabling health care providers to maintain contact with them and to identify individuals who may need additional support measures. In the Asia-Pacific region, current projects in Thailand, Philippines, and Bangladesh are assessing the feasibility and acceptability of these approaches as well as their effectiveness in relation to adherence and treatment outcomes with promising preliminary results [59–61]. In Thailand, the use of near field communication technology allowing migrants to store and share their digital treatment records, showed a 21% increase in treatment success rates in the intervention period compared to pre-intervention period.

TB programs cannot exist in a medicalized vacuum of vertical service delivery. To achieve elimination, TB programming must cut across other issues that are pertinent to communities impacted by TB. For example, malnutrition—a key symptom of poverty—can be addressed through TB programming. Interventions in Pakistan and Indonesia introduced food incentives and enablers to help people with TB and their families continue treatment and improve their overall nutritional status [37,42]. A TB REACH project in India is currently documenting the impact of India's direct benefit transfer program plus additional food support on treatment outcomes. A CBO in Pakistan worked in collaboration with transgender women and male sex worker community leaders to provide both social and nutritional support. The project tested over 7000 people for TB and initiated anti-TB treatment for more than 600 individuals, documenting high rates of both TB and HIV among these key populations [62].

Workplaces are another setting where interventions to improve TB detection and treatment can incorporate biosocial approaches. Some settings have crowded working conditions which can increase the risk of occupational exposure to TB. Many factory workers often lack time and resources to access health care. Employees found to have TB are often at risk for discrimination, stigma, and the potential for losing their job. TB REACH has supported ACF factory-based projects for garment workers in Bangladesh and is currently supporting projects in Myanmar and in Indonesia. These projects not only focus on identifying and treating people with TB, they also work to provide education on TB awareness, stigma, and confidentiality to help empower workers to seek care in a safe environment while being able to continue to work.

During the introduction of GeneXpert technology, TB REACH made large investments in not only the diagnostic tests, but also the infrastructure, electricity, and health systems to help reach more people. While the assay is a clear improvement over smear microscopy to diagnose TB and drug resistance, its implementation in settings that lack proper power supply, space, efficient laboratory networks, and/or functional health facilities was challenging and additional investments were needed [63]. A laboratory test alone will not reach more people who are ill, and results have shown that simply placing Xpert within the health system is not enough to increase TB diagnoses [64]. New diagnostics must be placed in a functional health system including community structures/involvement with organized outreach to expand access to the technology and benefit many people [65,66].

TB epidemiology in the Asia Pacific Region indicates a higher risk for males [67], but women often carry the burden of TB disease differently—through being the unpaid caretakers, having their healthcare deprioritized for the benefit of their male counterparts, and carrying a heavy burden of stigma associated with the disease [68]. In addition, in many high burden TB settings women also suffer from high rates of gender-based violence, HIV and other co-occurring biosocial phenomena [69,70]. In line with the Canada's Feminist International Assistance Policy [71] and the Sustainable Development Goals [72], TB REACH is currently working on cultivating the links between empowering women, development and TB—an initiative first of its kind for the TB community [73]. Notably, Asia-Pacific region already has examples of strong female leadership at community level that are challenging existing gender norms and promoting gender equality through TB programming. In India, women from the community are trained to be agents of change and conduct TB education and case finding activities, as well as link people with TB to private and public health facilities for treatment [74]. In Indonesia, grassroots mobilization of female community volunteers brought a significant increase in TB notifications [37], but also strengthened the status of women in communities. In another project in Pakistan, the Kiran Sitara program trains young schoolgirls leadership and communication skills, while also advancing the TB response [75].

7. Conclusions

Moving from TB control to ending TB is a large shift in global policy and ambition. The Asia Pacific Region has embraced these ideas at the highest political levels [76,77]. To work towards ending TB, the TB community needs to be innovative, bold, and try things that have never been done at scale by working to bring the highest standards of care to all of those who need it. We need to make targeted investments to reach populations missed by the current approaches. ACF will be a necessary part of reaching people with TB earlier, in greater numbers, and bending the downward curve of incidence globally. However, ACF, and other innovations must be accompanied by a scale up of TPT to stem new cases from developing among people who are infected. The TB community must also embrace interventions that address the biosocial aspects of the disease, as solely medicalized approaches are insufficient to end TB. TB REACH was envisioned to test and evaluate new approaches and set them on a path to scale. We applaud the efforts to end TB in the Asia Pacific, and globally, and will continue to support new ideas to move us closer to this goal.

Author Contributions: J.C. wrote the first draft, which was critically reviewed by A.K., M.I.B., M.B., V.V.K., C.M., O.R., M.S., Z.Z.Q., R.S., K.S.R., L.B., and J.C. All authors contributed to subsequent drafts and agreed upon and approved the final version. All authors have read and agreed to the published version of the manuscript.

Funding: The article received no external funding, but Stop TB Partnership's TB REACH initiative is provided foundational funding by Global Affairs Canada, with USAID and The Bill and Melinda Gates Foundation providing additional support.

Acknowledgments: The work of TB REACH is implemented by more than 100 different partners across more than 50 countries who bring new ideas to the TB community, and we are grateful for the enthusiasm and excellent work that they all have done. We would like to acknowledge Katy Addison for her review and edits.

Conflicts of Interest: None declared.

References

1. World Health Organization. *What is DOTS? A guide to Understanding the WHO-Recommended TB Control Strategy Known as DOTS*; WHO: Geneva, Switzerland, 1999.
2. World Health Organization. *The Stop TB Strategy: Building on and Enhancing DOTS to Meet the TB-Related Millennium Development Goals*; WHO: Geneva, Switzerland, 2006.
3. World Health Organization. *The End TB Strategy: Global Strategy and Targets for Tuberculosis Prevention, Care and Control after 2015*; WHO: Geneva, Switzerland, 2015.
4. Dowdy, D.W.; Basu, S.; Andrews, J.R. Is Passive Diagnosis Enough? *Am. J. Respir. Crit. Care Med.* **2013**, *187*, 543–551. [CrossRef] [PubMed]
5. Ho, J.; Fox, G.J.; Marais, B.J. Passive case finding for tuberculosis is not enough. *Int. J. Mycobacteriol.* **2016**, *5*, 374–378. [CrossRef] [PubMed]
6. Abebe, M.; Doherty, M.; Wassie, L.; Demissie, A.; Mihret, A.; Engers, H.; Aseffa, A. TB case detection: Can we remain passive while the process is active? *Pan. Afr. Med. J.* **2012**, *11*, 50.
7. Stop TB Partnership. *The Global Plan to End TB 2018—2022: The Paradigm Shift*; Stop TB Partnership: Geneva, Switzerland, 2019.
8. United Nations General Assembly. *Political Declaration of the High-Level Meeting of the General Assembly on the Fight against Tuberculosis*; United Nations General Assembly: New York, NY, USA, 2018.
9. Madhukar, P. To Eliminate TB We Need Imagination and Ambition. Available online: https://theconversation.com/to-eliminate-tb-we-need-imagination-and-ambition-103083 (accessed on 24 September 2020).
10. Cohen, J. Campaign against TB steps up its ambitions. *Science* **2015**, *350*, 1455. [CrossRef] [PubMed]
11. World Health Organization. *Global Tuberculosis Report 2019*; WHO: Geneva, Switzerland, 2019.
12. United Nations, Department of Economic and Social Affairs, Statistics Division. Standard Country or Area Codes for Statistical Use. Available online: https://unstats.un.org/unsd/methodology/m49/ (accessed on 24 September 2020).
13. Arinaminpathy, N.; Batra, D.; Khaparde, S.; Vualnam, T.; Maheshwari, N.; Sharma, L.; Nair, S.A.; Dewan, P. The number of privately treated tuberculosis cases in India: An estimation from drug sales data. *Lancet Infect Dis.* **2016**, *16*, 1255–1260. [CrossRef]

14. Marks, G.B.; Nguyen, N.V.; Nguyen, P.T.B.; Nguyen, T.A.; Nguyen, H.B.; Tran, K.H.; Nguyen, S.V.; Luu, K.B.; Tran, D.T.T.; Vo, Q.T.N.; et al. Community-wide Screening for Tuberculosis in a High-Prevalence Setting. *N. Engl. J. Med.* **2019**, *381*, 1347–1357. [CrossRef]
15. World Bank Open Data. Available online: https://data.worldbank.org/ (accessed on 24 September 2020).
16. Keshavjee, S.; Dowdy, D.; Swaminathan, S. Stopping the body count: A comprehensive approach to move towards zero tuberculosis deaths. *Lancet* **2015**, *386*, e46–e47. [CrossRef]
17. Stop TB Partnership. The TB REACH Initiative. Available online: http://www.stoptb.org/global/awards/tbreach/ (accessed on 24 September 2020).
18. Qin, Z.Z.; Pai, M.; Van Gemert, W.; Sahu, S.; Ghiasi, M.; Creswell, J. How is Xpert MTB/RIF being implemented in 22 high tuberculosis burden countries? *Eur. Respir. J.* **2015**, *45*, 549–554. [CrossRef]
19. Creswell, J.; Codlin, A.J.; Andre, E.; Micek, M.A.; Bedru, A.; Carter, E.J.; Yadav, R.P.; Mosneaga, A.; Rai, B.; Banu, S.; et al. Results from early programmatic implementation of Xpert MTB/RIF testing in nine countries. *BMC Infect Dis.* **2014**, *14*, 2. [CrossRef]
20. Chry, M.; Smelyanskaya, M.; Ky, M.; Codlin, A.J.; Cazabon, D.; Tan Eang, M.; Creswell, J. Can the High Sensitivity of Xpert MTB/RIF Ultra Be Harnessed to Save Cartridge Costs? Results from a Pooled Sputum Evaluation in Cambodia. *Trop. Med. Infect Dis.* **2020**, *5*, 27. [CrossRef]
21. Abdurrahman, S.T.; Mbanaso, O.; Lawson, L.; Oladimeji, O.; Blakiston, M.; Obasanya, J.; Dacombe, R.; Adams, E.R.; Emenyonu, N.; Sahu, S.; et al. Testing Pooled Sputum with Xpert MTB/RIF for Diagnosis of Pulmonary Tuberculosis To Increase Affordability in Low-Income Countries. *J. Clin. Microbiol.* **2015**, *53*, 2502–2508. [CrossRef] [PubMed]
22. Rahman, M.T.; Codlin, A.J.; Rahman, M.M.; Nahar, A.; Reja, M.; Islam, T.; Qin, Z.Z.; Khan, M.A.S.; Banu, S.; Creswell, J. An evaluation of automated chest radiography reading software for tuberculosis screening among public- and private-sector patients. *Eur. Respir. J.* **2017**, *49*, 1602159. [CrossRef] [PubMed]
23. Qin, Z.Z.; Sander, M.S.; Rai, B.; Titahong, C.N.; Sudrungrot, S.; Laah, S.N.; Adhikari, L.M.; Carter, E.J.; Puri, L.; Codlin, A.J.; et al. Using artificial intelligence to read chest radiographs for tuberculosis detection: A multi-site evaluation of the diagnostic accuracy of three deep learning systems. *Sci. Rep.* **2019**, *18*, 15000. [CrossRef]
24. Muyoyeta, M.; Maduskar, P.; Moyo, M.; Kasese, N.; Milimo, D.; Spooner, R.; Kapata, N.; Hogeweg, L.; van Ginneken, B.; Ayles, H.; et al. The Sensitivity and Specificity of Using a Computer Aided Diagnosis Program for Automatically Scoring Chest X-Rays of Presumptive TB Patients Compared with Xpert MTB/RIF in Lusaka Zambia. *PLoS ONE* **2014**, *9*, e93757. [CrossRef] [PubMed]
25. Wandwalo, E.; Creswell, J. TB REACH and the Global Fund: A Partnership to Find and Treat the "Missing Cases". Available online: https://www.theglobalfund.org/en/blog/2017-06-02-tb-reach-and-the-global-fund-a-partnership-to-find-and-treat-the-missing-cases/ (accessed on 4 October 2020).
26. Stop TB Partnership. TB REACH Presentation to the 32nd Board, Jakarta, Indonesia. 2019. Available online: http://www.stoptb.org/assets/documents/about/cb/meetings/32/32-08%20TB%20REACH%203.0/32-8.8%20TB%20REACH%203.0_Presentation.pdf (accessed on 30 September 2020).
27. Theron, G.; Jenkins, H.E.; Cobelens, F.; Abubakar, I.; Khan, A.J.; Cohen, T.; Dowdy, D.W. Data for action: Collection and use of local data to end tuberculosis. *Lancet* **2015**, *386*, 2324–2333. [CrossRef]
28. Rood, E.; Khan, A.H.; Modak, P.K.; Mergenthaler, C.; van Gurp, M.; Blok, L.; Bakker, M. A Spatial Analysis Framework to Monitor and Accelerate Progress towards SDG 3 to End TB in Bangladesh. *Int. J. Geo-Inf.* **2019**, *8*, 14. [CrossRef]
29. Vo, L.N.Q.; Vu, T.N.; Nguyen, H.T.; Truong, T.T.; Khuu, C.M.; Pham, P.Q.; Nguyen, L.H.; Le, G.T.; Creswell, J. Optimizing community screening for tuberculosis: Spatial analysis of localized case finding from door-to-door screening for TB in an urban district of Ho Chi Minh City, Vietnam. *PLoS ONE* **2018**, *13*, e0209290. [CrossRef]
30. Blok, L.; Creswell, J.; Stevens, R.; Brouwer, M.; Ramis, O.; Weil, O.; Klatser, P.; Sahu, S.; Bakker, M.I. A pragmatic approach to measuring, monitoring and evaluating interventions for improved tuberculosis case detection. *Int. Health* **2014**, *6*, 181–188. [CrossRef]
31. Cowan, J.; Michel, C.; Manhiça, I.; Mutaquiha, C.; Monivo, C.; Saize, D.; Beste, J.; Creswell, J.; Codlin, A.J.; Gloyd, S. Remote monitoring of Xpert® MTB/RIF testing in Mozambique: Results of programmatic implementation of GxAlert. *Int. J. Tuberc. Lung Dis.* **2016**, *20*, 335–341. [CrossRef]

32. Vo, L.N.Q.; Forse, R.J.; Codlin, A.J.; Vu, T.N.; Le, G.T.; Do, G.C.; Truong, V.V.; Dang, H.M.; Squire, B.; Levy, J.; et al. A comparative impact evaluation of two human resource models for community-based active tuberculosis case finding in Ho Chi Minh City, Vietnam. *BMC Public Health* **2020**, *20*, 934. [CrossRef]
33. Uplekar, M.; Creswell, J.; Ottmani, S.E.; Weil, D.; Sahu, S.; Lönnroth, K. Programmatic approaches to screening for active tuberculosis. *Int. J. Tuberc. Lung Dis.* **2013**, *17*, 1248–1256. [CrossRef] [PubMed]
34. National Center for Tuberculosis and Leprosy Control (CENAT). *National Strategic Plan for Control of Tuberculosis 2014–2020*; National Center for Tuberculosis and Leprosy Control: Phnom Penh, Cambodgia, 2014.
35. National Tuberculosis Programme, Myanmar. National Strategic Plan for Tuberculosis 2016–2020. Available online: https://www.aidsdatahub.org/sites/default/files/resource/myanmar-national-strategic-plan-tuberculosis-2016-2020.pdf (accessed on 19 September 2020).
36. Revised National Tuberculosis Control Programme. National Strategic Plan for Tuberculosis Elimination 2017–2025. Available online: https://tbcindia.gov.in/WriteReadData/NSP%20Draft%2020.02.2017%201.pdf (accessed on 19 September 2020).
37. Siahaan, E.S.; Bakker, M.I.; Pasaribu, R.; Khan, A.; Pande, T.; Hasibuan, A.M.; Creswell, J. Islands of tuberculosis elimination: An evaluation of community-based active case finding in North Sumatra, Indonesia. *Trop. Med. Infect. Dis* **2020**, *5*, 163. [CrossRef]
38. Malik, A.A.; Hussain, H.; Creswell, J.; Siddiqui, S.; FAhmed, J.; Madhani, F.; Habib, A.; Khan, A.J.; Amanullah, F. The Impact of Funding on Childhood TB Case Detection in Pakistan. *Trop. Med. Infect. Dis.* **2019**, *4*, 146. [CrossRef]
39. Malik, A.A.; Amanullah, F.; Codlin, A.J.; Siddiqui, S.; Jaswal, M.; Ahmed, J.F.; Saleem, S.; Khurshid, A.; Hussain, H. Improving childhood tuberculosis detection and treatment through facility-based screening in rural Pakistan. *Int. J. Tuberc. Lung Dis.* **2018**, *22*, 851–857. [CrossRef]
40. Codlin, A.J.; Monyrath, C.; Ky, M.; Gerstel, L.; Creswell, J.; Eang, M.T. Results from a roving, active case finding initiative to improve tuberculosis detection among older people in rural Cambodia using the Xpert MTB/RIF assay and chest X-ray. *J. Clin. Tuberc. Other Mycobact. Dis.* **2018**, *13*, 22–27. [CrossRef]
41. Blok, L.; Sahu, S.; Creswell, J.; Alba, S.; Stevens, R.; Bakker, M.I. Comparative Meta-Analysis of Tuberculosis Contact Investigation Interventions in Eleven High Burden Countries. *PLoS ONE* **2015**, *10*, e0119822. [CrossRef]
42. Shah, S.A.; Qayyum, S.; Abro, R.; Baig, S.; Creswell, J. Active contact investigation and treatment support: An integrated approach in rural and urban Sindh, Pakistan. *Int. J. Tuberc. Lung Dis.* **2013**, *17*, 1569–1574. [CrossRef]
43. Kranzer, K.; Afnan-Holmes, H.; Tomlin, K.; Golub, J.E.; Shapiro, A.E.; Schaap, A.; Corbett, E.L.; Lönnroth, K.; Glynn, J.R. The benefits to communities and individuals of screening for active tuberculosis disease: A systematic review. *Int. J. Tuberc. Lung Dis.* **2013**, *17*, 432–446. [CrossRef]
44. Vyas, A.; Creswell, J.; Codlin, A.J.; Stevens, R.; Rao, V.G.; Kumar, B.; Kharparde, S.; Sahu, S. Community-based active case-finding to reach the most vulnerable: Tuberculosis in tribal areas of India. *Int. J. Tuberc. Lung Dis.* **2019**, *23*, 750–755. [CrossRef]
45. Eang, M.T.; Satha, P.; Yadav, R.P.; Morishita, F.; Nishikiori, N.; van-Maaren, P.; Lambregts-van Weezenbeek, C. Early detection of tuberculosis through community-based active case finding in Cambodia. *BMC Public Health* **2012**, *12*, 469. [CrossRef]
46. Morishita, F.; Eang, M.T.; Nishikiori, N.; Yadav, R.-P. Increased Case Notification through Active Case Finding of Tuberculosis among Household and Neighbourhood Contacts in Cambodia. *PLoS ONE* **2016**, *11*, e0150405. [CrossRef] [PubMed]
47. Creswell, J.; Sahu, S.; Blok, L.; Bakker, M.I.; Stevens, R.; Ditiu, L. A Multi-Site Evaluation of Innovative Approaches to Increase Tuberculosis Case Notification: Summary Results. *PLoS ONE* **2014**, *9*, e94465. [CrossRef] [PubMed]
48. Mhimbira, F.A.; Cuevas, L.E.; Dacombe, R.; Mkopi, A.; Sinclair, D. Interventions to increase tuberculosis case detection at primary healthcare or community-level services. *Cochrane Datab. Syst. Rev.* **2017**, CD011432. [CrossRef] [PubMed]
49. Harries, A.D.; Kumar, A.M.V.; Satyanarayana, S.; Thekkur, P.; Lin, Y.; Dlodlo, R.A.; Khogali, M.; Zachariah, R. The Growing Importance of Tuberculosis Preventive Therapy and How Research and Innovation Can Enhance Its Implementation on the Ground. *Trop. Med. Infect. Dis.* **2020**, *5*, 61. [CrossRef] [PubMed]
50. Zero TB Initiative. Available online: https://www.zerotbinitiative.org/ (accessed on 24 September 2020).

51. Brostrom, R.; Largen, A.; Konelios-Langinlur, M.; Zachraias, Z.; Yadav, S.; Ko, E.; Dugan, G.; Hill, J.; Finlay, A.; Mermin, J. Voyage to TB elimination: A mass TB treatment and prevention campaign in the Marshall Islands. In Proceedings of the Union World Lung Conference, Hyderabad, India, 30 October–2 November 2019; 2019. Available online: https://hyderabad.worldlunghealth.org/wp-content/uploads/2019/11/20191101_UNION2019_Abstracts_Final.pdf (accessed on 24 September 2020).
52. Hargreaves, J.R.; Boccia, D.; Evans, C.A.; Adato, M.; Petticrew, M.; Porter, J.D. The social determinants of tuberculosis: From evidence to action. *Am. J. Public Health* **2011**, *101*, 654–662. [CrossRef]
53. Erlinger, S.; Stracker, N.; Hanrahan, C.; Nonyane, S.; Mmolawa, L.; Tampi, R.; Tucker, A.; West, N.; Lebina, L.; Martinson, N.A.; et al. Tuberculosis patients with higher levels of poverty face equal or greater costs of illness. *Int. J. Tuberc. Lung Dis.* **2019**, *23*, 1205–1212. [CrossRef] [PubMed]
54. Yellapa, V.; Devadasan, N.; Krumeich, A.; Pai, N.P.; Vadnais, C.; Pai, M.; Engel, N. How patients navigate the diagnostic ecosystem in a fragmented health system: A qualitative study from India. *Global Health Action* **2017**, *10*, 1350452. [CrossRef] [PubMed]
55. Garg, T.; Gupta, V.; Sen, D.; Verma, M.; Brouwer, M.; Mishra, R.; Bhardwaj, M. Prediagnostic loss to follow-up in an active case finding tuberculosis programme: A mixed-methods study from rural Bihar, India. *BMJ Open* **2020**, *10*, e033706. [CrossRef]
56. Garg, T.; Panibatla, V.; Bhardwaj, M.; Brouwer, M. Can Patient Navigators Help Potential TB Patients Navigate the Diagnostic and Treatment Pathway? In Proceedings of the Union World Lung Conference, Sevilla, Spain, 21–24 October 2020. (E-poster).
57. Gurung, S.C.; Dixit, K.; Rai, B.; Levy, J.W.; Malla, D.; Budhathoki, G.; Acharya, S.; Dhital, R.; Paudel, P.R.; Caws, M.; et al. The role of active case finding in reducing patient incurred catastrophic costs for tuberculosis in Nepal. *Infect. Dis. Poverty* **2019**, *8*, 99. [CrossRef]
58. Sagbakken, M.; Frich, J.C.; Bjune, G.A.; Porter, J.D. Ethical aspects of directly observed treatment for tuberculosis: A crosscultural comparison. *BMC Med. Ethics* **2013**, *14*, 25. [CrossRef]
59. Villanueva, A.; de Morales, M.; Alacapa, J.; Powers, R. Digital Adherence Technology in Action: 99DOTS as a Platform for quality TB Treatment by Private Providers in the Philippines. Available online: https://tbhealthtech.org/wp-content/uploads/2020/08/KNCV_99DOTS-in-the-Philippines_poster.jpg (accessed on 24 September 2020).
60. Gler, M.; Casalme, D.; Marcelo, D.; Frias, M. Feasibility and Acceptability of Video Observed Therapy Among Multi-Drug Resistant Tuberculosis Patients in Cavite, Philippines. Available online: https://tbhealthtech.org/wp-content/uploads/2020/08/DLSHSI_VOT_FINAL-POSTER.jpg (accessed on 24 September 2020).
61. Litner, R. The Potential of Near Field Communication Technology; Results and Lessons from a Digital Tuberculosis Management Program on the Thai-Myanmar Border. Available online: https://tbhealthtech.org/wp-content/uploads/2020/08/TB-Poster_D-treeInternational.jpg (accessed on 24 September 2020).
62. Shah, S. Active TB Case Finding Among Transgender and Male Sex Workers in Pakistan. In Oral Presentation in Reaching the Unreached to Find the Missing millions. In Proceedings of the World Lung Conference, The Hague, The Netherlands, 24–27 October 2018. SP46.
63. Abdurrahman, S.T.; Emenyonu, N.; Obasanya, O.J.; Lawson, L.; Dacombe, R.; Muhammad, M.; Oladimeji, O.; Cuevas, L.E. The hidden costs of installing Xpert machines in a tuberculosis high-burden country: Experiences from Nigeria. *Pan Afr. Med. J.* **2014**, *18*, 277. [CrossRef] [PubMed]
64. Creswell, J.; Rai, B.; Wali, R.; Sudrungrot, S.; Adhikari, L.M.; Pant, R.; Pyakurel, S.; Uranw, D.; Codlin, A.J. Introducing new tuberculosis diagnostics: The impact of Xpert® MTB/RIF testing on case notifications in Nepal. *Int. J. Tuberc. Lung Dis.* **2015**, *19*, 545–551. [CrossRef] [PubMed]
65. Lorent, N.; Choun, K.; Malhotra, S.; Koeut, P.; Thai, S.; Khun, K.E.; Colebunders, R.; Lynen, L. Challenges from Tuberculosis Diagnosis to Care in Community-Based Active Case Finding among the Urban Poor in Cambodia: A Mixed-Methods Study. *PLoS ONE* **2015**, *10*, e0130179. [CrossRef] [PubMed]
66. Morishita, F.; Garfin, A.M.C.G.; Lew, W.; Oh, K.H.; Yadav, R.-P.; Reston, J.C.; Infante, L.L.; Acala, M.R.C.; Palanca, D.L.; Kim, H.J. Bringing state-of-the-art diagnostics to vulnerable populations: The use of a mobile screening unit in active case finding for tuberculosis in Palawan, the Philippines. *PLoS ONE* **2017**, *12*, e0171310. [CrossRef] [PubMed]
67. Onozaki, I.; Law, I.; Sismanidis, C.; Zignol, M.; Glaziou, P.; Floyd, K. National tuberculosis prevalence surveys in Asia, 1990–2012: An overview of results and lessons learned. *Trop. Med. Int. Health* **2015**, *20*, 1128–1145. [CrossRef]

68. Daftary, A.; Furin, J.; Zelnick, J.; Venkatesan, N.; Steingart, K.; Smelyanskaya, M.; Seepamore, B.; Schoeman, I.; Reid, M.; Padayatchi, N.; et al. Tuberculosis and Women: A Call to Action. *Int. J. Tuberc. Lung Dis.* **2020**, In Press. [CrossRef]
69. Devries, K.M.; Mak, J.Y.; Garcia-Moreno, C.; Petzold, M.; Child, J.C.; Falder, G.; Lim, S.; Bacchus, L.J.; Engell, R.E.; Rosenfeld, L. The global prevalence of intimate partner violence against women. *Science* **2013**, *340*, 1527–1528. [CrossRef]
70. Singer, M.; Bulled, N.; Ostrach, B.; Mendenhall, E. Syndemics and the biosocial conception of health. *Lancet* **2017**, *389*, 941–950. [CrossRef]
71. Global Affairs Canada. Canada's Feminist International Assistance Policy; Ottawa, ON, Canada. 2017. Available online: https://www.international.gc.ca/world-monde/issues_development-enjeux_developpement/priorities-priorites/policy-politique.aspx?lang=eng (accessed on 24 September 2020).
72. Manandhar, M.; Hawkes, S.; Buse, K.; Nosrati, E.; Magar, V. Gender, health and the 2030 agenda for sustainable development. *Bull World Health Organ.* **2018**, *96*, 644–653. [CrossRef]
73. Stop TB Partnership. Framework for the Empowerment of Women and Girls in TB REACH Grants. 2019. Available online: http://stoptb.org/assets/documents/global/awards/tbreach/W7_WEmpowerment_TBREACHGrants.pdf (accessed on 24 September 2020).
74. Akundi, S. One Woman's Decade-Long Fight Against TB Stigma. The Hindu, 25 March 2019. Available online: https://www.thehindu.com/life-and-style/fitness/pharmacist-manjula-devi-has-been-raising-awareness-against-tuberculosis-for-the-last-one-decade/article26631725.ece (accessed on 24 September 2020).
75. Interactive Research and Development. The Kiran Sitara Leadership Program. Available online: http://ird.global/program/yepgap/projects/kiran-sitaraadolescent-girls-leadership-health-program/#detail (accessed on 19 September 2020).
76. Address by Prime Minister Narendra Modi, Vigyan Bhawan, New Delhi, The Delhi End TB Summit; Ministry of Health and Family Welfare, Government of India, Stop TB Partnership and WHO South-East Asia. 2018. Available online: http://www.stoptb.org/assets/documents/news/PM%20Modi%20speech%20on%2013%20March%202018%20in%20Vigyan%20Bhawan%20in%20Delhi.pdf (accessed on 24 September 2020).
77. Office of Assistant to Deputy Cabinet Secretary for State Documents & Translation. *Introductory Remarks of the President of the Republic of Indonesia in the Limited Cabinet Meeting on the Acceleration of Tuberculosis Elimination*; Jakarta, Indonesia. 2020. Available online: https://setkab.go.id/en/introductory-remarks-of-the-president-of-the-republic-of-indonesia-in-the-limited-cabinet-meeting-on-the-acceleration-of-tuberculosis-elimination-tuesday-21-july-2020-at-the-merdeka-palace-jakarta/ (accessed on 24 September 2020).

Publisher's Note: MDPI stays neutral with regard to jurisdictional claims in published maps and institutional affiliations.

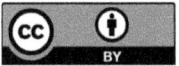

© 2020 by the authors. Licensee MDPI, Basel, Switzerland. This article is an open access article distributed under the terms and conditions of the Creative Commons Attribution (CC BY) license (http://creativecommons.org/licenses/by/4.0/).

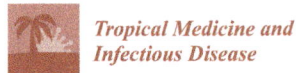 *Tropical Medicine and Infectious Disease*

Article

Enhanced Private Sector Engagement for Tuberculosis Diagnosis and Reporting through an Intermediary Agency in Ho Chi Minh City, Viet Nam

Luan Nguyen Quang Vo [1,2,*], **Andrew James Codlin [1]**, **Huy Ba Huynh [1]**, **Thuy Doan To Mai [1]**, **Rachel Jeanette Forse [1]**, **Vinh Van Truong [3]**, **Ha Minh Thi Dang [3]**, **Bang Duc Nguyen [3]**, **Lan Huu Nguyen [3]**, **Tuan Dinh Nguyen [4]**, **Hoa Binh Nguyen [4]**, **Nhung Viet Nguyen [4]**, **Maxine Caws [5,6]**, **Knut Lonnroth [7]** and **Jacob Creswell [8]**

1 Friends for International TB Relief, Ha Noi 100000, Vietnam; andrew.codlin@tbhelp.org (A.J.C.); huy.huynh@tbhelp.org (H.B.H.); thuy.mai@tbhelp.org (T.D.T.M.); rachel.forse@tbhelp.org (R.J.F.)
2 Interactive Research and Development, Singapore 189677, Singapore
3 Pham Ngoc Thach Hospital, Ho Chi Minh City 700000, Vietnam; drvinhpnt2020@gmail.com (V.V.T.); hadtm2018@gmail.com (H.M.T.D.); mmdbang@gmail.com (B.D.N.); nguyenhuulan1965@gmail.com (L.H.N.)
4 Viet Nam National Lung Hospital, Ha Noi 100000, Vietnam; tuandinh10@yahoo.com (T.D.N.); nguyenbinhhoatb@yahoo.com (H.B.N.); vietnhung@yahoo.com (N.V.N.)
5 Liverpool School of Tropical Medicine, Department of Clinical Sciences, Liverpool L3 5QA, UK; maxine.caws@lstmed.ac.uk
6 BNMT Nepal, Lazimpat, Ward No. 2, Kathmandu 44600, Nepal
7 Karolinska Institutet, Department of Public Health Sciences, 171 77 Solna, Sweden; knut.lonnroth@ki.se
8 Stop TB Partnership, 1218 Geneva, Switzerland; jacobc@stoptb.org
* Correspondence: luan.vo@tbhelp.org; Tel.: +84-902908004

Received: 31 July 2020; Accepted: 1 September 2020; Published: 14 September 2020

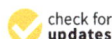

Abstract: Under-detection and -reporting in the private sector constitute a major barrier in Viet Nam's fight to end tuberculosis (TB). Effective private-sector engagement requires innovative approaches. We established an intermediary agency that incentivized private providers in two districts of Ho Chi Minh City to refer persons with presumptive TB and share data of unreported TB treatment from July 2017 to March 2019. We subsidized chest x-ray screening and Xpert MTB/RIF testing, and supported test logistics, recording, and reporting. Among 393 participating private providers, 32.1% (126/393) referred at least one symptomatic person, and 3.6% (14/393) reported TB patients treated in their practice. In total, the study identified 1203 people with TB through private provider engagement. Of these, 7.6% (91/1203) were referred for treatment in government facilities. The referrals led to a post-intervention increase of +8.5% in All Forms TB notifications in the intervention districts. The remaining 92.4% (1112/1203) of identified people with TB elected private-sector treatment and were not notified to the NTP. Had this private TB treatment been included in official notifications, the increase in All Forms TB notifications would have been +68.3%. Our evaluation showed that an intermediary agency model can potentially engage private providers in Viet Nam to notify many people with TB who are not being captured by the current system. This could have a substantial impact on transparency into disease burden and contribute significantly to the progress towards ending TB.

Keywords: tuberculosis; private sector; intermediary agency; referral; notification; Viet Nam

1. Introduction

Tuberculosis (TB) is a curable disease, yet an estimated 10 million people develop active TB and 1.5 million people succumb to TB each year [1]. It remains the deadliest disease caused by a single infectious agent and a major source of avoidable deaths worldwide. Over the first 6 months of 2020, an estimated 867,000 persons died of TB as a negative consequence of the Covid-19 pandemic [2]. Moreover, it is estimated that about one-quarter of the world's population is infected with subclinical, noninfectious TB [3].

Viet Nam has a well-organized National Tuberculosis Control Programme (NTP). TB treatment is provided free of charge at all public sector sites and reported TB treatment outcomes are high. In 2014, Viet Nam committed to reduce TB prevalence to 20 per 100,000 by 2030 [4]. However, following the second national prevalence survey in 2018 [5], the country's estimated TB incidence rate was revised upward from 124 to 174 per 100,000, suggesting that just 57% of the estimated burden was captured by the NTP's official TB case notification statistics [6].

In 1986, the government initiated a package of reforms [7] that shifted Viet Nam's centralized, public healthcare sector towards neoliberalism and later to New Public Management, which resulted in the rapid development of a private healthcare sector [8]. Fueled by the country's strong economic growth and rising population welfare, demand for private sector services due to greater convenience and quality perceptions has similarly increased [9].

People often prefer to seek care with non-NTP facilities owing to their flexibility regarding diagnostic procedures, drug regimens and treatment observation methods, more convenient operating hours and locations, and lower administrative burden [10]. Studies have shown that pharmacies and private clinics represent the initial point of health care seeking for 50–70% of people with TB in Viet Nam [11–13]. Despite the existence of a mandatory notification law since 2007 [14], the implementation of this policy has been suboptimal. As such, the private healthcare sector is a major driver of 'missed people with TB' and loss to follow-up (LTFU) [15].

The Ministry of Health subsequently passed a law in 2013 (Circular 02/2013/TT-BYT) to enable systematic inclusion of private providers and public institutions outside of the NTP via four public-private mix (PPM) engagement models: (1) referral; (2) diagnosis; and referral; (3) directly observed treatment (DOT) provider and (4) full-service TB care facility [16]. The law has resulted in roughly 10% of TB case notifications at the national-level coming from PPM initiatives. Yet over 80% of these PPM notifications originate from public institutions, such as general care, military, and police hospitals that are not specialized in TB care and thereby are outside of the technical supervision of the NTP. This implies that private providers contribute only 2% to annual notifications nationwide. Meanwhile, it is estimated that about half of Viet Nam's 'missing cases' are taking their TB treatment outside of the NTP network [17]. More importantly, there is evidence that private sector TB care is often of substandard quality. Patients may suffer diagnostic delays with no bacteriological confirmation and receive inappropriate or inadequate treatment regimens. Poor adherence support has resulted in loss to follow-up rates of up to 65% [18–21].

A key reason for the limited engagement of private providers is the restrictive nature of Circular 02/2013/TT-BYT. Providers that wish to retain their clientele are expected to participate as a full-service TB facility and fulfill associated diagnostic and reporting requirements, while submitting to close oversight and supervision by the NTP. Meanwhile, benefits of participation, such as capacity building, free medicines, and eligibility for monetary stipends at government rates, may be insufficiently powered or implemented [16]. This has proven untenable for many non-NTP providers apart from large public tertiary care facilities. As a result, it is critical to develop and evaluate engagement schemes, which take into account the economic interests of smaller private providers.

One such scheme is the Private Provider Interface Agency (PPIA) model that has subsequently been scaled through the Joint Effort for Elimination of Tuberculosis (JEET) to 23 states of India [22,23]. This model employs intermediary agencies [15,24] that aim to offer a tangible value proposition with bottom-line impact rather than appeal to altruistic motivations [25,26]. This value proposition includes free or discounted access to nucleic acid amplification testing (NAAT) and medicines at pre-negotiated price-points for providers and patients and, perhaps most importantly, the option for private providers to retain their customers and thereby their livelihoods [27]. The implementation of PPIA's showed promising results in multiple sites throughout India [28,29] and has been recognized as one avenue of sustainably scaling private sector engagement for TB worldwide [30].

In 2017, Friends for International TB Relief piloted a private-sector engagement initiative called Proper Care Private Sector (PCPS), modeled after the successful PPIA pilots from India [27]. This pilot investigated the feasibility of building a portfolio of private providers and measured the outputs of incentivizing and supporting referral and reporting of private TB treatment.

2. Materials and Methods

2.1. Study Setting

This pilot was conducted in two districts of Ho Chi Minh City (HCMC), Viet Nam—District 10 and Go Vap—between July 2017 and March 2019. The intervention area had a combined population of 1.2 million people and notified 1070 people with All Forms of TB in the 12 months preceding the study. In each district, there is a District TB Unit (DTU) responsible for managing diagnosis, treatment and notification of TB according to NTP guidelines and for coordinating patient management with primary health facilities. There were no official private sector TB-reporting entities in the evaluation area before this study's implementation.

2.2. Private Provider Engagement

We obtained lists of licensed private healthcare providers from each intervention district's regulatory authority. These providers included pharmacies, single-doctor practices and multi-doctor clinics. In collaboration with licensing, health, and TB authorities, through consensus we conducted a mapping exercise to identify priority providers with a high likelihood of encountering people who had pulmonary TB, while categorically excluding certain specialists, such as dermatologists, obstetricians, and gynecologists. Through repeated in-person and telephonic engagement, we recruited eligible providers. Interested providers were invited to capacity building events organized in collaboration with the Pham Ngoc Thach provincial lung hospital (PNT). The scope of these training events included new diagnostic tests for TB and specifically Xpert MTB/RIF (Xpert) and the newly recommended MTB/RIF Ultra assay [31], standardized TB treatment regimens, and follow-up schedules according to NTP guidelines. We complemented these formal training events with one-on-one provider detailing activities [32] to elaborate on the study's procedures, the provider's role and responsibilities, and the benefits of participation. Providers were eligible to participate through two principal strategies: diagnostic referral and private TB treatment reporting (Figure 1).

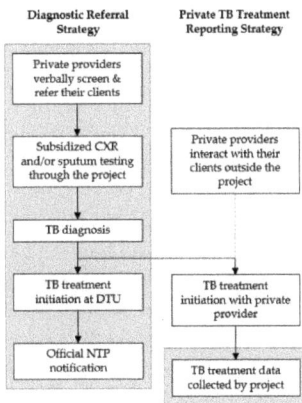

Figure 1. Schematic of the two private sector engagement strategies; the grey boxes show in which parts of the tuberculosis (TB) care cascade private providers were engaged by the study.

2.3. Diagnostic Referral Strategy

In this strategy, participating providers verbally screened their customers for TB symptoms and distributed referral vouchers to anyone reporting at least one TB symptom, i.e., (productive) cough or hemoptysis, weight/appetite loss, fatigue, fever, night sweats, chest pain, dyspnea. Symptomatic persons could use the voucher to access a chest X-ray (CXR) subsidy of VND 50,000 (USD 2.20 at an exchange rate of VND 22,700 = USD 1) at one of the study's 12 participating radiology sites. As the cost per CXR charged by these radiology sites ranged from VND 80,000 (USD 3.52) to VND 120,000 (USD 5.29), the radiography site collected the balance payment from the health-seeking person. In comparison, the price for one CXR at the District TB Unit was VND 49,000 (USD 2.16) at the start of the study and was subsequently raised to VND 69,000 (USD 3.04). Patients who elected to take their TB treatment with a private provider were charged a consultation fee of between VND 80,000 and VND 150,000 (USD 6.61) in addition to drugs and other services. According to field staff estimates, the approximate average cost per visit per person at private facilities was VND 200,000 (USD 8.81).

Persons assessed with parenchymal abnormalities on CXR by the X-ray technician and verified by the attending radiologist at the radiography site provided a sputum sample for free follow-on testing with the Xpert assay. At selected sites, health-seeking persons also underwent smear microscopy, in which case these results were requested from the participating provider as well. Sputum was collected at the radiography site or by the referring private provider. Study staff collected sputum specimens for transport to a designated government Xpert laboratory in Go Vap district. People with Xpert-positive results were encouraged to take treatment at their closest DTU, or at PNT if their Xpert result showed rifampicin resistance. When an individual was diagnosed and treated for TB via this strategy, the private provider making the initial referral received a VND 500,000 (USD 22.07) payment or approximately 2.5x the estimated average cost per visit per person. If the person chose to take TB treatment with a private provider, the treatment was recorded through the study's second strategy.

2.4. Private TB Treatment Reporting Strategy

The second strategy focused on documenting private TB treatment practices. Once a month, study staff collected TB treatment information from participating private providers. This information included individuals diagnosed through the diagnostic referral strategy above that elected treatment outside of the NTP. Providers were paid VND 500,000 (USD 22.07) for each complete patient report, which included the patient's name, age, sex, address, CXR results, sputum test results (Xpert, smear, culture, other), type of TB (pulmonary, extra-pulmonary), treatment regimen, and initiation dates. Treatment outcomes were not systematically assessed in this pilot study due to resource limitations and data provided by providers were sparse as providers did not conduct post-treatment follow-up with patients.

Despite the attempts to characterize these treatment reports in detail, they were not recognized by the NTP for official notification for several reasons. The primary reason was that these providers were not registered as official PPM model 4 participants in accordance to 02/2013/TT-BYT and therefore had not undergone required capacity building and site assessment by the NTP.

2.5. Statistical Analyses

We tabulated descriptive statistics for private provider engagement and participation, the number and proportion of referred people progressing through the study's TB care cascade by intervention district and the private TB treatment reported to our study. We calculated the ratio of bacteriologic confirmation over the number of successful CXR referrals. Official TB notifications were collected from the two intervention districts for three years prior to the study and during the study period to analyze trends of official TB notifications before and during the pilot. Additional notifications and percent change from baseline were calculated using a pre-/post-intervention comparison of official notification data in the intervention districts. Due to barriers outlined above, the collected private TB treatment cases were not included in the official NTP notification statistics, so that a second additionality model was constructed to assess the impact of including these privately treated individuals in official TB statistics for the intervention districts. Statistical analyses were performed on Stata version 13 (StataCorp, College Station, TX, USA).

2.6. Ethical Considerations

The Institutional Review Boards of Pham Ngoc Thach Hospital (155/NCKH-PNT) and the Hanoi School of Public Health (324/2019/YTCC-HD3) granted scientific and ethical approval for this study. The Ho Chi Minh City Provincial People's Committee approved the implementation of the intervention (4699/QD-UBND). Participating private providers granted permission to use data for the analyses based on the terms and conditions of their practice. All personally identifying information was removed prior to analysis.

3. Results

3.1. Private Provider Engagement and Participation

The study enumerated 1107 licensed private providers in the two intervention districts (Table 1). Of these, 67.0% (742/1107) were targeted for recruitment based on the initial mapping exercise and 53.0% (393/742) of those targeted agreed to participate. Among participants, at least one staff member of 48.6% of centers (191/393) attended a capacity building event. By the end of the study, we recorded at least one referral for CXR from 32.1% (126/393).

Table 1. Summary of provider recruitment and participation referral yields by district (2017-Q3 to 2019-Q1).

	Go Vap	District 10	Total
All licensed private providers	626	481	1107
# deemed eligible for recruitment	469 (74.9%)	273 (56.8%)	742 (67.0%)
# who signed a participation agreement	139 (22.2%)	254 (52.8%)	393 (35.5%)
# trained by provincial lung hospital	119 (19.0%)	72 (15.0%)	191 (17.3%)
# with at least one referral	105 (16.8%)	21 (4.4%)	126 (11.4%)
# reporting private TB treatment	5 (0.8%)	9 (1.9%)	14 (1.3%)

Of the 126 private providers with at least one successful CXR referral (Table 2), 58.7% were multi-doctor clinics and 25.4% were single-doctor practices. These two provider types accounted for 70.0% and 18.9% of referrals, respectively. The remaining referrals were from pharmacies, hospitals or could not be traced to the source. The bacteriologic positivity rate among successful CXR referrals was highest among single pulmonologist practices at 58.6%, followed by multi-doctor clinics at 21.9% and single-doctor practices with no specialty focus at 11.2%. Eighty-two point two percent of the people diagnosed with TB via the diagnostic referral strategy were referred by just ten private providers constituting 7.9% (10/126) of those making at least one successful CXR referral and 2.5% (10/393) of those signing participation agreements.

The study received TB diagnosis and treatment data from 3.6% (14/393) of participating private providers. These consisted of 71.4% (10/14) single-doctor practices and 28.6% (4/14) multi-doctor clinics. The top five providers supplying TB diagnosis and treatment data reported 81.7% (907/1112) of patients on private TB treatment.

Table 2. Summary of chest X-ray (CXR) referrals and Bac(+) TB detection by type of private provider (2017-Q3 to 2019-Q1).

	Providers with Signed Participation Agreement	Providers with 1+ Successful CXR Referral	Successful CXR Referrals	Bac(+) TB Detection
Single doctor clinics	62 (15.8%)	32 (25.4%)	943 (18.9%)	118 (69.8%)
-Pulmonologists	17 (4.3%)	17 (13.5%)	144 (2.9%)	99 (58.6%)
-General practitioners	45 (11.5%)	15 (11.9%)	799 (16.0%)	19 (11.2%)
Multiple doctor clinics	111 (28.2%)	74 (58.7%)	3489 (70.0%)	37 (21.9%)
-Pulmonology specialists	3 (0.8%)	3 (2.4%)	48 (1.0%)	0 (0%)
-Other specialists	108 (27.5%)	71 (56.3%)	3441 (69.0%)	37 (21.9%)
Hospitals	2 (0.5%)	2 (1.6%)	4 (0.1%)	4 (2.4%)
Pharmacies	218 (55.5%)	18 (14.3%)	86 (1.7%)	5 (3.0%)
Community referrals [1]	N/A	N/A	17 (0.3%)	5 (3.0%)
Undefined provider type	N/A	N/A	445 (8.9%)	0 (0%)
Total	393 (100%)	126 (100%)	4984 (100%)	169 (100%)

[1] Indicates referrals from a separate community-based ACF initiative that accessed a private sector radiology site for CXR screening.

3.2. Detection and Reporting Yield

The study identified 1203 people with TB of whom 7.6% (91/1203) were referred and linked to care with the NTP (Figure 2), while 92.4% (1112/1203) consisted of private TB treatment reports and remained un-notified (Table 3). All 91 TB patients linked to care with the NTP were bacteriologically confirmed. Among persons treated in the private sector, the proportion with bacteriologic confirmation was 30.5% (339/1112). Together, the total proportion of TB patients with bacteriologic confirmation was 35.7% (430/1203). Overall, 1.2% (15/1203) were people with Multi-drug resistant TB (MDR-TB). Patients diagnosed with rifampicin resistance were largely referred by private providers to NTP facilities. Particularly, diagnostic referrals generated 93.3% (14/15) of persons detected with rifampicin resistance (Figure 2). Meanwhile, private TB treatment reports included one MDR-TB case (Table 3). In addition to persons treated for active TB, four persons were treated for latent TB infection by private providers.

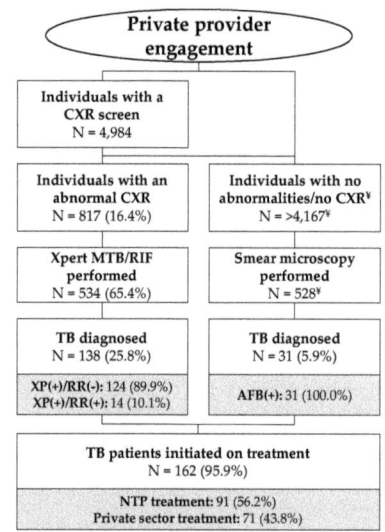

¥ The sample of smear microscopy result includes persons for whom no chest radiography was performed. These persons were not systematically recorded, so that it was not possible to estimate a denominator or calculate a proportion.

Figure 2. Care cascade among persons screened and referred (2017-Q3 to 2019-Q1).

Table 3. Summary characteristics of reported private TB treatment by district.

	Go Vap	District 10	Total
Private providers reporting private TB treatment	5	9	14
Private TB treatment reported	507	605	1112
Average number of privately treated TB patients reported per provider per quarter (range)	14.5 (0–54)	9.6 (0–59)	11.3 (0–59)
Provider type			
Single-doctor practice	263 (51.9%)	389 (64.3%)	652 (58.6%)
Multi-doctor clinic	244 (48.1%)	216 (35.7%)	460 (41.4%)
Diagnosis			
Bacteriologically-confirmed	172 (33.9%)	167 (27.6%)	339 (30.5%)
Clinically diagnosed	335 (66.1%)	438 (72.4%)	773 (69.5%)
Type of TB			
Pulmonary drug susceptible TB	372 (73.4%)	471 (77.9%)	843 (75.7%)
Extra-pulmonary drug susceptible TB	110 (21.7%)	133 (22.0%)	243 (21.9%)
Pulmonary Multi-drug resistant TB	0 (0.0%)	1 (0.2%)	1 (0.1%)
Not reported	25 (4.9%)	0 (0.0%)	25 (2.2%)
Reported residency			
Living in Go Vap or District 10	241 (47.5%)	81 (13.4%)	322 (29.0%)
Living in another district of HCMC	167 (32.9%)	290 (47.9%)	457 (41.1%)
Living outside of HCMC	99 (19.5%)	220 (36.4%)	319 (28.7%)
Not reported	0 (0.0%)	14 (2.3%)	14 (1.3%)
Treatment regimen			
Standard first-line regimen	261 (51.5%)	498 (82.3%)	759 (68.3%)
Modified first-line regimen/no duration	244 (48.1%)	63 (10.4%)	307 (27.6%)
Streptomycin-containing regimen	0 (0.0%)	33 (5.5%)	33 (3.0%)
Levofloxacin-containing regimen [1]	2 (0.4%)	10 (1.6%)	12 (1.1%)
None reported	0 (0.0%)	1 (0.2%)	1 (0.1%)

[1] Includes second-line regimen.

The results of the study's diagnostic referral strategy are in Figure 2. The 12 radiology centers recorded 4984 CXR results, of which 817 were abnormal (16.4% of those with CXR results). Sputum specimens were collected from 65.4% (534/817) of these individuals and tested on the Xpert assay with a positivity of 25.8% (138/534) including 14 individuals with rifampicin-resistant TB (14/138 = 10.1%). An additional 528 smear microscopy tests were conducted for individuals who did not get a CXR or presented no radiographic abnormalities suggestive of TB but still reported TB symptoms, resulting in the detection of 31 (31/528 = 5.9%) people with smear-positive TB. Of the total 169 people diagnosed with bacteriologically-confirmed TB, 95.9% (162/169) were linked to care, corresponding to a ratio of 3.2% among successfully referred persons with a CXR screen. Among patients linked to care, 56.2% (91/162) were initiated on treatment at a NTP facility, while 43.8% (71/162) elected to take treatment with the initially referring private provider. These patients are included in the private TB treatment reports.

The characteristics of the privately-treated, un-notified 1112 individuals are in Table 3. Of these, 30.5% (339/1112) had either a positive smear microscopy, Xpert, and/or culture result. Just 29.0% (322/1112) of those taking private TB treatment lived inside the study's intervention area, with another 41.1% (455/1112) living in one of HCMC's other 22 districts. About 28.7% (319/1112) of privately treated persons were registered residents of other provinces, while the remaining 1.3% (14/1112) of people had no documented address. Overall, 68.3% (759/1112) of people privately treated for TB were prescribed a standard first-line regimen as per NTP guidelines, while the records for another 27.6% (307/1112) of people showed the correct drugs but were modified from the standard regimen or missing information on duration. Three percent (33/1112) of treatments included streptomycin, and 1.1% (12/1112) included levofloxacin.

3.3. Notification Impact

Table 4 and Figure 3 summarize changes in the NTP's TB case notifications in the study's intervention area and present the modeled impact of including private TB treatment on official notification statistics. Bacteriologically-confirmed and All Forms TB notifications increased by +17.0% (+177 TB cases) and +8.5% (+158 TB cases), respectively, over six quarters of implementation. If private TB treatment had been eligible for inclusion in the official notification statistics, bacteriologically-confirmed and All Forms of TB notifications would have increased by +49.7% (+516 TB cases) and +68.3% (+1270 TB cases), respectively.

Table 4. Changes in public-sector TB case notification and private TB treatment by district and type of TB.

	Bac(+) TB	All Forms TB
Go Vap		
Baseline period public-sector TB notifications	703	1315
Intervention period public-sector TB notifications	885	1493
Additional public-sector TB notifications	+182 (+25.9%)	+178 (+13.5%)
Private TB treatment reported during the intervention period	+172 (+24.5%)	507 (+38.6%)
Theoretical additional TB notifications (public & private)	+354 (+50.4%)	+685 (+52.1%)
District 10		
Baseline period public-sector TB notifications	336	544
Intervention period public-sector TB notifications	331	524
Additional public-sector TB notifications	−5 (−1.5%)	−20 (−3.7%)
Private TB treatment reported during the intervention period	+167 (+49.7%)	+605 (+111.2%)
Theoretical additional TB notifications (public & private)	+162 (+48.2%)	+585 (+107.5%)
Both Intervention Districts		
Baseline period public-sector TB notifications	1039	1859
Intervention period public-sector TB notifications	1216	2017
Additional public-sector TB notifications	+177 (+17.0%)	+158 (+8.5%)
Private TB treatment reported during the intervention period	+339 (+32.6%)	+1112 (+59.8%)
Theoretical additional TB notifications (public & private)	+516 (+49.7%)	+1270 (+68.3%)

Baseline period = (2016-Q3 to 2017-Q2)*2 + 2017-Q3. Intervention period = 2017-Q3 to 2019-Q1.

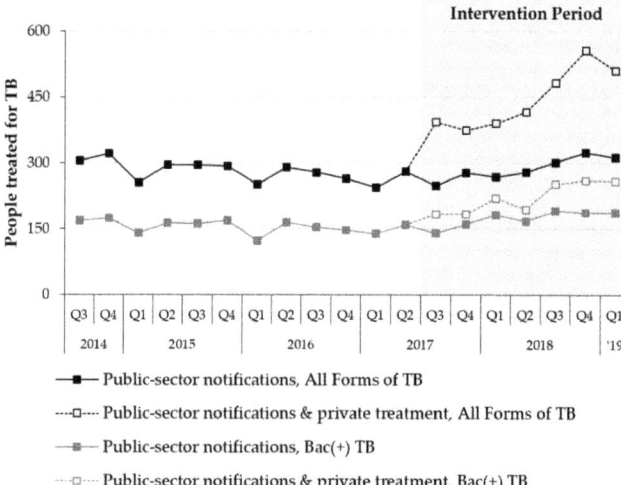

Figure 3. Pre- and post-intervention trends in public-sector TB case notifications and private TB treatment in the study area.

4. Discussion

Our pilot study showed that the PPIA model was effective in engaging a large number of private providers in the Vietnamese urban setting to contribute to TB care and prevention efforts. We found a substantial number of persons treated for TB in the private sector of HCMC, the vast majority of whom were not known to the NTP. This indicates that creating enabling mechanisms, as well as further scale-up and evaluation of private TB treatment reporting approaches, should be a critical component of the TB response in Viet Nam's urban areas.

Numerous studies have shown that effective engagement of private providers to screen for TB and refer presumptive cases for diagnostic testing can be an efficient way to close the detection gap [33–35]. This was corroborated by the results of our study and particularly by the increase in All Forms TB notifications compared to the baseline period. Moreover, this share of private provider contribution to notifications (+8.5%) was over five times Viet Nam's 2017 national average private sector contribution rate (1727/105,733 = 1.6%) [36]. Lastly, and perhaps most telling, un-notified private TB treatment reports corresponded to about 70% of the officially notified patient load in these two districts managed by the NTP. Even though these districts are not representative of the average district in Viet Nam, they present a compelling argument to expand novel private provider engagement models in the country's urban areas.

Meanwhile, the efficiency of this approach was evidenced by the high ratio of positively detected cases among those successfully referred. This high ratio suggests a pre-screening step performed by these healthcare professionals or self-selection by patients. The high ratio consequently implies the risk of false-negative assessments and missed opportunities to engage persons with TB. Therefore, more advocacy for providers and the general population to raise top-of-mind awareness about TB is warranted.

As observed on our study and documented by PPM projects in other settings, a referral strategy in isolation remains limited in both novelty and impact [37]. A more comprehensive engagement strategy is required to identify TB patients accessing treatment via the private sector. Including the reported private TB treatments into the NTP's routine surveillance would have represented a substantial increase in case notifications in the two study districts. However, since these providers did not complete the NTP's registration process as an accredited PPM partner, the private TB treatment records were not recognized as official notifications. The registration process is arduous and accompanied by external inspections and laborious reporting requirements, which can inhibit PPM participation for TB in Viet Nam [16]. This suggests the need for bold policies that promote private provider participation. This need is well-understood and has shown substantial impact in other settings once addressed [38,39].

Notification gains represent only the initial milestone. While all people with TB detected and notified through the referral strategy were bacteriologically confirmed, we observed low levels of bacteriologic confirmation among private-sector TB treatments, as only one-third was substantiated by a positive sputum test. We further observed that clinical diagnoses and follow-up testing for bacteriologically-confirmed patients oftentimes did not follow national treatment guidelines. As this study focused on case detection, treatment outcomes were optional to report and sparse when collected. Private providers did not employ a systematic follow-up process but also did not permit the study to directly engage their customers for household contact investigations due to fears of reputational damages from breaching patient confidentiality. This has also been observed in other settings [35] and represents a crucial opportunity to improve quality of private-sector TB care. This is particularly the case in light of the low attendance rate on the capacity building sessions offered by the study, as they were not mandatory for study participation. Consequently, while the goal of policy reform should be to remove unnecessary bureaucratic barriers to promote private provider participation, this reform should be designed with the long-term goal of improving quality of care among all stakeholders in mind.

Meanwhile, access to Xpert testing constituted a unique selling proposition of the PPIA to these providers, which they could pass on to their clientele. This study was the first to enable commercial access to Xpert testing for non-PPM providers in Viet Nam, so that the consistent message across size and geography of providers was that the ability to offer NAAT to their clients was a critical catalyst for participation. While this dynamic may be a temporary effect until market access is established through registration and formalization of a commercial distribution channel, intermediary agencies in other settings should leverage these dynamics to build the private provider network. Increased acceptance of Xpert testing has also been observed to result in a reduction of clinical diagnosis [40], so that increasing private-sector Xpert uptake could substantially reduce the rate of over-diagnosis and contribute to improved individual and public health outcomes. Efforts to optimize NAAT access have proven effective in several settings through the Initiative for Promoting Affordable, Quality TB tests [24,38,41].

An important lesson across both strategies was the need to sufficiently power monetary and non-monetary incentives. Evidence suggests that referral and notification incentives can represent a welcome income generation opportunity [42,43]. However, determining the appropriate threshold at which the individual cost-benefit analysis turns favorable is critical. The level of USD 22.07 proved sufficient to elicit private TB treatment reports among some, but it is safe to say that the 14 reporting providers in our study did not constitute the entire spectrum of private TB treatment. For example, risk-averse providers and those with a small caseload may have found the incentive to be insufficient to offset the risk exposure and expected value of penalties of un-notified TB treatment. These incentives may have also created inefficiencies whereby pulmonologists referred persons with TB through our study that would also have been referred in our absence as this level of incentive was high compared to traditionally paid amounts in Viet Nam [19,44,45]. Nevertheless, the costs of incentives paid by our study to detect a person with TB were a fraction of estimated total costs of detecting a new case through other systematic screening strategies [46] and warrant further optimization and evaluation.

A key success factor of the study was the broad coverage and participation of a diverse set of private providers. This was evidenced by the fact that we received referrals from all types of providers listed above and detected TB cases from most provider types. This effectiveness in generating leads and detecting TB patients also suggests that we were able to target the right providers. One reason for this was likely the detailed a priori landscaping and targeting, which allows implementers to have a better sense of the options people have for care seeking and coverage of their interventions [22,47].

Our study faced several limitations. With respect to private-sector TB treatment, our study was observational in nature, so that we did not attempt to change clinical practices. Similarly, we did not systematically incentivize and collect treatment outcomes in this study, but we intend to do so in future engagements. As such, provider willingness to alter behavior to meet international standards of TB care and the extent to which previously mentioned aspiration of improving diagnostic and treatment quality are feasible remain critical research questions to be answered on future studies. Another limitation was that we were only able to verify private TB treatment through reviews and abstractions of data, which were only available in patient records, as private providers did not permit direct engagement of their customers. The study's implementation area was limited, so that it is necessary to test the model at a greater scale to strengthen the generalizability of these results. Lastly, it also remains unclear, if this model or an adaptation thereof were appropriate in non-urban areas.

Nevertheless, this pilot study has elucidated the potential gains inherent in effective private sector engagement to national and provincial stakeholders in Viet Nam. As has been noted elsewhere, future work should focus on strengthening data systems, including the use of direct electronic data capture to track referrals and loss to follow up between referral and CXR [38]. This work should also employ mechanisms to verify that private TB treatment reports are genuine individuals who have not already been reported elsewhere in the TB notification system. Finally, policy changes are required to facilitate the scale-up of this approach.

5. Conclusions

Private providers in HCMC are treating many people with TB who are not reported to the national program, and it is critical to improve engagement approaches that arrive at a system, which allows private providers to notify through the NTP. To achieve public health targets, this system will also need to ensure the highest level of care adherent to national standards. Scaling effective private-sector engagement efforts, such as this enhanced intermediary model, could have a strong impact on the progress towards ending TB, and we recommend the NTP to scale up the model and through it to build capacity for improvements in quality of TB diagnosis and care.

Author Contributions: Conceptualization and protocol development, L.N.Q.V., R.J.F., H.M.T.D. and M.C.; data collection, H.B.H., B.D.N. and R.J.F.; data analysis and interpretation, L.N.Q.V., T.D.T.M. and A.J.C.; writing—original draft preparation, L.N.Q.V. and A.J.C.; writing—review and editing, L.N.Q.V., A.J.C., R.J.F., M.C., K.L. and J.C.; supervision, V.V.T., L.H.N., T.D.N., H.B.N., N.V.N.; funding acquisition, L.N.Q.V. All authors have read and agreed to the published version of the manuscript.

Funding: This research was supported by the TB REACH initiative of the Stop TB Partnership, grant number STBP/TBREACH/GSA/W5-25, with funding from the Global Affairs Canada. Additional support for its evaluation was provided by the European Commission Horizon 2020 Programme IMPACT TB grant number 733174.

Acknowledgments: The authors express their sincere gratitude to the Viet Nam National Tuberculosis Control Programme, the Pham Ngoc Thach Hospital and the staff working at the District TB Units in the study's intervention areas (District 10 and Go Vap) for their participation. The authors also wish to thank Giang T. Le, Thanh N. Vu and the Ho Chi Minh City Public Health Association and all participating private providers.

Conflicts of Interest: The authors declare no conflict of interest. The funders had no role in the design of the study; in the collection, analyses, or interpretation of data; in the writing of the manuscript, or in the decision to publish the results.

References

1. World Health Organization. *Global Tuberculosis Report 2019*; World Health Organization: Geneva, Switzerland, 2019.
2. Stop TB Partnership. *Potential Impact of the Covid-19 Response on Tuberculosis in High-Burden Countries: A Modelling Analysis*; Stop TB Partnership: Geneva, Switzerland, 2020.
3. Houben, R.M.; Dodd, P.J. The Global Burden of Latent Tuberculosis Infection: A Re-estimation Using Mathematical Modelling. *PLoS Med.* **2016**, *13*, 1–13. [CrossRef] [PubMed]
4. Office of the Prime Minister. *Approval of the National Strategy for TB Prevention and Control until 2020 with Vision to 2030 [Vietnamese]*; 374/QĐ-TTg; Viet Nam Office of the Prime Minister: Hanoi, Vietnam, 2014.
5. Nguyen, H.V.; Tiemersma, E.W.; Nguyen, H.B.; Cobelens, F.G.J.; Finlay, A.; Glaziou, P.; Dao, C.H.; Mirtskhulava, V.; Van Nguyen, H.; Pham, H.T.T.; et al. The second national tuberculosis prevalence survey in Vietnam. *PLoS ONE* **2020**, *15*, 1–15. [CrossRef]
6. World Health Organization. *Global Tuberculosis Report 2018*; World Health Organization: Geneva, Switzerland, 2018.
7. Ladinsky, J.L.; Nguyen, H.T.; Volk, N.D. Changes in the Health Care System of Vietnam in Response to the Emerging Market Economy. *Palgrave Macmillan J.* **2000**, *21*, 82–98. [CrossRef]
8. Adams, S.J. Vietnam's Health Care System: A Macroeconomic Perspective. In Proceedings of the International Symposium on Health Care Systems in Asia, Tokyo, Japan, 21–22 January 2005.
9. Nguyen, M.P.; Wilson, A. Perspective How Could Private Healthcare Better Contribute to Healthcare Coverage in Vietnam ? *Int. J. Health Policy Manag.* **2017**, *6*, 305–308. [CrossRef] [PubMed]
10. Lönnroth, K.; Thuong, L.M.; Linh, P.D.; Diwan, V. Risks and benefits of private health care: Exploring physicians' views on private health care in Ho Chi Minh City, Vietnam. *Health Policy* **1998**, *45*, 81–97. [CrossRef]
11. Hoa, N.B.; Sy, D.N.; Nhung, N.V.; Tiemersma, E.W.; Borgdorff, M.W.; Cobelens, F.G. National survey of tuberculosis prevalence in Viet Nam. *Bull. World Health Organ.* **2010**, *88*, 273–280. [CrossRef]
12. Lonnroth, K.; Lambregts, K.; Nhien, D.T.T.; Quy, H.T.; Diwan, V.K. Private pharmacies and tuberculosis control: A survey of case detection skills and reported anti-tuberculosis drug dispensing in private pharmacies in Ho Chi Minh City, Vietnam. *Int. J. Tuberc. Lung Dis.* **2000**, *4*, 1052–1059.

13. Nguyen, B.H.; Cobelens, F.G.J.; Dinh, N.S.; Nguyen, V.N.; Borgdorff, M.W.; Tiemersma, E.W. Diagnosis and Treatment of Tuberculosis in the Private Sector, Vietnam. *Emerg. Infect. Dis.* **2011**, *17*, 562–563.
14. Viet Nam National Assembly. *Law on the Management and Prevention of Infectious Diseases [Vietnamese]*; 03/2007/QH12; Viet Nam National Assembly: Hanoi, Vietnam, 2007; p. 23.
15. World Health Organization. *First Meeting of the Public–Private Mix Subgroup for DOTS Expansion. Public-Private Mix for DOTS Expansion*; World Health Organization: Geneva, Switzerland, 2003.
16. Ministry of Health. *Circular about the Decision on Coordination between Health Care Providers in the Management of TB [Vietnamese]*; 02/2013/TT-BYT; Ministry of Health: Hanoi, Vietnam, 2013; 02/2013/TT-BYT.
17. Hennig, C. *Progress and Plans Viet Nam. PPM Progress and Plans Viet Nam*; World Health Organization: Kuala Lumpur, Malaysia, 2012; p. 14.
18. Lönnroth, K.; Thuong, L.M.; Lambregts, K.; Quy, H.T.; Diwan, V.K. Private tuberculosis care provision associated with poor treatment outcome: Comparative study of a semi-private lung clinic and the NTP in two urban districts in Ho Chi Minh City, Vietnam. *Int. J. Tuberc. Lung Dis.* **2003**, *7*, 165–171.
19. Quy, H.T.; Lan, N.T.N.; Lönnroth, K.; Buu, T.N.; Dieu, T.T.N.; Hai, L.T. Public-private mix for improved TB control in Ho Chi Minh City, Vietnam: An assessment of its impact on case detection. *Int. J. Tuberc. Lung Dis.* **2003**, *7*, 464–471.
20. Van Maaren, P. Progress and Plans for PPM in the Western Pacific Region. In Proceedings of the Fifth PPM DOTS Subgroup Meeting, Cairo, Egypt, 3–5 June 2008; p. 15.
21. Lönnroth, K.; Thuong, L.M.; Linh, P.D.; Diwan, V.K. Delay and discontinuity—A survey of TB patients' search of a diagnosis in a diversified health care system. *Int. J. Tuberc. Lung Dis.* **1999**, *3*, 992–1000. [PubMed]
22. Shah, D.; Vijayan, S.; Chopra, R.; Salve, J.; Gandhi, R.K.; Jondhale, V.; Kandasamy, P.; Mahapatra, S.; Kumta, S. Map, know dynamics and act; a better way to engage private health sector in TB management. A report from Mumbai, India. *Indian J. Tuberc.* **2019**. [CrossRef]
23. Wells, W.A. Scale and ambition in the engagement of private providers for tuberculosis care and prevention. *Glob. Health Sci. Pract.* **2019**, *7*, 3–5. [CrossRef] [PubMed]
24. Anand, T.; Babu, R.; Jacob, A.G.; Sagili, K.; Chadha, S.S. Enhancing the role of private practitioners in tuberculosis prevention and care activities in India. *Lung India* **2017**, *34*, 538–544. [CrossRef]
25. Ashraf, N.; Bandiera, O. Altruistic capital. *Am. Econ. Rev.* **2017**, *107*, 70–75. [CrossRef]
26. Dewan, P.K.; Lal, S.S.; Lonnroth, K.; Wares, F.; Uplekar, M.; Sahu, S.; Granich, R.; Chauhan, L.S. Improving tuberculosis control through public-private collaboration in India: Literature review. *Br. Med. J.* **2006**, *332*, 574–577. [CrossRef]
27. PATH. Private sector engagement for TB control in Mumbai—Private Provider Interface Agency (PPIA). In *South Asian Public-Private Initiative Experience Sharing*; PATH: Negombo, Sri Lanka, 2016.
28. World Health Partners. Universal Access to TB Care: PPIA Patna. In *South Asian Public-Private Initiative Experience Sharing*; World Health Partners: Negombo, Sri Lanka, 2016.
29. Shibu, V.; Daksha, S.; Rishabh, C.; Sunil, K.; Devesh, G.; Lal, S.; Jyoti, S.; Kiran, R.; Bhavin, V.; Amit, K.; et al. Tapping private health sector for public health program? Findings of a novel intervention to tackle TB in Mumbai, India. *Indian J. Tuberc.* **2020**, *67*, 189–201. [CrossRef]
30. Wells, W.A.; Uplekar, M.; Pai, M. Achieving Systemic and Scalable Private Sector Engagement in Tuberculosis Care and Prevention in Asia. *PLoS Med.* **2015**, e1001842. [CrossRef]
31. World Health Organization. *Meeting Report of a Technical Expert Consultation: Non-Inferiority Analysis of Xpert MTB/RIF Ultra Compared to Xpert MTB/RIF*; World Health Organization: Geneva, Switzerland, 2017; pp. 1–11.
32. Worthington, H.; Cheng, L.; Majumdar, S.R.; Morgan, S.J.; Raymond, C.B.; Soumerai, S.B.; Law, M.R. The impact of a physician detailing and sampling program for generic atorvastatin: An interrupted time series analysis. *Implement. Sci.* **2017**, *12*, 141. [CrossRef]
33. Lönnroth, K.; Uplekar, M.; Blanc, L. Hard gains through soft contracts: Productive engagement of private providers in tuberculosis control. *Bull. World Health Organ.* **2006**, *84*, 876–883. [CrossRef]
34. Lönnroth, K.; Uplekar, M.; Arora, V.K.; Juvekar, S.; Lan, N.T.N.; Mwaniki, D.; Pathania, V. Public-private mix for DOTS implementation: What makes it work? *Bull. World Health Organ.* **2004**, *82*, 580–586. [CrossRef]
35. Creswell, J.; Khowaja, S.; Codlin, A.; Hashmi, R.; Rasheed, E.; Khan, M.; Durab, I.; Mergenthaler, C.; Hussain, O.A.; Khan, F.; et al. An evaluation of systematic tuberculosis screening at private facilities in Karachi, Pakistan. *PLoS ONE* **2014**, *9*. [CrossRef] [PubMed]

36. Viet Nam National TB Control Programme. *NTP Year-End Report 2017 [Vietnamese]*; Viet Nam National TB Control Programme: Hanoi, Vietnam, 2018; p. 160.
37. Sulis, G.; Pai, M. Missing tuberculosis patients in the private sector: Business as usual will not deliver results. *Public Health Action* **2017**, *7*, 80–81. [CrossRef] [PubMed]
38. Uplekar, M. Public-private mix for tuberculosis care and prevention. What progress? What prospects? *Int. J. Tuberc. Lung Dis.* **2016**, *20*, 1424–1429. [CrossRef]
39. World Health Organization. *Global Tuberculosis Report 2016*; World Health Organization: Geneva, Switzerland, 2016; ISBN 978 92 4 156539 4.
40. Creswell, J.; Rai, B.; Wali, R.; Sudrungrot, S.; Adhikari, L.M.; Pant, R.; Pyakurel, S.; Uranw, D.; Codlin, A.J. Introducing new tuberculosis diagnostics: The impact of Xpert MTB/RIF testing on case notifications in Nepal. *Int. J. Tuberc Lung Dis.* **2015**, *19*, 545–551. [CrossRef]
41. Dabas, H.; Deo, S.; Sabharwal, M.; Pal, A.; Salim, S.; Nair, L.; Chauhan, K.; Maheshwari, P.; Parulkar, A.; Singh, R.; et al. Initiative for Promoting Affordable and Quality Tuberculosis Tests (IPAQT): A market-shaping intervention in India. *BMJ Glob. Health* **2019**, *4*, e001539. [CrossRef]
42. Ashraf, R.; Naureen, F.; Noor, A.; Ilyas, J.; Fatima, R.; Yaqoob, A.; Wali, S.; Haq, M.U.; Latif, A.; Hussain, S. Does Cash Incentive Effect TB Case Notification by Public Private Mix-General Practitioners Model in Pakistan? *J. Tuberc. Res.* **2018**, *6*, 166–174. [CrossRef]
43. Khan, A.J.; Khowaja, S.; Khan, F.S.; Qazi, F.; Lotia, I.; Habib, A.; Mohammed, S.; Khan, U.; Amanullah, F.; Hussain, H.; et al. Engaging the private sector to increase tuberculosis case detection: An impact evaluation study. *Lancet Infect. Dis.* **2012**, *12*, 608–616. [CrossRef]
44. Revised National Tuberculosis Control Programme. *National Strategic Plan for Tuberculosis Elimination 2017–2025*; Revised National Tuberculosis Control Programme: New Delhi, India, 2017.
45. Deo, S.; Jindal, P.; Gupta, D.; Khaparde, S.; Rade, K.; Sachdeva, K.S.; Vadera, B.; Shah, D.; Patel, K.; Dave, P.; et al. What would it cost to scale-up private sector engagement efforts for tuberculosis care? Evidence from three pilot programs in India. *PLoS ONE* **2019**, *14*, e0214928. [CrossRef]
46. Azman, A.S.; Golub, J.E.; Dowdy, D.W. How much is tuberculosis screening worth? Estimating the value of active case finding for tuberculosis in South Africa, China, and India. *BMC Med.* **2014**, *12*, 216. [CrossRef]
47. World Health Organization. Guide to Develop a National Action Plan on Public-Private Mix for Tuberculosis Prevention and Care [Internet]. 2017. Available online: https://www.who.int/tb/publications/2017/PPMActionPlanGuide/en/ (accessed on 1 September 2020).

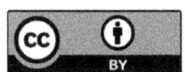

© 2020 by the authors. Licensee MDPI, Basel, Switzerland. This article is an open access article distributed under the terms and conditions of the Creative Commons Attribution (CC BY) license (http://creativecommons.org/licenses/by/4.0/).

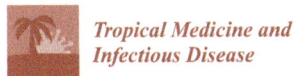

Article

Does Drug-Resistant Extrapulmonary Tuberculosis Hinder TB Elimination Plans? A Case from Delhi, India

Sheelu Lohiya [1,*], Jaya Prasad Tripathy [2], Karuna Sagili [3], Vishal Khanna [1], Ravinder Kumar [4], Arun Ojha [1], Anuj Bhatnagar [5] and Ashwani Khanna [1]

1 Lok Nayak Hospital, New Delhi 110002, India; dr.vishalkhanna@rediffmail.com (V.K.); dpsdllnc@rntcp.org (A.O.); stodl@rntcp.org (A.K.)
2 All India Institute of Medical Sciences, Nagpur 441108, India; ijay.doc@gmail.com
3 International Union Against Tuberculosis and Lung Disease, The Union South East Asia Office, New Delhi 110016, India; KSagili@theunion.org
4 All India Institute of Medical Sciences, New Delhi 110029, India; dpsdlndm@rntcp.org
5 Rajan Babu Institute of Pulmonary Medicine and Tuberculosis, New Delhi 110009 India; dpsdlkcc@rntcp.org
* Correspondence: dtodllnc@rntcp.org

Received: 11 March 2020; Accepted: 28 May 2020; Published: 1 July 2020

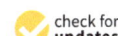

Abstract: Extrapulmonary drug-resistant tuberculosis (DR-EPTB) poses a formidable diagnostic and therapeutic challenge.Besides associated with high morbidity, it is a major financial burden for the patient and the health system. In spite of this, it has often been neglected as it does not "pose" a visible public health threat. We study clinical profiles, treatment outcomes, and factors associated with unfavourable outcomes among DR-EPTB patients under programmatic settings in New Delhi, India, and evaluate how this could impact TB elimination. A retrospective analysis of all DR-EPTB patients registered at three nodal DR-TB centres in Delhi in 2016 was carried out. Of the 1261 DR-TB patients registered, 203 (16%) were DR-EPTB, with lymph nodes (118, 58%) being the most common site, followed by bone (69, 34%). Nearly 29% ($n = 58$) experienced adverse drug reactions with severe vomiting (26, 13 %), joint pain (21, 10%) and behavioral disorder (15, 7%). History of previous TB treatment was observed in a majority of the cases (87.7%). Nearly one-third of DR-EPTB cases (33%) had unfavourable treatment outcomes, with loss-to-follow-up ($n = 40$, 58%) or death ($n = 14$, 20%) being the most common unfavourable outcomes. In the adjusted analysis, weight band 31–50 kilograms (aRR = 1.8, 1.2–3.4) and h/o previous TB (aRR = 2.1, 1.1–4.8) were mainly associated with unfavourable outcomes. TB elimination efforts need to focus on all forms of TB, including DR-EPTB, leaving no one behind, in order to realise the dream of ending TB.

Keywords: adverse drug reactions; unfavourable outcome; lymph node TB; bone TB; TB elimination; extrapulmonary tuberculosis

1. Introduction

Tuberculosis (TB) remains the top infectious killer, ranking above HIV/AIDS, with 10.0 million cases and 1.4 million deaths in 2018 [1]. *Mycobacterium tuberculosis* (MTB), the causative agent, usually affects the lungs (pulmonary TB/PTB). However, MTB may spread through lymphatic or hematogenous routes to virtually any organ in the body, resulting in extrapulmonary TB (EPTB). The most common sites of EPTB infection include peripheral lymph nodes, pleura, genitourinary sites, bones and joints, abdomen (peritoneum and gastrointestinal tract), and the central nervous system.

While EPTB has existed for millennia, pulmonary TB has remained the prime focus of global TB control programmes. EPTB is often less contagious than PTB, and is therefore overlooked even though it constitutes about 15% of all forms of TB, amounting to nearly 1 million incident cases notified in 2018, as per the WHO Global TB report [1]. Additionally, EPTB results in significant morbidity and mortality due to various diagnostic and therapeutic challenges that lead to delayed care.

In the present era of HIV pandemic coupled with global emergence of multidrug-resistant TB (MDR TB) and extensively drug-resistant TB (XDRTB), drug-resistant EPTB (DR-EPTB) presents a real and new public health challenge that has yet to receive serious attention. While drug resistance in PTB has been extensively studied, DR-EPTB has been neglected. Several systematic reviews and individual patient meta-analysis have reported treatment outcomes of MDR-TB, without disaggregated outcomes of DR-EPTB [2–5]. The WHO MDR-TB update, as per the global TB report, shows treatment success of 55%, a death rate of 15%, 14% lost to follow up, 8% of failed treatment and 7% of the patients not evaluated [6]. However, there is little information on outcomes disaggregated by type of TB, especially DR-EPTB. Interestingly, the National Tuberculosis Program of India does not report treatment outcomes separately for PTB and EPTB in DRTB reports.

India continues to have the highest number of TB cases in the world, with nearly 2.69 million cases in 2018 [7]. It also features among the top 10 high MDR-TB burden countries, with nearly 130,000 MDR/RR-TB cases notified in 2018 [1]. The Revised National Tuberculosis Control Programme (RNTCP) has reported poor treatment outcomes of successive MDR-TB cohorts [5,8]. Previous studies in four large states of India also reported poor overall treatment outcomes (40%–56%) among DR-TB patients, with high rates of death and lost-to-follow-up (LTFU) [9,10]. However, there is scarce information in the country on the profile and treatment outcomes of DR-EPTB patients and their associated risk factors. While it may be expected that treatment outcomes and associated risk factors of DR-EPTB are different from those of DR-PTB, there is no scientific evidence to support this.

India aims to eliminate TB by 2025; however, this goal will remain unachieved if EPTB, especially the drug-resistant cases, continues to be ignored [11]. Compared to the rest of the country, the situation is different in Delhi, with 42% EPTB among all TB cases, probably due to better availability of diagnostic services [8]. However, there are no estimates of the burden of DR-EPTB since disaggregate figures are not routinely reported in the programme. A previous study by Kant et al. in North India has reported a 13.4% prevalence of drug resistance among all EPTB cases [12]. Another study in Mumbai showed resistance in 29% of Mycobacterium isolates in extrapulmonary specimens [13]. A similar study from Chennai found that 37/189 (19%) of extrapulmonary TB specimens were multidrug-resistant, while one was extensively drug-resistant (XDR) [14].

A better understanding of this small yet significant group of patients is necessary to design effective interventions that might help reduce morbidity and mortality and improve treatment success rates. When the global community talks about TB elimination, it talks about TB per se; however, most interventions and strategies are focused on pulmonary TB. The strategy and milestones to end the global TB epidemic include all diagnosed TB cases and latent TB cases [7], hence we need specific interventions to focus on extrapulmonary TB, both sensitive and resistant.

Indicators such as TB treatment coverage, treatment success rates, the percentage of TB-affected households that experience catastrophic costs due to TB and drug-susceptibility testing (DST) coverage for TB patients is difficult to measure, and sustainable development goals (SDGs) cannot be achieved without giving due importance to DR-EPTB [15].

To address these gaps, we carried out this operational research in order to study the demographics, clinical profiles, and treatment outcomes of patients with DR-EPTB registered at three selected DR-TB nodal centres in Delhi in 2016, and explored risk factors associated with unfavourable treatment outcomes.

2. Methods

2.1. Study Design

This is a retrospective cohort study involving a record review of routine program data.

2.2. Setting

General Setting

Delhi is the capital of India inhabited by 18.6 million people, with a large number of migrants. It has one of the highest population densities of 11,320 persons per square km, and a literacy rate of 86% [16]. Delhi has the highest rate of TB notification in the country, probably due to better diagnostic facilities in tertiary care hospitals [17].

The Programmatic Management of Drug-Resistant TB (PMDT) services were launched in India in 2006 and obtained full geographical coverage in 2013. PMDT services started in Delhi in 2008 with a culture and drug susceptibility testing (C & DST) laboratory located at the state-owned Intermediate Reference Laboratory (IRL). Other tests, such as the cartridge-based nucleic acid amplification test (CBNAAT) and line probe assay (LPA), are also available at the IRL. PMDT services are provided through 25 chest clinics and four Nodal DR-TB centres in Delhi. Since 2018, all the chest clinics in Delhi have been designated as district DR-TB centres.

Microbiological confirmation of disease for DR-EPTB patients is preferred for diagnosis. This is done using either CBNAAT or culture or both. However, clinical diagnosis is also reached with the help of fine needle aspiration cytology (FNAC), histopathology findings, or interferon gamma release assays (IGRA), along with other signs and symptoms of TB, especially among those not responding to the WHO drug-sensitive ATT regimen. The patients are usually diagnosed at the district DR-TB centres or nodal DR-TB centres, and a sample, if available, is sent to the IRL along with a filled form requesting C&DST. Patients are started on the conventional MDR regimen at the Nodal DR-TB centres after pretreatment evaluation, as per NTP guidelines. Further follow-up and management is done at the district DR-TB centres. The diagnostic algorithm, which is common for both pulmonary and EPTB, is given in Figure 1 [18].

The conventional RNTCP regimen for MDR-TB is given to the patients with DR-EPTB, i.e., intensive phase with six drugs for 6–9 months (kanamycin, ofloxacin, ethionamide, cycloserine, pyrazinamide, ethambutol and pyridoxine), followed by a continuous phase with four drugs for 18 months (ofloxacin, ethionamide, cycloserine and ethambutol) as per RNTCP PMDT guidelines 2016 [7]. The patients found to be fluoroquinolone-resistant or resistant to other injectable drugs are started on the pre-XDRTB regimen (switched to high dose moxifloxacin and PAS).

Clinical monitoring is mainly based on clinical parameters such as weight gain, change in the size of lymph nodes/lesions, the appearance of new lymph nodes/lesions and monitoring of other EP sites located deep in the body by ultrasound, magnetic resonance imaging, computed tomography scan, and ESR (erythrocyte sedimentation rate). Surgery is considered in the absence of response to chemotherapy despite 6–9 months of treatment [18,19].

Treatment outcome definitions used by the RNTCP are given in Box 1. They are similar for pulmonary and extrapulmonary DR-TB patients. After the completed course of treatment, outcomes are assessed based on the response to treatment in terms of the resolution of symptoms and healing of lesions assessed through culture reports of specimens taken from discharging sinuses (if available) and investigation reports (e.g., ultrasonography, bone X-ray and magnetic resonance imaging).

Regular monitoring of side effects of drugs is done by blood tests (complete blood count, serum urea, creatinine, electrolytes, blood glucose, alkaline phosphatases, transaminases, total bilirubin), audiometry, thyroid function tests, ocular examinations, ECG for QT prolongation and other tests, if needed.

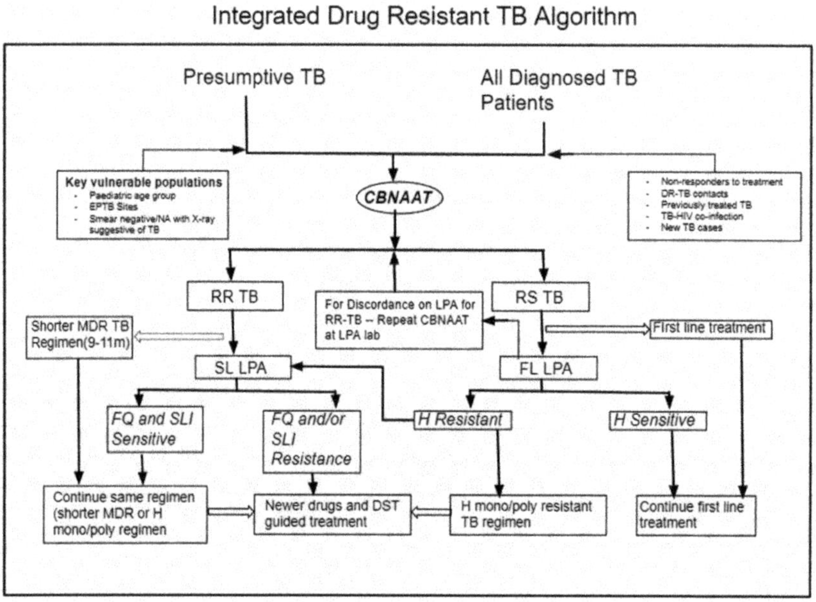

Figure 1. Diagnostic algorithm of drug-resistant tuberculosis as per PMDT India 2017. RR-TB, rifampicin-resistant tuberculosis; RS-TB, rifampicin-sensitive tuberculosis. SL-LPA, second line, line probe assay; FL-LPA, first line, line probe assay. FQ, fluoroquinolone; SLI, second line injectable; H, isoniazid; DRTB, drug-resistant TB; EPTB, extrapulmonary TB.

Box 1. Operational definitions for treatment outcomes in patients with multidrug-resistant TB (MDR TB).

Cure: Treatment completed as recommended by the national policy without evidence of failure, and three or more consecutive cultures taken at least 30 days apart during CP are negative, including culture at the end of treatment.
Treatment completed: Treatment completed as recommended by the national policy without evidence of failure, but no record that three or more consecutive cultures taken at least 30 days apart are negative after the intensive phase.
Treatment success: This is a combination of cure plus treatment completed.
Treatment failure: Treatment terminated or a need for permanent regimen change of at least two or more anti-TB drugs in CP because of the lack of microbiological conversion by the end of the extended intensive phase or microbiological reversion in the continuation phase after conversion to negative or evidence of additional acquired resistance to FQ or SLI drugs or adverse drug reactions (ADR).
Death: A patient who dies for any reason during the course of treatment.
Treatment lost-to-follow-up: A patient whose treatment was interrupted for one month or more for any reasons prior to being declared as failed.
Not evaluated: A patient for whom no treatment outcome is assigned.
Regimen changed: A TB patient's need for permanent regimen change of at least one or more anti-TB drugs prior to being declared as failed.
Treatment stopped due to adverse drug reactions: A patient who develops adverse drug reactions and cannot continue the M/XDR-TB treatment in spite of the management of adverse drug reactions as per the defined protocols and a decision has been taken by the DR-TB Centre committee to stop treatment.

2.3. Study Site

The study was conducted in three designated Nodal DR-TB centres under RNTCP in the state of Delhi.

2.4. Study Population

The study population included all DR-EPTB patients registered from 1 January 2016 to 31 December 2016 in the three selected nodal DR-TB centres in Delhi. These patients were admitted to a common TB hospital and initiated on a conventional MDR-TB regimen.

Those with associated pulmonary TB or on ITR (individualised treatment protocol) or XDR treatment regimen were excluded from the study; there were only three cases of associated pulmonary TB.

2.4.1. Data Variables, Sources of Data and Data Collection

A list of all eligible DR-EPTB patients registered in 2016 at the selected nodal DR-TB centres was prepared. The principal investigator (SL) extracted data from the patient treatment cards and PMDT registers from September 2018 to February 2019 into a structured data collection instrument.

Socio-demographic and clinical variables like PMDT TB number, date of registration, nodal DR-TB centre, age, sex, type of disease (primary/secondary MDR), site/s involved, history of previous TB treatment, site involved in previous TB episode, basis of diagnosis, resistance to drugs, comorbidities like HIV, diabetes, initial weight (in kilograms), final weight (in kilograms), adverse drug reaction, number of missed doses, treatment outcome (see Box 1) and date of outcome were included. Primary and secondary MDR was based on the previous TB treatment history.

2.4.2. Data Analysis and Statistics

Data collected were double-entered and validated using EpiData version 3.1, and discrepancies were corrected by referring to the data collection forms or the original patient files. Data analysis was carried out using EpiData analysis version 2.2.2.183 (EpiData Association, Odense, Denmark) and STATA version 13.0. Number and proportion were used to summarise categorical variables, and mean (standard deviation) or median (interquartile ranges (IQR)), as applicable, were used to summarise continuous variables. A chi-square test was performed to find the association of various socio-demographic and clinical variables with the treatment outcome. Binomial regression was done to explore the predictors of unfavourable treatment outcomes after controlling for confounders. The strength of association was expressed using relative risks (RRs) and 95% confidence intervals (95% CI). Variables with $p < 0.2$ on univariable analysis were included in the final regression model. Unfavourable outcomes were defined as death, loss to follow-up, treatment failure, not evaluated, regimen change, or stopped treatment due to reasons other than adverse drug reactions. Favourable outcome was defined as treatment completed and cured.

3. Ethics Approval

Administrative approval was obtained from the State TB Office, Delhi, India. Ethics approval was obtained from the Ethics Advisory Group of the International Union Against Tuberculosis and Lung Disease, Paris, France. Names of patients were not captured. The PMDT registration number was used to identify patients.

4. Results

4.1. Patient Characteristics

Of the total 1261 DR-TB patients registered in the three selected DR-TB sites in Delhi in 2016, 1058 (84%) were pulmonary and 203 (16%) were DR-EPTB cases, all of whom were included in the study.

Most patients were female (111, 54.7%), aged 15–44 years (147, 72.4%). Around two-thirds of the patients (134, 66.0%) weighed less than 50 kilograms. Lymph node (118, 58.1%) was the most common site of involvement, followed by bone and joint (69, 34.0%). A large majority of patients had a previous history of TB (178, 87.7%). CBNAAT was the basis of diagnosis in 173 patients (85.2%) and LPA in 20 (9.9%) cases (Table 1).

Table 1. Baseline demographic and clinical characteristics of drug-resistant extrapulmonary TB patients in Delhi in 2016 ($n = 203$).

	Characteristics	Number	(%)
Sex	Male	92	(45.3)
	Female	111	(54.7)
Age (years)	< 15	50	(24.6)
	15–44	147	(72.4)
	45 and above	06	(3.0)
Weight (in kilograms)	< 30	41	(20.2)
	31–50	93	(45.8)
	Above 50	69	(34.0)
DR-TB Centre	Centre 1	56	(27.6)
	Centre 2	59	(29.1)
	Centre 3	88	(43.3)
Site of disease	Peripheral lymph node	108	(53.2)
	Deep lymph node	10	(4.9)
	Brain	09	(4.4)
	Bone	69	(34.0)
	Pleural effusion	19	(9.4)
	Abdomen	10	(4.9)
	Heart	0	(0)
	Genital	02	(1.0)
Basis of diagnosis	CBNAAT	173	(85.2)
	Culture	2	(1.0)
	Line Probe Assay	20	(9.9)
	Clinical	8	(3.9)
Drug Resistance	HR	19	(9.4)
	Rifampicin	195	(96.1)
	Fluoroquinolone	05	(2.5)
	Other injectables	02	(1.0)

Table 1. *Cont.*

	Characteristics	Number	(%)
History of TB	Yes	178	87.7
	No	24	11.8
	Not recorded	01	(0.5)
HIV status	Negative	200	(98.5)
	Positive	03	(1.5)
Diabetes	Yes	05	(2.5)
	No	198	(97.5)
Severe adverse reaction	Yes	58	(28.6)
	No	145	(71.4)

TB: tuberculosis; HR: isoniazid, rifampicin CBNAAT: cartridge-based nucleic acid amplification test; DR-TB: drug-resistant tuberculosis. All CBNAAT-negative, culture-positive samples were subjected to second-line DST and put on LPA for first-line DST.

4.2. Adverse Drug Reactions (ADRs)

Nearly 28.6% (*n* = 58) experienced at least one ADR, with severe vomiting (26, 12.8%), joint pain (21, 10.3%), behavioral disorder (15, 7.4%) and hearing loss (7, 3.4%) being the most commonly observed ADRs (Table 2).

Table 2. Adverse drug reactions among drug-resistant extrapulmonary TB cases in Delhi in 2016 (*n* = 58).

Adverse Drug Reactions	Number	(%)
Severe vomiting	26	12.8
Behavior disorder	15	7.4
Hearing loss	7	3.4
Severe joint pain	21	10.3
Renal disturbance	03	1.5
Allergic reaction	04	2.0
Recurrent hepatitis	01	0.5
Gynaecomastia	02	1.0
Thyroid disturbance	02	1.0
Peripheral neuropathy	01	0.5
Vision loss	01	0.5
Others	02	1.0

Others include ocular disturbance, hemiparesis.

4.3. Delay in Treatment Initiation

The median (IQR) number of days from diagnosis to registration for treatment was 15 [9–25] days, whereas from diagnosis to initiation of treatment was 14 days [8–24].

4.4. Treatment Outcomes

Overall treatment success was 66% (*n* = 134). Of the 69 (34%) patients with unfavourable treatment outcomes, most of them were due to LTFU (*n* = 40, 58.0%) or death (*n* = 14, 20.3%) (Table 3).

Table 3. Treatment outcomes of drug-resistant extrapulmonary TB cases in Delhi, 2016.

Adverse Drug Reactions	Number	(%)
Treatment success	134	66.0
Unfavourable treatment outcome	69	34.0
Death	14	6.9
Treatment failure	1	0.5
Lost to follow up	40	19.7
Regimen changed	3	1.5
Treatment stopped d/t ADR	0	0.0
Not evaluated	11	5.4

ADR = adverse drug reaction.

In the adjusted analysis, weight band 31–50 kilograms (aRR = 1.8, 1.2–3.4, p-value = 0.02), DR-TB centre (aRR = 1.5, 1.0–2.5, p-value = 0.05) and history of previous TB (aRR = 2.1, 1.1–4.8, p-value = 0.03) were significantly associated with unfavourable treatment outcomes (Table 4).

Table 4. Socio-demographic and clinical factors associated with unfavourable treatment outcomes among drug-resistant extrapulmonary TB cases in Delhi, 2016.

Variables		Total N	Unfavourable n	%	RR (95% CI)	p-Value	aRR (95% CI)	p-Value
Sex	Male	92	35	(38.0)	1.2 (0.8–1.8)	0.2	1.3 (0.9–1.9)	0.13
	Female	111	34	(30.6)	1.0		1.0	
Age (years)	≥ 15 years	153	57	(37.3)	1.6 (0.9–2.7)	0.08	1.6 (0.8–3.0)	0.14
	< 15 years	50	12	(24.0)	1.0		1.0	
Weight (in Kilograms)	< 30	41	8	(19.5)	1.0		1.0	
	31–50	93	37	(39.8)	2.0 (1.1–4.0)	0.02	1.8 (1.2–3.4)	**0.02**
	Above 50	69	24	(34.8)	1.8 (0.9–3.6)	0.09	1.6 (0.8–3.0)	0.1
DR-TB Centre	Centre 1	59	16	(27.1)	1.0		1.0	
	Centre 2	88	37	(42.0)	1.6 (1.0–2.5)	0.06	1.5 (1.0–2.5)	**0.05**
	Centre 3	56	16	(28.6)	1.05 (0.6–1.9)	0.8	1.0 (0.7–2.0)	0.8
Site of disease	Others	104	38	(36.5)	1.2 (0.8–1.7)	0.4		
	Lymph node	99	31	(31.3)	1.0			
Basis of diagnosis	Others	30	10	(33.3)	1.0 (0.6–1.7)	0.9		
	CBNAAT	173	59	(34.1)	1.0			
History of previous TB	Yes	178	65	(36.5)	2.3 (1.0–5.7)	0.04	2.1 (1.1–4.8)	**0.03**
	No	25	4	16.0)	1.0		1.0	
HIV status	Negative	200	67	(33.5)	1.0	0.3		
	Positive	3	2	(66.7)	2.0 (0.9–4.5)			
Diabetes	Yes	5	3	(60.0)	1.8 (0.9–3.8)	0.2	1.9 (0.9–3.4)	0.18
	No	198	66	(33.3)	1.0		1.0	
Severe adverse reaction	Yes	58	16	27.6	1.0	0.2	1.0	
	No	145	53	36.6	1.3 (0.8–2.1)		1.4 (0.9–2.2)	0.15

TB: tuberculosis; HR: isoniazid, rifampicin; ADR: adverse drug reaction; CBNAAT: cartridge-based nucleic acid amplification test.

Stratified analysis was conducted to study the associations with unfavorable treatment outcomes in two different age groups (< 15 years and ≥ 15 years; Tables S1 and S2 in supplementary materials) Weight was not associated with unfavourable treatment outcomes among both children (< 15 years) and adults. Type of DR-TB centre was associated with the outcome among children and age ≥ 45 years was a significant predictor of unfavourable treatment outcome.

5. Discussion

The key findings of our study are: (i) one in every six registered DR-TB patients has DR-EPTB, (ii) lymph node is the most common site of involvement, followed by bone, in DR-EPTB patients, (iii) one-third of all DR-EPTB cases had unsuccessful treatment outcomes, and (iv) baseline weight, DR-TB centre and history of previous TB were significantly associated with unsuccessful treatment outcomes.

Of all DR-TB patients registered, 16% were DR-EPTB cases. These figures are comparable to the prevalence of EP disease in drug-sensitive cases [20]. This is probably due to the availability and scale-up of rapid TB diagnostics (CBNAAT) in the region. With universal access to DST, DR-EPTB is an important and clinically challenging subgroup to tackle. A 10-year epidemiological study in China observed a higher proportion of MDR TB among patients with EPTB [21]. They observed a large increase in MDR TB, from 17.3% to 35.7%, for pleural TB cases. A similar high proportion of drug resistance has also been observed from extrapulmonary specimens in India [12–14]. The increasing drug resistance among EPTB highlights the need for drug susceptibility testing and the formulation of more effective regimens for extrapulmonary TB treatment.

Lymph node involvement is the most common EPTB, in general. We encountered a similar pattern in the DR-EPTB cases in the previous literature from the Netherlands (39%), the United States (40%), and the United Kingdom (37%) [11,22]. Pleural TB is the most prevalent form of extrapulmonary TB in Poland (36%) and Romania (58%), and bone TB (41%) is the most common site in China [21]. This study shows that bone TB (includes musculoskeletal TB) is the second most common site of DR-EPTB, accounting for nearly one-third of the cases. This finding is supported by other studies in the literature [23,24].

Nearly two-thirds of DR-EPTB cases (66%) had favourable treatment outcomes. This is better than the outcomes of the overall national DR-TB cohort (47%) notified between the 3rd quarter of 2014 to the 2nd quarter of 2015, which ranged between 36%–61% across all states [8]. Similarly, previous studies from India have also reported lower success rates among different DR-TB cohorts [5,9,10].

A recent study at a DR-TB centre in Mumbai reported a much higher completion rate of 82% among DR-EPTB patients, probably because it was a single centre study with different patient profiles and the use of a shorter regimen, which showed much better treatment completion rates [23].

A review found that the death rates among DR-EPTB patients were widely ranged from 0%–80% in different studies across the globe [11]. This wide variation in death rates could be due to various factors such as patient profiles, delayed diagnosis, comorbidities, severity of the disease, and type of regimen/treatment protocol. The present study reports 14 deaths (6.9%), probably because of treatment with suboptimal regimens. Culture DST or 2nd line LPA is not always possible, either due to insufficient clinical samples or inability to obtain samples from an inaccessible site, which renders resistance profiling difficult. Newer treatment options with newer drugs may be tried.

LTFU is common, which was seen among one-fifth of the patients. However, newer initiatives such as mobile adherence support, online web-based platform (Nikshay) for real-time reporting, efficient referral systems using Nikshay ID and newer treatment guidelines (all-oral H mono-resistant DRTB regimens, shorter MDR TB regimens, all-oral longer MDR TB regimens) could contribute to a decrease in LTFU.

The risk factors for unfavourable treatment outcomes help in stratifying patients for additional monitoring and improving outcomes. Patients with a previous history of TB have worse outcomes, which supports the findings in other studies [9,11]. This calls for more aggressive monitoring of treatment in such patients.

Patients registered at DR-TB Centre 2 had a higher risk of unfavourable treatment outcomes, mostly LTFU or transferred out, because the centre receives a large number of patients from regions outside Delhi, who are eventually lost to follow-up. This calls for close monitoring, and better linkages and tracking of such patients.

A weight band between 31–50 kg at baseline was found to be significantly associated with unfavourable treatment outcomes compared to a weight band of < 30 kg. This has to be interpreted with caution as the role of unexplained confounders cannot be ruled out. A stratified analysis was conducted to study the association of weight bands on treatment outcomes in different age groups (children < 15 years and adults > 15 years). Although statistical significance was not seen, the proportion of outcomes among the 31–50 kg weight band was higher compared to other weight bands. Statistical nonsignificance could be due to small numbers and fewer numbers of outcomes in exposure categories, especially among children. This warrants a better understanding of the role of initial weight in determining treatment outcomes. We also need to explore whether a change in weight during the course of treatment or body mass index are better indicators compared to baseline weight in predicting outcomes.

The strength of this study is that it was conducted within the routine programmatic setting in three designated Nodal DR-TB centres under RNTCP in Delhi. All the cases of DR-EPTB registered during the study period from three out of four nodal DR TB centres (covering 21 out of 25 chest clinics) in Delhi were included in the study without any exclusion, which covered nearly 90% of all such cases during the study period. This lends generalizability to the study findings. The study also adhered to Strengthening the Reporting of Observational studies in Epidemiology (STROBE) guidelines for conducting and reporting on observational studies [25]. There were some limitations as well. First, as this is a retrospective study using programmatic data, information on other possible predictors for TB treatment outcomes, such as socio-economic status, adherence to treatment, smoking and alcohol intake status, were not available. Second, a large majority of the cases were bacteriologically confirmed, thus indicating that many clinically diagnosed cases may have been missed. Third, the MDR-TB treatment regimens have changed in the last couple of years, such as the replacement of ofloxacin with levofloxacin or moxifloxacin, which might affect treatment outcomes. This requires similar analysis of the successive cohorts.

The study results have four important programmatic implications. First, high rates of death and LTFU among DR-EPTB patients need to be addressed urgently. Besides the risk factors identified in this study, some of which are non-modifiable, a shorter and easier-to-follow DR-TB treatment regimen with newer oral drugs such as bedaquiline or delamanid is probably the answer to reducing mortality and LTFU in this patient group. With the recent evidence from trials and large observational cohorts, the WHO stance has also departed from conventional treatment approaches for MDR TB in favour of shorter regimens with noninjectables [14,26,27]. However, newer drugs are being given only for pulmonary DRTB at present in India. The high LTFU could also well be due to the fact that a large chunk of the residents in the study area are mobile migrants. Delhi, being the capital city and a medical hub with modern health care facilities, receives patients from all over the country for diagnosis, who do not usually remain in the city to complete their treatment. Thus, close monitoring of the transfer-out-policy is necessary in order to understand the referral system, identify any loopholes within, and address them accordingly. Nikshay is a welcome step in this regard, wherein a unique ID is given to each patient to enable tracking. However, the objective of Nikshay ID is far from being achieved. More operational research is needed to identify the gaps in the referral mechanism and streamline the process to minimise leakages.

Second, low weight was also one of the risk factors for unfavourable treatment outcomes, which require tailored interventions to improve treatment outcomes for these patient sub-groups, especially those with poor weight at baseline and with a previous history of TB. The national program has initiated "Nikshay Poshan Yojana" which provides incentives for nutritional support to TB patients, which is a welcome step; however, studies have reported poor implementation of this [7]. Proper implementation of such schemes, with further customised options such as packaged groceries, would be more beneficial.

Third, the proportion of DR EP-TB diagnosed clinically stands at a dismal 4% in this study. The diagnosed drug-sensitive EP-TB cases in Delhi constitute about 40%–45% of all TB cases, as per the India TB Report, while DR EP-TB is usually 15% to 20% of all DR-TB cases. It shows that we are probably missing clinically diagnosed EP-DRTB cases. Clinical nonresponders of EP-TB need to be reported too. In addition, there is over-reliance on bacteriological confirmation and drug sensitivity testing for the diagnosis of DR EP-TB, which is resulting in the underestimation of clinically diagnosed cases. Thus, diagnosis should be based on clinical judgement supported by culture/Xpert results, and not solely on bacteriological tests, as is common practice.

Fourth, those with a previous history of TB could be followed-up for at least two years to document relapse-free survival. For this, an aggressive strategy of follow-up and monitoring needs to be in place.

6. Conclusions

DR-EPTB constitutes a significant subgroup of the DR-TB cases that needs urgent attention. Every third DR-EPTB patient has unfavourable treatment outcomes, with high rates of LTFU that needs to be tackled if we are to realise the goal of ending TB. The use of shorter regimens and close monitoring/tracking of the migrant population and the transfer-out cases are required to minimise LTFU. Those with a previous history of TB need to be monitored closely for compliance to treatment. Further studies are needed to understand the operational reasons for the low proportion of clinically diagnosed DR EP-TB and explore the role of baseline weight or other proxy indicators, such as body mass index or weight gain during the treatment, in predicting treatment outcomes.

Supplementary Materials: The following are available online at http://www.mdpi.com/2414-6366/5/3/109/s1.

Author Contributions: Conceptualization, S.L., J.P.T. and K.S.; methodology, S.L., J.P.T., K.S. and A.K.; data collection, S.L., V.K., R.K., A.O. and A.B.; data curation and analysis, S.L., J.P.T., K.S.; resources, S.L., V.K., R.K., A.O., A.B., A.K.; writing—original draft preparation, S.L., J.P.T. and K.S.; writing—review and editing, S.L., V.K., R.K., A.O., A.B. and A.K.; supervision, S.L., V.K., R.K., A.O., A.B. and A.K.; project administration, S.L., V.K., R.K., A.O., A.B. and A.K. All authors have read and agreed to the published version of the manuscript.

Funding: No funding was obtained for this study. The training course under which this research was conducted and the open access publication charges were funded by The Global Fund to Fight AIDS, Tuberculosis and Malaria (GFATM). The funders had no role in study design, data collection and analysis, decision to publish, or preparation of the manuscript.

Acknowledgments: This research was conducted as a part of the "National Operational Research Training Course 2018–2019" organised by Project Axshya, funded by The Global Fund and implemented by The International Union Against Tuberculosis and Lung Diseases (The Union), South-East Asia Regional Office, New Delhi, India. The training course was conducted in collaboration with Revised National Tuberculosis Control Program, Ministry of Health and Family Welfare, Government of India, and National Institute for TB and Respiratory Diseases, New Delhi, India. The training is based on "The Union/Medécins sans Frontières (MSF)" model OR course and has been acknowledged/accredited by the Special Programme for Research and Training in Tropical Diseases at the World Health Organization (WHO/TDR) under SORT IT (Structured Operational Research and Training Initiative). Mentorship and facilitation for this course was provided through The Union South-East Asia Office, New Delhi; the Centre for Operational Research, The Union, Paris, France; Baroda Medical College, Vadodara; Médecins Sans Frontières, New Delhi; ESIC Medical College and PGIMSR, Bengaluru; North Delhi Municipal Corporation Medical College, Hindu Rao Hospital, New Delhi; GMERS Medical College, Vadodara; Postgraduate Institute of Medical Education and Research, Chandigarh, India; Yenepoya Medical College, Mangalore. We acknowledge the support of S.M. Abbas, Rashmi, Mahesh and Hitesh for their assistance in data collection.

Conflicts of Interest: The authors declare no conflict of interest. The funders had no role in the design of the study; in the collection, analyses, or interpretation of data; in the writing of the manuscript, or in the decision to publish the results.

References

1. World Health Organization. Global Tuberculosis Report 2019 [Internet]. [Cited 8 March 2020]. Available online: https://www.who.int/tb/global-report-2019 (accessed on 28 May 2020).
2. Bastos, M.L.; Hussain, H.; Weyer, K.; Garcia-Garcia, L.; Leimane, V.; Leung, C.C.; Narita, M.; Penã, J.M.; Ponce-de-Leon, A.; Seung, J.K.; et al. Treatment outcomes of patients with multidrug-resistant and extensively drug-resistant tuberculosis according to drug susceptibility testing to first- and second-line drugs: An individual patient data meta-analysis. *Clin. Infect. Dis.* **2014**, *59*, 1364–1374. [CrossRef] [PubMed]
3. Ahuja, S.D.; Ashkin, D.; Avendano, M.; Banerjee, R.; Bauer, M.; Bayona, J.N.; Becerra, M.C.; Benedetti, A.; Burgos, M.; Centis, R.; et al. Multidrug Resistant Pulmonary Tuberculosis Treatment Regimens and Patient Outcomes: An Individual Patient Data Meta-analysis of 9,153 Patients. *PLoS Med.* **2012**, *9*, e1001300. [CrossRef]
4. Ahmad, N.; Ahuja, S.D.; Akkerman, O.W.; Alffenaar, J.-W.C.; Anderson, L.F.; Baghaei, P.; Bang, D.; Barry, P.M.; Bastos, M.L.; Behera, D.; et al. Treatment correlates of successful outcomes in pulmonary multidrug-resistant tuberculosis: An individual patient data meta-analysis. *Lancet* **2018**, *392*, 821–834. [CrossRef]
5. Parmar, M.; Sachdeva, K.S.; Dewan, P.K.; Rade, K.; Nair, S.A.; Pant, R.; Khaparde, S.D. Unacceptable treatment outcomes and associated factors among India's initial cohorts of multidrug-resistant tuberculosis (MDR-TB) patients under the revised national TB control programme (2007–2011): Evidence leading to policy enhancement. *PLoS ONE* **2018**, *13*, e0193903. [CrossRef] [PubMed]
6. World Health Organization. Multi-Drug Resistant Tuberculosis (MDR-TB) 2018 Update [Internet]. World Health Organization (WHO), 2020. [Cited 20 May 2020]. Available online: https://www.who.int/tb/areas-of-work/drug-resistant-tb/MDR-RR_TB_factsheet_2018_Apr2019.pdf?ua=1 (accessed on 28 May 2020).
7. Central TB Division. *National Strategic Plan for Tuberculosis Elimination 2017–2025*; Ministry of Health with Family Welfare: New Delhi, India, 2017.
8. Central TB Division Directorate General of Health Services. *India TB Report 2018 Revised National TB Control Programme*; Ministry of Health with Family Welfare: New Delhi, India, 2018.
9. Nair, D.; Velayutham, B.; Kannan, T.; Tripathy, J.P.; Harries, A.D.; Natrajan, M.; Swaminathan, S. Predictors of unfavourable treatment outcome in patients with multidrug-resistant tuberculosis in India. *Public Health Action* **2017**, *7*, 32–38. [CrossRef] [PubMed]
10. Suryawanshi, S.L.; Shewade, H.D.; Nagaraja, S.B.; Nair, S.A.; Parmar, M. Unfavourable outcomes among patients with MDR-TB on the standard 24-month regimen in Maharashtra, India. *Public Health Action* **2017**, *7*, 116–122. [CrossRef] [PubMed]
11. Singh, P.K.; Jain, A. Epidemiological perspective of drug resistant extrapulmonary tuberculosis. *World J. Clin. Infect. Dis.* **2015**, *5*, 77. [CrossRef]
12. Kant, S.; Maurya, A.K.; Nag, V.L.; Bajpai, J. Rising trend of drug resistance among extra pulmonary TB in Northern India. *Tuberculosis* **2018**, *52*, PA3681. [CrossRef]
13. Vadwai, V.; Shetty, A.; Supply, P.J.; Rodrigues, C. Evaluation of 24-locus MIRU-VNTR in extrapulmonary specimens: Study from a tertiary centre in Mumbai. *Tuberculosis* **2012**, *92*, 264–272. [CrossRef] [PubMed]
14. Swaminathan, S.; Dusthackeer, A.; Sekar, G.; Chidambaram, S.; Kumar, V.; Mehta, P. Drug resistance among extrapulmonary TB patients: Six years experience from a supranational reference laboratory. *Indian J. Med Res.* **2015**, *142*, 568–574. [CrossRef] [PubMed]
15. World Health Organization. *Global Tuberculosis Report 2018*; World Health Organization: Geneva, Switzerland, 2018.
16. Density of Population Census 2011 [Internet]. [Cited 20 May 2020]. Available online: https://censusindia.gov.in/2011-prov-results/data_files/india/Final_PPT_2011chapter7.pdf (accessed on 28 May 2020).
17. Central TB Division Ministry of Health and Family Welfare. *India TB Report 2019 Revised National TB Control Programme Annual Report*; Ministry of Health and Family Welfare: New Delhi, India, 2019.
18. Central TB Division Ministry of Health and Family Welfare. Guidelines for Programmatic Management of Drug Resistant Tuberculosis in India 2017 [Internet]. 2017. Available online: https://tbcindia.gov.in/index1.php?lang=1&level=2&sublinkid=4780&lid=3306 (accessed on 28 May 2020).
19. Lee, J.Y. Diagnosis and Treatment of Extrapulmonary Tuberculosis. *Tuberc. Respir. Dis.* **2015**, *78*, 47–55. [CrossRef] [PubMed]

20. Central TB Division Ministry of Health and Family Welfare. TB India 2017 Revised National Tuberculosis Control Programme Annual Status Report [Internet]. Available online: https://tbcindia.gov.in/index1.php?lang=1&level=1&sublinkid=4160&lid=2807 (accessed on 28 May 2020).
21. Pang, Y.; An, J.; Shu, W.; Huo, F.; Chu, N.; Gao, M.; Qin, S.; Huang, H.; Chen, X.; Xu, S. Epidemiology of Extrapulmonary Tuberculosis among Inpatients, China, 2008–2017. *Emerg. Infect. Dis.* **2019**, *25*, 457–464. [CrossRef] [PubMed]
22. Arora, V.K.; Rajnish, G. Trends of extra-pulmonary tuberculosis under Revised National Tuberculosis Control Programme: A study from South Delhi. *Indian J. Tuberc.* **2006**, *53*, 77–83.
23. Joshi, J.M.; Desai, U. Extrapulmonary drug-resistant tuberculosis at a drug-resistant tuberculosis center, Mumbai: Our experience – Hope in the midst of despair! *Lung India* **2019**, *36*, 3–7. [CrossRef] [PubMed]
24. Tuli, S.; Jvn, J.; Gupta, N.; Raju, S.; Indrani, T.; Padhiary, K.; Madala, B. *Tuberculosis of the Skeletal System*; Jaypee Brothers Medical Publishing: New Delhi, India, 2004.
25. von Elm, E.; Altman, D.G.; Egger, M.; Pocock, S.J.; Gøtzsche, P.C.; Vandenbroucke, J.P. Strengthening the Reporting of Observational Studies in Epidemiology (STROBE) statement: Guidelines for reporting observational studies. *BMJ* **2007**, *335*, 806–808. [CrossRef] [PubMed]
26. Van Deun, A.; Maug, A.K.J.; Salim, A.H.; Das, P.K.; Sarker, M.R.; Daru, P.; Rieder, H.L. Short, Highly Effective, and Inexpensive Standardized Treatment of Multidrug-resistant Tuberculosis. *Am. J. Respir. Crit. Care Med.* **2010**, *182*, 684–692. [CrossRef] [PubMed]
27. World Health Organization. *WHO Updates Its Treatment Guidelines for Multidrug- and Rifampicin-Resistant Tuberculosis*; WHO: Geneva, Switzerland, 2019.

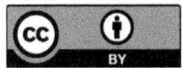

© 2020 by the authors. Licensee MDPI, Basel, Switzerland. This article is an open access article distributed under the terms and conditions of the Creative Commons Attribution (CC BY) license (http://creativecommons.org/licenses/by/4.0/).

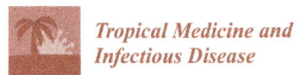 *Tropical Medicine and Infectious Disease*

Article

Combined Tuberculosis and Diabetes Mellitus Screening and Assessment of Glycaemic Control among Household Contacts of Tuberculosis Patients in Yangon, Myanmar

Nyi-Nyi Zayar [1,2], Rassamee Sangthong [1], Saw Saw [3], Si Thu Aung [4] and Virasakdi Chongsuvivatwong [1,*]

1. Epidemiology Unit, Faculty of Medicine, Prince of Songkla University, Hat Yai 90110, Thailand; nyinyi1987@gmail.com (N.-N.Z.); rassamee.s@psu.ac.th (R.S.)
2. Epidemiology Research Division, Department of Medical Research, Yangon 11191, Myanmar
3. Department of Medical Research (Pyin Oo Lwin Branch), Pyin Oo Lwin 05085, Myanmar; sawsawsu@gmail.com
4. Department of Public Health, Ministry of Health and Sports, Nay Pyi Taw 15015, Myanmar; sithuaung@mohs.gov.mm
* Correspondence: cvirasak@medicine.psu.ac.th; Tel.: +66-74-451165; Fax: +66-74-429754

Received: 4 May 2020; Accepted: 19 June 2020; Published: 29 June 2020

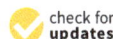

Abstract: Background: This study aimed to identify the prevalence of diabetes mellitus (DM) and tuberculosis (TB) among household contacts of index TB patients in Yangon, Myanmar. Method: Household contacts were approached at their home. Chest X-ray and capillary blood glucose tests were offered based on World Health Organization and American Diabetes Association guidelines. Crude prevalence and odds ratios of DM and TB among household contacts of TB patients with and without DM were calculated. Results: The overall prevalence of DM and TB among household contacts were (14.0%, 95% CI: 10.6–18.4) and (5%, 95% CI: 3.2–7.6), respectively. More than 25% of DM cases and almost 95% of TB cases among household contacts were newly diagnosed. Almost 64% of known DM cases among household contacts had poor glycaemic control. The risk of getting DM among household contacts of TB patients with DM was significantly higher (OR—2.13, 95% CI: 1.10–4.12) than those of TB patients without DM. There was no difference in prevalence of TB among household contacts of TB patients with and without DM. Conclusion: Significant proportions of the undetected and uncontrolled DM among household contacts of index TB patients indicate a strong need for DM screening and intervention in this TB–DM dual high-risk population.

Keywords: screening; tuberculosis; diabetes mellitus; contact investigation; TB-DM

1. Introduction

Globally, approximately 15% of tuberculosis (TB) patients are comorbid with diabetes mellitus (DM) [1]. Meanwhile, patients with DM have almost a three times higher risk of developing TB than the general population [2]. It is estimated that stopping the increasing prevalence of DM could prevent 6 million TB cases and 1.1 million TB deaths in 13 countries over 20 years [3]. Myanmar is ranked 10th among high TB burden countries, with an estimated annual TB incidence of 181,000 (95% CI: 119,000–256,000) [4]. The country is also ranked 9th among countries with the highest incidence of TB with DM comorbidity [5]. The TB incidence in the Yangon Region was 506/100,000 of the population, which was significantly higher than the global average 132/100,000 [6,7]. The prevalence of DM in the Yangon urban area was 12.1% [8], which was also higher than the global and regional averages [9].

It was found that the adjusted hazard ratio of TB was 2.09 among patients with DM over three years [10]. Therefore, the burden of TB is predicted to increase in the future, with an increased prevalence of DM in the Yangon Region.

It is known that the risks of getting TB and DM are higher among household contacts and family members. The prevalence of TB among household contacts was 4.5% in low and middle income countries [11]. Additionally, close blood relatives and spouses of patients with DM have more than a two times higher risk of developing DM due to sharing genetic susceptibility and/or sharing lifestyles, including physical inactivity, dietary habits associated with BMI, and central obesity [12–14]. Previous studies reported that DM is more prevalent among patients with TB compared to the general population [15]. Therefore, the prevalence of both TB and DM might be increased among household contacts of TB patients because of the high prevalence of DM among patients with TB.

In Myanmar, household contact investigation of TB, implemented since 2011, is an effective screening method for undiagnosed TB among household contacts of patients with TB [16]. Screening of DM was launched in 2018, according to a WHO recommendation, among patients with TB aged 40 years and above in 32 townships in 23 districts of Myanmar [17]. However, there is no guidance on screening of DM among household contacts of index TB patients. Without appropriate intervention, the burden of future TB might be higher among household contacts with DM living in the same household with patients with TB in Yangon. In addition, the risk of TB is especially higher among patients with poorly controlled DM who are exposed to patients with active TB [18]. Therefore, integration of DM screening and glycaemic monitoring of DM in household contact investigations could uncover not only hidden TB patients but also the undiagnosed DM and poor glycaemic control DM patients who are at high risk of developing TB. Comparing the TB and DM prevalence among household contacts of TB index cases with and without DM allows us to examine whether the two groups had different risks and different levels of needs in screening. This study intended to examine the prevalence of DM and of TB among household contacts of patients with TB and compare this prevalence based on the DM status of index TB patients. The proportion of poor glycaemic control of known cases of DM among these contacts was also assessed.

2. Materials and Methods

2.1. Study Design and Setting

A cross-sectional study was conducted in the Insein and North Okkalapa townships in the Yangon urban area from March to December 2018. These areas were selected for two reasons. First, they had the highest TB case notification rates in the Yangon region, with 387 and 248 per 100,000 population, respectively. Second, Yangon Region had the highest DM prevalence (12.1%) in Myanmar [8].

More than 80% of patients with TB living in the study townships are registered in the Township TB clinics and take regular treatment, while others are registered in clinics supported by local and international non-government organizations [19]. Existing routine household contact investigation for TB in these areas is carried out by basic health staff at the township level. The screening of signs and symptoms of TB followed by sputum smear and chest radiography (CXR) to confirm the diagnosis and a gene Xpert test to detect multidrug resistant TB (MDR-TB) were done in Township TB clinics. The findings from this study may give a clue to the situation on a larger scale throughout the country.

2.2. Study Sample

The study included newly diagnosed sputum smear positive index TB patients, aged ≥ 25 years, registered in township TB clinics. The study recruited only patients with newly diagnosed TB who had never received TB treatment to avoid hyperglycaemia due to the TB treatment [20]. Pregnant women, HIV positive TB patients, MDR-TB patients and those who had no family members were excluded. The exclusion criteria were based on some medical conditions that may affect blood sugar or risk of having DM. Pregnant women may have gestational DM [21]. Consistently, people living with HIV and receiving treatment for HIV may have increased risk of type 2 DM [22]. Furthermore, patients with DM have lower risk of developing MDR-TB compared to drug sensitive TB [2,23]. Therefore, the study excluded them to maintain homogeneity among the index cases. Family members living in the same households with an index TB patient for at least 3 months before having diagnosis of TB were invited for a contact investigation of TB. Among them, household contacts aged < 25 years were excluded for DM screening because the prevalence of DM increases steadily from age 25 years [24].

2.3. Sample Size Calculation

The sample size was calculated to test that the prevalence of TB among household contacts with DM (28%) was higher than that without DM (13%) [25]. At least 259 household contacts of index TB patients without DM and 65 household contacts of index TB patients with DM were required.

2.4. Data Collection Tools

A set of structured questionnaires was modified from previous research on household contact investigation in Myanmar [25] and a manual for WHO STEPwise approach to surveillance of non-communicable diseases and their risk factors [26].

The questionnaire included (1) Sociodemographic characteristics, such as age, gender, education, employment status and daily income per household member. Daily income per household member was converted from Myanmar kyats into United States dollars (USD) and cut off values for income level were 1.9 and 3.1 USD/day based on the poverty level defined by the World Bank [27]. (2) Signs and symptoms of TB, including evening rise in temperature, cough, coughing up blood, breathlessness, chest pain and weight loss. (3) Previous history of TB and DM (history of TB and/or DM diagnosed by a medical doctor). (4) Risk factors of TB (closeness with index TB patients including sharing the same room, sleeping in the same bed and taking care of index TB patients) and risk factors of DM (family history of DM, low physical activity: defined as <3 days of vigorous-level activity (e.g., carrying heavy loads, running, etc.,) of at least 20 min/week, or <5 days of moderate-level activity (e.g., walking very briskly, performing domestic chores, etc.,) using standard metabolic equivalents [28].

A physical examination including body mass index (BMI) was calculated using weight and height (kg/m^2) and classified < 18.5 kg/m^2 as underweight, 18.5–24.9 as normal, 25.0–29.9 kg/m^2 as overweight and ≥30 kg/m^2 as obese [29], and central obesity defined for those with waist circumference ≥ 94 cm in men and ≥80 cm in women [30], were also done during household visits.

2.5. Diagnosis of DM in Index TB Patients and Household Contacts

Both index TB patients and their household contacts were asked about their previous history of DM diagnosed by a medical doctor. The diagnosis was used as a confirmation of DM. They were also tested for their glycaemic control by fasting capillary blood glucose (FBG). Those without history of DM were tested by random capillary blood glucose (RBG) followed by FBG on the following day for TB index patients, and within 2 weeks for household contacts at township TB clinics. In case a contact did not revisit the clinics within 2 weeks, researchers then visited them at their home within 4 weeks to perform an FBG test. Any single positive test result was repeated on a separate day. All blood tests were done by an Accu-Chek® Performa glucometer [31].

Based on the American Diabetes Association [32], DM was defined as subjects with known DM or newly diagnosed DM with RBG ≥ 200 mg/dl and FBG ≥ 126 mg/dl (or) RBG ≥ 200 mg/dl for two times on separate days (or) FBG ≥ 126 mg/dl for two times on separate days. Poor glycaemic control was defined as FBG ≥ 130 mg/dl among known cases of DM [33].

All participants were duly informed of their results. New patients with DM were referred to DM clinics for further management.

2.6. Diagnosis of TB among Household Contacts

Household contacts were firstly screened by (1) asking about signs and symptoms of TB and (2) taking CXR at township TB clinics.

For household contacts with at least one signs and symptoms of TB (or) abnormal CXR suggested of TB, smear microscopy test was done by collecting one spot sputum specimen at the time of visit to TB clinic and next-day early morning sputum specimen. Gene Xpert test was done for those who had at least one positive sputum smear microscopy result.

For those who could not produce sputum, a 2-week trial of broad-spectrum antibiotics was prescribed. Disappearance of abnormalities on CXR would indicate non-TB. Otherwise, the subject was classified as TB. All contacts who were deemed to have positive TB were invited to register in the township TB clinics, where treatment would be provided according to the National TB treatment guideline.

Confirmation of TB could be made by 2 criteria. First, bacteriological confirmation using either a sputum smear or GeneXpert tests [34]. Second, a clinical diagnosis for those who did not meet the first criteria but had abnormal CXR. All contacts with newly diagnosed TB were asked to receive a full course of treatment [34].

2.7. Data Collection Procedure

Eligible patients registered in each township's TB clinic were invited to participate in the study. After informed consent, a face-to-face interview and a blood investigation for DM were done. Participants were then asked for their permission to visit their home and screen their household contacts for TB and DM.

2.8. Data Analysis

Epidata version 3.1 was used for data entry and R software was used for data analysis. The prevalence of TB or DM among household contacts was calculated by dividing the number of contacts with TB or DM by the number of household contacts screened for TB or DM. Chi-square test and Fisher's exact test were used to test differences between the prevalence of TB or DM among household contacts of TB patients with and without DM.

Multivariate logistic regression models were done to determine the odds ratios of getting DM and TB among household contacts based on the DM status of index TB patients, adjusted for covariates identified in previous studies [14,35–37]. Covariates included age, gender, socioeconomic status (SES), low physical activity, BMI, central obesity for risk of DM, age, gender, SES and closeness to index TB patient for risk of TB. These covariates were added cumulatively into each model. The model with the lowest Akaike's information criterion (AIC) value indicated the best fitting model. All p values < 0.05 were taken as statistically significant.

2.9. Ethical Approval

Ethical approval was obtained by the Ethics Review Committee at Prince of Songkla University (33/2017) and the Ethics Review Committee at the Department of Medical Research, Myanmar (023/2018).

3. Results

3.1. Investigation for DM among Index TB Patients

Prevalence of DM among Index TB Patients

Figure 1 shows a flow chart of the study. A total of 235 index TB patients were registered in the township TB clinics during the study period. Among them, 16 were excluded for various reasons. A total of 219 patients were invited and 193 agreed to participate (88% response rate). Among the 193 index TB patients, the prevalence with 95% confidence interval (CI) of known DM, newly diagnosed DM and overall DM were 24.9% (18.9–31.5), 7.8% (4.4–12.5) and 32.6% (26.1–39.7), respectively. Eight (12.7%) patients were aged between 29 and 39 years.

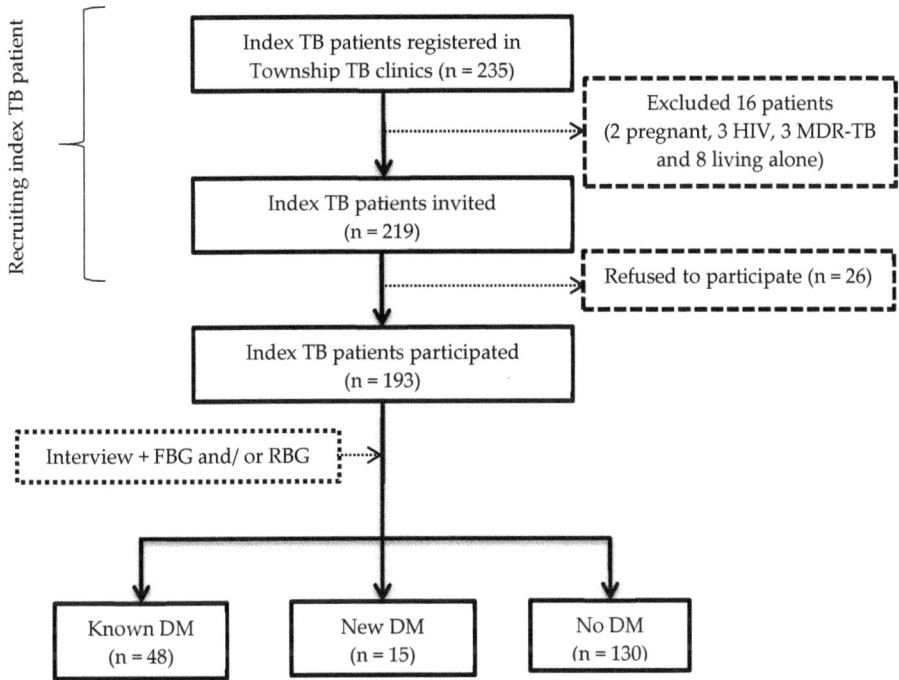

Figure 1. Flow chart of recruiting and investigation for diabetes mellitus (DM) among newly diagnosed index tuberculosis (TB) patients. MDR-TB—Multidrug resistant TB; RBG—Random capillary blood glucose; FBG—Fasting capillary blood glucose; Known DM—Patients with previous history of DM diagnosed by a medical doctor; New DM—Newly diagnosed DM patients (RBG ≥ 200 mg/dl & FBG ≥ 126 mg/dl (or) RBG ≥ 200 mg/dl for two times on separate days (or) FBG ≥ 126 mg/dl for two times on separate days).

3.2. Prevalence and Glycaemic Control of DM among Household Contacts

Figure 2 shows a flow chart of the 347 household contacts aged 25 years and above who were investigated for DM. Among them, 33 had history of diagnosed with DM. Among the 314 household contacts without a history of DM and invited to have an FBG test in township TB clinics, 139 (44.3%) attended. The remaining 156 contacts (49.7%) had their FBG tested at their home during the household revisit.

In total, 328 contacts completed all DM investigations. Among these, 33 (10.1%) were known to have DM and 13 (4.0%) were newly diagnosed, resulting in an overall prevalence of DM among household contacts of 14.0%. Most (94%) of the contacts with DM were aged 40 years and above. Among the 33 known cases, 21 (63.6%) had poor glycaemic control.

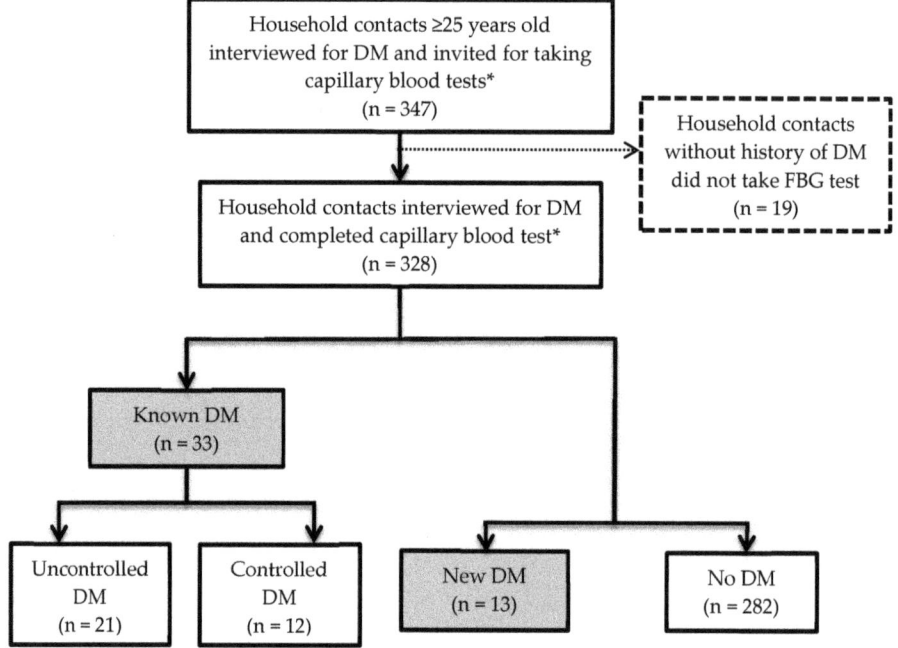

Figure 2. Flow chart for investigation for diabetes mellitus (DM) among household contacts. * Capillary blood test—Only fasting capillary blood glucose (FBG) test was done for known DM; and both random capillary blood glucose (RBG) test and FBG test were done for contacts without history of DM; Known DM—Household contacts with previous history of DM diagnosed by a health care personnel; Uncontrolled DM—FBG ≥ 130 mg/dl among known DM; New DM—Newly diagnosed DM (RBG ≥ 200 mg/dl & FBG ≥ 126 mg/dl (or) RBG ≥ 200 mg/dl for two times on separate days (or) FBG ≥ 126 mg/dl for two times on separate days).

3.3. Prevalence of TB among Household Contacts

Figure 3 shows a flow chart of the 553 household contacts who were investigated for TB. One household contacts among them was known case of TB. All household contacts, except the known case of TB, were invited to township TB clinics to have CXR regardless of having signs and symptoms of TB. Among them, 249 (45.1%) complied after the 1st home visit and 190 (34.4%) complied after the 2nd visit.

Overall, 439 (79.4%) completed all TB investigation. One (0.2%) was a known case and 21 (4.8%) were newly diagnosed, resulting in an overall TB prevalence of 5.0% among household contacts. MDR-TB was not detected.

3.4. Comparing Prevalence of DM and TB among Household Contacts of Index TB Patients with and without DM

Table 1 compares the prevalence of DM and TB among household contacts of TB patients with and without DM. The prevalence of DM, including known and newly diagnosed cases, was higher among household contacts of index TB with DM, although the difference was statistically significant only for the overall prevalence of DM. The prevalence of TB among household contacts, however, was comparable between the index TB with DM and without DM groups.

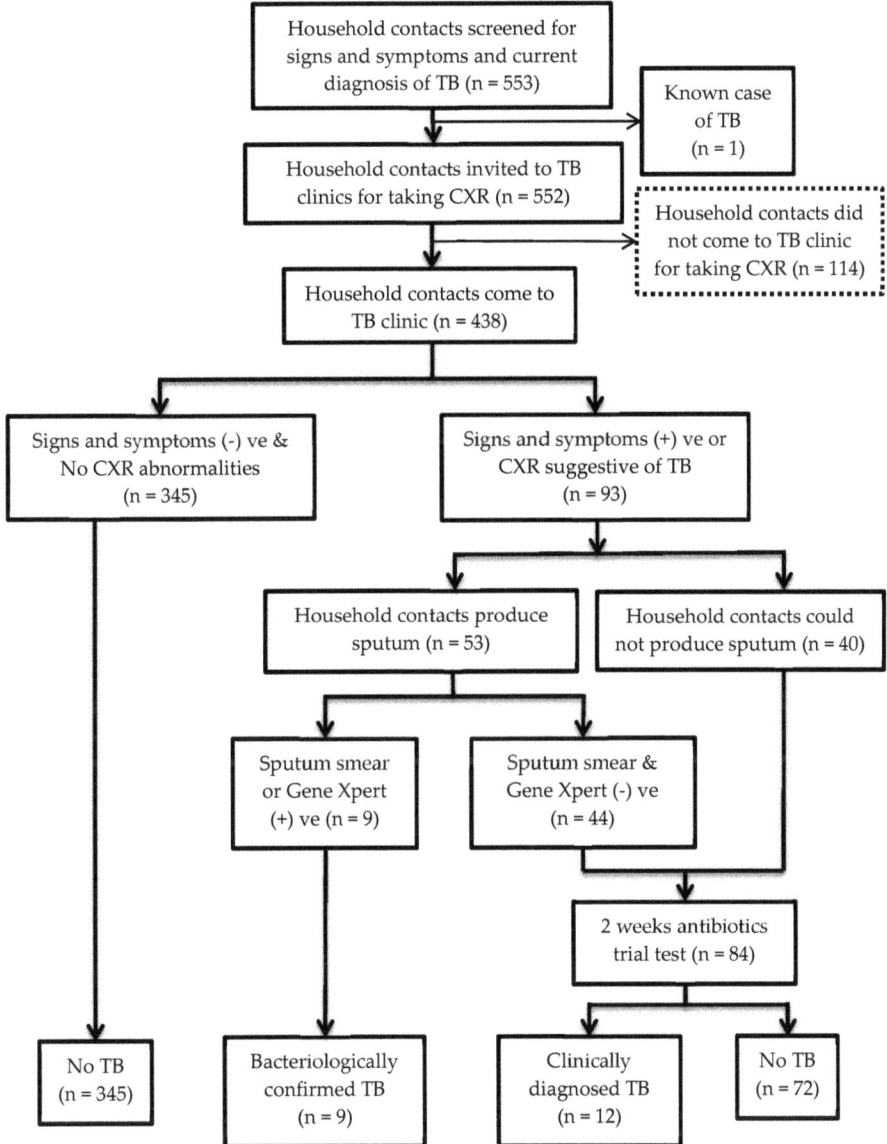

Figure 3. Flow chart for investigation for tuberculosis (TB) among household contacts.

Table 1. Comparison of prevalence of overall and newly diagnosed DM and TB among household contacts of TB patients with and without DM.

DM Screening in Household Contacts	Total	Household Contacts of Index TB with DM	Household Contacts of Index TB without DM	p Value
Number of household and household contact				
Total number of households visited (a)	193	63	130	N/A
Total number of household contacts screened for DM * (b)	328	104	224	N/A
Number of DM patients				
Known case of DM (c)	33	15	18	N/A
Newly diagnosed DM (d)	13	6	7	N/A
Prevalence of DM among household contacts, % (95%CI)				
Overall DM ((c + d)/b)	14.0 (10.6–18.4)	20.2 (13.2–29.4)	11.2 (7.5–16.2)	0.03
Known case of DM (c/b)	10.1 (7.1,13.9)	14.4 (8.6–22.9)	8.0 (4.9–12.6)	0.07
Newly diagnosed DM (d/b)	4.0 (2.2–6.9)	5.8 (2.4–12.6)	3.1 (1.4–6.6)	0.36 [†]
TB Screening in Household Contacts	**Total**	**Household Contacts of Index TB with DM**	**Household Contacts of Index TB without DM**	**p Value**
Number of household and household contact				
Total number of households visited (a)	193	63	130	N/A
Total number of household contacts screened for TB (b)	439	134	305	N/A
Number of TB patient				
Known case of TB (c)	1	0	1	N/A
Newly diagnosed TB (d)	21	6	15	N/A
Prevalence of TB among household contacts, % (95%CI)				
Overall TB prevalence ((c + d)/b)	5.0 (3.2–7.6)	4.5 (1.8–9.9)	5.3 (3.1–8.6)	0.73
Newly diagnosed TB (d/b)	4.8 (3.1–7.3)	4.5 (1.9–10.0)	4.9 (2.9–8.2)	0.84

N/A–Not applicable; * including both existing DM and household contacts who completed both RBG and FBG tests; CI—confidence interval; [†] Fisher's exact test.

3.5. Number of Patients with DM among Household Contacts ≥ 25 Years Old

Among household contacts aged ≥ 25 years without TB, 32 (12.1%) were diagnosed with DM, including all newly diagnosed cases.

Among household contacts aged ≥ 25 years with TB, one case was found to have existing DM with poor glycaemic control.

3.6. Odds Ratio of Getting DM and TB among Household Contacts Based on DM Status of Index TB Patients

Table 2 shows the odds ratios of obtaining DM and TB among household contacts, based on the DM status of index TB patients adjusted for covariates. From models D1 to D7, household contacts of index TB patients with DM had significantly higher risks of getting DM than household contacts of index TB patients without DM. Among these models, D2 had the lowest AIC. Based on this model, household contacts of index TB–DM patients had 2.13 times higher risk of getting DM than household contacts of index TB patients without DM.

From models T1 to T5, the risk of getting TB was lower in household contacts of index TB patients with DM, although the risk was not significantly different.

Table 2. Odds of getting DM and TB among household contacts based on the DM status of index TB patients in combination with various covariates.

	Outcome—DM Status of Household Contacts								
Model	Main Hypothesis Exposure	Covariate Included in the Model						OR (95% CI)	AIC
	DM in Index TB Patient	Age	Gender	SES	Low Physical Activity	BMI	Central Obesity		
D1	+	-	-	-	-	-	-	2.01 (1.07–3.79) *	265.4
D2	+	+	-	-	-	-	-	2.13 (1.10–4.12) *	248.1
D3	+	+	+	-	-	-	-	2.24 (1.15–4.35) *	248.3
D4	+	+	+	+	-	-	-	2.39 (1.22–4.72) *	254.0
D5	+	+	+	+	+	-	-	2.37 (1.19–4.69) *	253.5
D6	+	+	+	+	+	+	-	2.27 (1.13–4.56) *	253.5
D7	+	+	+	+	+	+	+	2.28 (1.13–4.57) *	254.6
	Outcome—Active TB Status of Household Contacts								
Model	Main Hypothesis Exposure	Covariate Included in the Model						OR (95% CI)	AIC
	DM in Index TB Patient	Age	Gender	SES	Closeness to Index TB Patient				
T1	+	-	-	-	-			0.85 (0.32–2.21)	178.5
T2	+	+	-	-	-			0.85 (0.33–2.23)	178.1
T3	+	+	+	-	-			0.82 (0.31–2.17)	175.3
T4	+	+	+	+	-			0.81 (0.30–2.21)	174.4
T5	+	+	+	+	+			0.87 (0.31–2.39)	175.7

OR—odds ratio; CI—confidence interval; AIC—Akaike's information criterion; * p value < 0.05; SES—Socioeconomic status including formal education, employment and daily income per household member; Closeness with TB patients—sharing same room, sleeping in same bed and taking care of index TB patients.

4. Discussion

In this study, comorbidity with DM among 32.6% of index TB patients highlighted the increased double burden of TB and DM in Yangon. The adherence to DM and TB screening among household contacts was increased with repeated home visits. Among household contacts, the prevalence of DM and TB were 14.0 and 5.0%, respectively, and more than a quarter of DM and 95% of TB were newly diagnosed. Among household contacts with existing DM, almost 63.6% had poor glycaemic control. The risk of DM among household contacts of index TB patients with DM was two times higher than those of TB patients without DM. There was no difference in the prevalence of TB among household contacts of both index TB patient groups.

The adherence to having an FBG test in a TB clinic after the 1st home visit was 44.3% and an additional 49.7% were tested in their homes during the 2nd revisit. Therefore, testing FBG during household visits increased the screening coverage of household contacts. The adherence of household contacts to TB investigation in clinics after the 1st home visit was similar to a study conducted in South Africa (45.1%) [38]. The adherence rate in our study was increased up to 79.5% after the 2nd visit. Therefore, repeated home visits achieved more than 30% adherence to TB investigation.

Among index TB patients, the prevalence of DM, 32.6% (95% CI: 26.1–39.7) was significantly higher than that in the general population 12.1% (95% CI: 8.4–17.0) [8]. After adjustment for age, the risk of DM among index TB patients was 2.8 times greater than the risk of DM in the general population. This finding is similar to the results of a meta-analysis, where the risk of DM was found to be three times higher in TB patients [2]. In the current study, the prevalence of newly diagnosed DM among 29 to 39 year old TB patients was almost 13% of all newly diagnosed DM cases. The current Myanmar guideline on screening for DM confined to those aged ≥ 40 years for TB patients would miss nearly 13% of the DM cases among TB patients in the Yangon Region.

Among household contacts who were aged 25 years or older, 14.0% (95% CI: 10.6–18.4) had DM, which was slightly higher than the 12.1% (95% CI: 8.4–17.0) prevalence in the general population [8]. After adjustment for age, no significant difference was found between the risk of DM among household contacts of TB patients and the risk of DM in the general population. Around 94% of patients with DM among household contacts were aged 40 years or over, which was similar with a previous Indian study, where household contacts aged 35 years and above comprised almost 93% of total DM patients [39]. Household contacts of TB–DM patients were more likely to have DM than those of TB patients without DM. This could be explained by genetic linkage similarity in risk behaviours among subjects in the same household.

Our contact investigation could identify around 4.0% of new DM. In a survey in the Yangon urban area, 7.6% of the participants were identified as new DM based on a one time FBG test [8]. In our study, confirmation of DM was defined based on results of both RBG and FBG tests. Therefore, the specificity of the test is higher than that of either test [40]. The prevalence of DM among household contacts without TB was 12.1%, including all newly diagnosed DM patients. These newly diagnosed DM patients comprised almost 25% of all DM patients among household contacts. Although integration of DM screening in household contacts of TB patients increases the case detection rate of a relatively small percentage of hidden DM cases in a community, newly detected DM cases are more at risk to TB than those detected by other screening methods.

Our overall prevalence of TB among household contacts (5.0%) was similar with a systematic review of contact investigation done in low and middle-income countries [11]. The prevalence was higher than studies done in China (3.8%) estimated by the same method [41], but lower than the 13.8% found in a study done in Mandalay region, Myanmar [25]. The difference in prevalence of TB among household contacts can be explained by different TB backgrounds in different populations, and the lifestyles and living conditions of people in each area [42]. There was no significant difference in prevalence of TB among household contacts of index TB patients with and without DM. This result is similar to a previous one reported from India [39].

In the current study, nearly two-thirds of known DM cases among household contacts had poor glycaemic control. The corresponding percentage was 54% among the general population but the cut off value for poor glycaemic control was FBG ≥ 126 mg/dl, which was lower than FBG ≥ 130 mg/dl in our study [8]. A previous study conducted in the US found that uncontrolled DM patients continued to have a significantly elevated risk of TB infection (OR, 2.6; 95% CI, 1.5–4.6) compared to nondiabetics [43]. A study conducted in Taiwan reported that DM patients with poor glycaemic control had a significantly higher hazard of TB than those without DM during a median follow-up time of 4.6 years [18]. In the current study, screening of DM was done among household contacts of recently diagnosed TB patients and only one TB case was identified among household contacts with poorly controlled DM. Therefore, these DM patients need good follow up to improve their DM conditions and reduce the risk of developing TB in the future.

5. Limitations

Our screening of DM was based on the finger prick method due to limited resources. The prevalence of DM may be different had the standard glucose concentrations in plasma been used [31,44]. Screening using CXR without sputum culture among those whose sputum could not be obtained might have led to an overestimated prevalence of TB among our contacts.

6. Conclusions

Despite these limitations, our findings indicate that screening of DM during household visits increased feasibility and repeated household visits improved the adherence of TB screening using CXR among household contacts. In a high TB and DM co-prevalent area, DM screening and glycaemic control assessment for TB household contacts aged 40 years or over should be integrated with routine TB screening programmes.

Author Contributions: N.-N.Z. completed this article as part of his Ph.D. thesis project supervised by V.C. and R.S. All authors contributed equally to this manuscript. N.-N.Z., V.C. and R.S. designed this study. N.-N.Z. collected and analysed the data, and prepared the first draft. S.S. and S.T.A. supervised the data collection. V.C. and R.S. supervised the data analysis. V.C. and R.S. reviewed the literature, contributed to interpretation of the results and reviewed the final manuscript. All authors gave equal contribution on revising and preparing the final version. All authors have read and agreed to the published version of the manuscript.

Funding: This study was a part of the PhD/Master thesis of the first author to fulfil the requirement for the TB/MDR-TB research training program at Epidemiology Unit, Prince of Songkla University under the support of Fogarty International Center, National Institutes of Health—Grant number D43TW009522. Additional funding also supported from the Department of Medical Research, Myanmar and the Graduate School Scholarship from Prince of Songkla University.

Acknowledgments: We would like to acknowledge all the respondents, research assistants, Township Tuberculosis Coordinators, Township Health Officers, and Basic Health Staff in research townships and responsible persons in Yangon Regional Tuberculosis Program, Department of Public Health, Myanmar.

Conflicts of Interest: The authors declare no conflict of interest.

References

1. Girardi, E.; Sañé Schepisi, M.; Goletti, D.; Bates, M.; Mwaba, P.; Yeboah-Manu, D.; Ntoumi, F.; Palmieri, F.; Maeurer, M.; Zumla, A.; et al. The global dynamics of diabetes and tuberculosis: The impact of migration and policy implications. *Int. J. Infect. Dis.* **2017**, *56*, 45–53. [CrossRef]
2. Jeon, C.Y.; Murray, M.B. Diabetes Mellitus Increases the Risk of Active Tuberculosis: A Systematic Review of 13 Observational Studies. *PLoS Med.* **2008**, *5*, e152. [CrossRef]
3. Pan, S.-C.; Ku, C.-C.; Kao, D.; Ezzati, M.; Fang, C.-T.; Lin, H.-H. Effect of diabetes on tuberculosis control in 13 countries with high tuberculosis: A modelling study. *Lancet Diabetes Endocrinol.* **2015**, *3*, 323–330. [CrossRef]
4. World Health Organization. *World Health Organization Global Tuberculosis Report 2019*; World Health Organization: Geneva, Switzerland, 2019; ISBN 978-92-4-156571-4.
5. Lönnroth, K.; Roglic, G.; Harries, A.D. Improving tuberculosis prevention and care through addressing the global diabetes epidemic: From evidence to policy and practice. *Lancet Diabetes Endocrinol.* **2014**, *2*, 730–739. [CrossRef]
6. Yangon Region Plans Two-Year Campaign against Tuberculosis. Available online: https://www.mmtimes.com/news/yangon-region-plans-two-year-campaign-against-tuberculosis.html (accessed on 26 May 2020).
7. Incidence of Tuberculosis (per 100,000 People) Data. Available online: https://data.worldbank.org/indicator/SH.TBS.INCD (accessed on 26 May 2020).
8. Aung, W.P.; Htet, A.S.; Bjertness, E.; Stigum, H.; Chongsuvivatwong, V.; Kjøllesdal, M.K.R. Urban–rural differences in the prevalence of diabetes mellitus among 25–74 year-old adults of the Yangon Region, Myanmar: Two cross-sectional studies. *BMJ Open* **2018**, *8*, e020406. [CrossRef]
9. International Diabetes Federation. Diabetes Atlas—2017 Atlas. Available online: https://diabetesatlas.org/resources/2017-atlas.html (accessed on 30 October 2019).
10. Baker, M.A.; Lin, H.-H.; Chang, H.-Y.; Murray, M.B. The Risk of Tuberculosis Disease among Persons with Diabetes Mellitus: A Prospective Cohort Study. *Clin. Infect. Dis.* **2012**, *54*, 818–825. [CrossRef]
11. Morrison, J.; Pai, M.; Hopewell, P.C. Tuberculosis and latent tuberculosis infection in close contacts of people with pulmonary tuberculosis in low-income and middle-income countries: A systematic review and meta-analysis. *Lancet Infect. Dis.* **2008**, *8*, 359–368. [CrossRef]
12. Hemminki, K.; Li, X.; Sundquist, K.; Sundquist, J. Familial Risks for Type 2 Diabetes in Sweden. *Diabetes Care* **2010**, *33*, 293–297. [CrossRef]

13. Khan, A.; Lasker, S.S.; Chowdhury, T.A. Are Spouses of Patients with Type 2 Diabetes at Increased Risk of Developing Diabetes? *Diabetes Care* **2003**, *26*, 710–712. [CrossRef]
14. Nielsen, J.; Bahendeka, S.K.; Whyte, S.R.; Meyrowitsch, D.W.; Bygbjerg, I.C.; Witte, D.R. Household and familial resemblance in risk factors for type 2 diabetes and related cardiometabolic diseases in rural Uganda: A cross-sectional community sample. *BMJ Open* **2017**, *7*. [CrossRef]
15. Viswanathan, V.; Kumpatla, S.; Aravindalochanan, V.; Rajan, R.; Chinnasamy, C.; Srinivasan, R.; Selvam, J.M.; Kapur, A. Prevalence of Diabetes and Pre-Diabetes and Associated Risk Factors among Tuberculosis Patients in India. *PLoS ONE* **2012**, *7*, e41367. [CrossRef]
16. Aye, S.; Majumdar, S.S.; Oo, M.M.; Tripathy, J.P.; Satyanarayana, S.; Kyaw, N.T.T.; Kyaw, K.W.Y.; Oo, N.L.; Thein, S.; Thu, M.K. Evaluation of a tuberculosis active case finding project in peri-urban areas, Myanmar: 2014–2016. *Int. J. Infect. Dis.* **2018**, *70*, 93–100. [CrossRef]
17. Kyaw Soe, T.; Soe, K.T.; Satyanarayana, S.; Saw, S.; San, C.C.; Aung, S.T. Gaps in Implementing Bidirectional Screening for Tuberculosis and Diabetes Mellitus in Myanmar: An Operational Research Study. *Trop. Med. Infect. Dis.* **2020**, *5*, 19. [CrossRef] [PubMed]
18. Lee, P.-H.; Fu, H.; Lai, T.-C.; Chiang, C.-Y.; Chan, C.-C.; Lin, H.-H. Glycemic Control and the Risk of Tuberculosis: A Cohort Study. *PLoS Med.* **2016**, *13*, e1002072. [CrossRef] [PubMed]
19. *Annual Report 2016—National Tuberculosis Programme*; Ministry of Health and Sports: Nay Pyi Taw, Myanmar, 2016.
20. Takasu, N.; Yamada, T.; Miura, H.; Sakamoto, S.; Korenaga, M.; Nakajima, K.; Kanayama, M. Rifampicin-induced Early Phase Hyperglycemia in Humans. *Am. Rev. Respir. Dis.* **1982**, *125*, 23–27. [CrossRef] [PubMed]
21. Ben-Haroush, A.; Yogev, Y.; Hod, M. Epidemiology of gestational diabetes mellitus and its association with Type 2 diabetes. *Diabet. Med.* **2004**, *21*, 103–113. [CrossRef]
22. Lin, S.P.; Wu, C.-Y.; Wang, C.-B.; Li, T.-C.; Ko, N.-Y.; Shi, Z.-Y. Risk of diabetes mellitus in HIV-infected patients receiving highly active antiretroviral therapy: A nationwide population-based study. *Medicine* **2018**, *97*, e12268. [CrossRef]
23. Liu, Q.; Li, W.; Xue, M.; Chen, Y.; Du, X.; Wang, C.; Han, L.; Tang, Y.; Feng, Y.; Tao, C.; et al. Diabetes mellitus and the risk of multidrug resistant tuberculosis: A meta-analysis. *Sci. Rep.* **2017**, *7*, 1090. [CrossRef]
24. Feltbower, R.G.; McKinney, P.A.; Campbell, F.M.; Stephenson, C.R.; Bodansky, H.J. Type 2 and other forms of diabetes in 0–30 year olds: A hospital based study in Leeds, UK. *Arch. Dis. Child.* **2003**, *88*, 676–679. [CrossRef]
25. Htet, K.K.K.; Liabsuetrakul, T.; Thein, S.; McNeil, E.B.; Chongsuvivatwong, V. Improving detection of tuberculosis among household contacts of index tuberculosis patients by an integrated approach in Myanmar: A cross-sectional study. *BMC Infect. Dis.* **2018**, *18*. [CrossRef]
26. World Health Organization NCDs STEPS Manual. Available online: http://www.who.int/ncds/surveillance/steps/manual/en/ (accessed on 25 June 2019).
27. Ferreira, F.H.G.; Chen, S.; Dabalen, A.L.; Dikhanov, Y.M.; Hamadeh, N.; Jolliffe, D.M.; Narayan, A.; Prydz, E.B.; Revenga, A.L.; Sangraula, P. *A Global Count of the Extreme Poor in 2012: Data Issues, Methodology and Initial Results*; The World Bank: Washington, DC, USA, 2015; pp. 1–66.
28. World Health Organization. NCDs STEP Wise Approach to Chronic Disease Risk Factor Surveillance. Available online: http://www.who.int/ncds/surveillance/steps/myanmar/en/ (accessed on 21 May 2019).
29. World Health Organization. Obesity: Preventing and Managing the Global Epidemic. Available online: http://www.who.int/entity/nutrition/publications/obesity/WHO_TRS_894/en/index.html (accessed on 23 June 2019).
30. World Health Organization. *Waist Circumference and Waist-Hip Ratio: Report of a WHO Expert Consultation, GENEVA, 8–11 December 2008*; World Health Organization: Geneva, Switzerland, 2011; ISBN 978-92-4-150149-1.
31. Accu-Chek Performa. Available online: https://www.accu-chek.com.au/meter-systems/performa (accessed on 21 May 2019).
32. American Diabetes Association. 2. Classification and Diagnosis of Diabetes: Standards of Medical Care in Diabetes—2019. *Diabetes Care* **2019**, *42*, S13–S28. [CrossRef] [PubMed]
33. American Diabetes Association. 6. Glycemic Targets: Standards of Medical Care in Diabetes—2019. *Diabetes Care* **2019**, *42*, S61–S70. [CrossRef]

34. World Health Organization. *Chest Radiography in Tuberculosis Detection: Summary of Current WHO Recommendations and Guidance on Programmatic Approaches*; World Health Organization: Geneva, Switzerland, 2016; ISBN 978-92-4-151150-6.
35. Soh, A.Z.; Chee, C.B.E.; Wang, Y.-T.; Yuan, J.-M.; Koh, W.-P. Alcohol drinking and cigarette smoking in relation to risk of active tuberculosis: Prospective cohort study. *BMJ Open Respir. Res.* **2017**, *4*, e000247. [CrossRef]
36. Acuña-Villaorduñ, C.; Jones-López, E.C.; Fregona, G.; Marques-Rodrigues, P.; Gaeddert, M.; Geadas, C.; Hadad, D.J.; White, L.F.; Molina, L.P.D.; Vinhas, S.; et al. Intensity of exposure to pulmonary tuberculosis determines risk of tuberculosis infection and disease. *Eur. Respir. J.* **2018**, *51*. [CrossRef]
37. Triasih, R.; Rutherford, M.; Lestari, T.; Utarini, A.; Robertson, C.F.; Graham, S.M. Contact Investigation of Children Exposed to Tuberculosis in South East Asia: A Systematic Review. *J. Trop. Med.* **2012**. [CrossRef]
38. Kigozi, N.G.; Heunis, J.C.; Engelbrecht, M.C. Yield of systematic household contact investigation for tuberculosis in a high-burden metropolitan district of South Africa. *BMC Public Health* **2019**, *19*. [CrossRef]
39. Shivakumar, S.V.B.Y.; Chandrasekaran, P.; Kumar, A.M.V.; Paradkar, M.; Dhanasekaran, K.; Suryavarshini, N.; Thomas, B.; Kohli, R.; Thiruvengadam, K.; Kulkarni, V.; et al. Diabetes and pre-diabetes among household contacts of tuberculosis patients in India: Is it time to screen them all? *Int. J. Tuberc. Lung Dis.* **2018**, *22*, 686–694. [CrossRef] [PubMed]
40. Weinstein, S.; Obuchowski, N.A.; Lieber, M.L. Clinical Evaluation of Diagnostic Tests. *Am. J. Roentgenol.* **2005**, *184*, 14–19. [CrossRef]
41. Xu, C.; Hu, B. Prevalence of active pulmonary tuberculosis among household contacts of recently diagnosed pulmonary tuberculosis patients with positive sputum-smear. *Zhonghua Liu Xing Bing Xue Za Zhi* **2008**, *29*, 693–695.
42. Nishikiori, N.; Weezenbeek, C.V. Target prioritization and strategy selection for active case-finding of pulmonary tuberculosis: A tool to support country-level project planning. *BMC Public Health* **2013**, *13*, 1–10. [CrossRef]
43. Martinez, L.; Zhu, L.; Castellanos, M.E.; Liu, Q.; Chen, C.; Hallowell, B.D.; Whalen, C.C. Glycemic Control and the Prevalence of Tuberculosis Infection: A Population-based Observational Study. *Clin. Infect. Dis.* **2017**, *65*, 2060–2068. [CrossRef] [PubMed]
44. Freckmann, G.; Schmid, C.; Baumstark, A.; Pleus, S.; Link, M.; Haug, C. System Accuracy Evaluation of 43 Blood Glucose Monitoring Systems for Self-Monitoring of Blood Glucose according to DIN EN ISO 15197. *J. Diabetes Sci. Technol.* **2012**, *6*, 1060. [CrossRef] [PubMed]

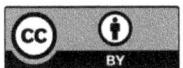

© 2020 by the authors. Licensee MDPI, Basel, Switzerland. This article is an open access article distributed under the terms and conditions of the Creative Commons Attribution (CC BY) license (http://creativecommons.org/licenses/by/4.0/).

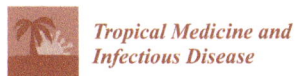

Perspective

An Opportunity to END TB: Using the Sustainable Development Goals for Action on Socio-Economic Determinants of TB in High Burden Countries in WHO South-East Asia and the Western Pacific Regions

Srinath Satyanarayana [1,2,*], Pruthu Thekkur [1,2], Ajay M. V. Kumar [1,2,3], Yan Lin [2,4], Riitta A. Dlodlo [2], Mohammed Khogali [5], Rony Zachariah [5] and Anthony David Harries [2,6]

1. The Union South-East Asia (The USEA) Office, C-6 Qutub Institutional Area, New Delhi 110016, India; pruthu.tk@theunion.org (P.T.); akumar@theunion.org (A.M.V.K.)
2. International Union against Tuberculosis and Lung Disease, 68 Boulevard Saint Michel, 75006 Paris, France; ylin@theunion.org (Y.L.); rdlodlo@theunion.org (R.A.D.); adharries@theunion.org (A.D.H.)
3. Yenepoya Medical College, Yenepoya (Deemed to be University), University Road, Deralakatte, Mangalore 575018, India
4. International Union against Tuberculosis and Lung Disease, No.1 Xindong Road, Beijing 100600, China
5. Special Programme for Research and Training in Tropical Disease (TDR), World Health Organization, Avenue Appia 20, 1211 Geneva, Switzerland; khogalim@who.int (M.K.); zachariahr@who.int (R.Z.)
6. London School of Hygiene and Tropical Medicine, Keppel Street, London WC1E 7HT, UK
* Correspondence: ssrinath@theunion.org; Tel.: +91-931-344-0973

Received: 12 May 2020; Accepted: 12 June 2020; Published: 18 June 2020

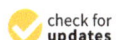

Abstract: The progress towards ending tuberculosis (TB) by 2035 is less than expected in 11 high TB burden countries in the World Health Organization South-East Asia and Western Pacific regions. Along with enhancing measures aimed at achieving universal access to quality-assured diagnosis, treatment and prevention services, massive efforts are needed to mitigate the prevalence of health-related risk factors, preferably through broader actions on the determinants of the "exposure-infection-disease-adverse outcome" spectrum. The aim of this manuscript is to describe the major socio-economic determinants of TB and to discuss how there are opportunities to address these determinants in an englobing manner under the United Nations Sustainable Development Goals (SDGs) framework. The national TB programs must identify stakeholders working on the other SDGs, develop mechanisms to collaborate with them and facilitate action on social-economic determinants in high TB burden geographical areas. Research (to determine the optimal mechanisms and impact of such collaborations) must be an integral part of this effort. We call upon stakeholders involved in achieving the SDGs and End TB targets to recognize that all goals are highly interlinked, and they need to combine and complement each other's efforts to end TB and the determinants behind this disease.

Keywords: tuberculosis; End TB; sustainable development goals; South-East Asia; Western Pacific Region; national TB program; socio-economic determinants

1. Introduction

Tuberculosis (TB), caused by the bacteria *Mycobacterium tuberculosis* (Mtb), is one of the top 10 leading causes of death world-wide and the leading cause of death from a single infectious agent [1]. Mtb spreads from person to person through airborne droplet nuclei. When a person with active TB of the lungs or throat, coughs or sneezes, droplets containing Mtb are expelled into the air and inhalation of this contaminated air may cause TB infection [2]. Once infected, about 5–15% of the people develop active TB disease in their lifetime, with the risk of developing the disease being highest in the first two years of infection [3,4]. About 1.7 billion people or 23% of the world's population are estimated to be infected with Mtb, of which 55.5 million (0.8% of the world's population) are estimated to be recently infected and at high risk of progression to active TB [5]. The aim of this manuscript is to describe the major socio-economic determinants of TB and to discuss how there are opportunities to address these determinants in an englobing manner.

2. TB Burden: Globally and in the WHO South-East Asia and Western Pacific Regions

Globally, about 10 million people developed TB in 2018, with this number being relatively stable in recent years. The annual TB incidence rate ranged from less than 5 people per 100,000 population to more than 500 people per 100,000 population, with the global average of 130 people per 100,000 population. In 2018, an estimated 1.2 million HIV-negative people and an additional 251,000 HIV-positive people died from TB. Although these numbers are large, the number of deaths among HIV-negative people has reduced by 27% from 1.7 million in 2000 to 1.2 million in 2018. Similarly, the number of deaths among HIV-positive people has reduced by 60%, from 620,000 in 2000 to 251,000 in 2018.

Geographically, in 2018, the TB burden varied across the six regions of the World Health Organization (WHO): this comprised 44% in the South-East Asia region [6], 24% in the Africa region, 18% in the Western Pacific region, 8% in the Eastern Mediterranean region, and 3% each in the Americas and Europe. Globally, 30 high TB burden countries accounted for 87% of the world's patients, with 11 of these being in the South-East Asia and Western Pacific regions (Table 1). Five countries in the South-East Asia and Western Pacific regions accounted for more than half of the global total: India—27%, China—9%, Indonesia—8%, the Philippines—6%, and Bangladesh—4%. Even within countries, the distribution of the TB burden is highly heterogeneous [7].

Table 1. List of high TB burden countries in the WHO South-East Asia and Western Pacific Regions.

Country	Annual TB Incidence in Thousands (Uncertainty Intervals)	The Approximate Annual Number of TB Deaths in Thousands (Best Estimates)
Bangladesh	357 (260–469)	47.2
Cambodia	49 (27–77)	6.7
China	866 (740–1000)	39.4
DPR Korea	131 (114–149)	20.0
India	2690 (1840–3700)	449.7
Indonesia	845 (770–923)	98.3
Myanmar	181 (119–256)	24.7
Papua New Guinea	37 (30–45)	4.7
Philippines	591 (332–924)	26.6
Thailand	106 (81–136)	11.5
Vietnam	174 (111–251)	13.2

Source: WHO Global TB Report 2019 [6].

3. End TB Strategy

In 2014, to rid mankind of the enormous burden of TB, the 67th World Health Assembly adopted a resolution to make the world free of TB by the year 2035. WHO's "End TB Strategy" provides a holistic overview of this resolution and has four principles and three pillars [8]. The three high-level target indicators of the End TB Strategy are reductions in TB deaths by 95%, reductions in the TB incidence rate by 90% and the percentage of TB patients and their households experiencing catastrophic costs being maintained at zero. These indicators and targets are relevant to all countries, with interim milestones to be achieved by 2020, 2025 and 2030.

Progress towards the 2020 Milestones of the End TB Strategy

By the end of 2019, at the global level, most of the WHO regions and many high TB burden countries were not on track to reach the End TB Strategy's 2020 milestones (20% reduction in TB incidence rate, 35% reduction in the number of TB deaths and reduction in the households experiencing catastrophic costs to 0%). The reduction in the cumulative global TB incidence rate between 2015 and 2018 was only 6.3%, and the reduction in the total number of TB deaths between 2015 and 2018 was 11% [6]. Table 2 shows the reduction in the TB incidence rate, TB mortality, and catastrophic costs in the 11 high TB burden countries in the Asia Pacific region (which comprises South-East Asia and the Western Pacific). However, with this rate of decline in incidence and mortality, and with the data on catastrophic costs unavailable, it is unlikely that any of the countries in the Asia Pacific region will be able to reach all the End TB Strategy's 2020 milestones.

Table 2. High TB burden countries in the WHO South-East Asia and Western Pacific Regions and the relative change in crucial indicators between 2015 and 2018.

Country	TB Incidence Rate (Per 100,000 Population)			Number of TB Deaths (in Thousands)			Proportion of TB Patients Experiencing Catastrophic Costs (in 2018)
	2015	2018	Reduction *	2015	2018	Reduction *	
Bangladesh	221	221	0%	66.0	47.0	29%	NA
Cambodia	367	302	18%	3.8	3.4	11%	NA
China	65	61	6%	43.0	40.0	7%	NA
DPR Korea	513	513	0%	10.0	20.0	−100%	NA
India	217	199	8%	470.0	449.0	4%	NA
Indonesia	325	316	3%	102.0	98.0	4%	NA
Myanmar	391	338	14%	36.0	25.0	31%	NA
Papua New Guinea	432	432	0%	4.3	4.7	−9%	NA
Philippines	550	554	−1%	28.0	26.0	7%	NA
Thailand	163	153	6%	15.0	11.0	27%	NA
Vietnam	199	182	9%	17.0	13.0	24%	NA

Source: Point estimates from WHO Global TB Report 2019 [6]; NA = Data Not available; * negative sign indicates an increase in the TB incidence rate or number of TB deaths.

4. Factors Influencing the Risk of Exposure to Mycobacterium tuberculosis (Mtb), Infection, the Progression from Infection to Disease and Adverse Treatment Outcomes

There are two important aspects to understanding the TB epidemiology. First, Mtb infection in humans results in a spectrum of clinical presentations. As mentioned earlier, most infections are subclinical and asymptomatic, with Mtb replication contained by the host immunity—a condition called latent TB infection (LTBI)—and only a small subset of infected individuals presenting with symptomatic, active TB disease. Even within and between these two states, there is a wide ranging spectrum of Mtb bacterial load, immune responses, pathologies and clinical presentations [9]. Second, like all other infectious diseases, the risk of infection and disease is dependent on the characteristics and interaction of the bacteria, the human host and the environment [7]. A good understanding of these factors and their unique complex interactions—at both the population level and the individual level—is crucial for designing the intervention strategies to mitigate the TB burden.

The factors that influence the risk of exposure to Mtb, infection, the progression of infection to disease, and adverse treatment outcomes (such as death) are shown in Box 1 [10,11]. The factor that is essential for TB infection and disease is close contact with a person with a person with infectious TB disease; the greater the closeness, bacterial load and duration of contact, the higher the chances of infection. Other factors such as age, sex, tobacco use, alcohol use, malnutrition, human immunodeficiency virus (HIV) infection, diabetes mellitus and silicosis increase the risk of infection, the progression from infection to disease and adverse TB treatment outcomes, and are therefore called major health-related risk factors. Factors such as poverty, socio-economic and/or gender inequality, food and/or job insecurity and weak health systems affect not only all aspects of the "exposure-infection-disease-adverse outcome" spectrum, but also several aspects of the health of populations in general, and are therefore called the critical underlying 'determinants' or the 'root causes' of TB. While age and sex are not modifiable, all the other factors listed in Box 1 can be modified by human interventions. Table 3 shows the health-related risk factors and the corresponding lifetime increase in the risk of TB disease and the 'population attributable fraction (PAF)' of these factors [12–18].

Table 3. Health-related risk factors and the corresponding lifetime increase in the risk of TB disease and their corresponding population attributable fraction.

Risk Factor	Relative Risk of TB (95% Confidence Intervals) *	Estimated Prevalence of Risk Factor in the South-East Asia and Pacific Region **	Estimated Population Attributable Fraction (PAF) ***
HIV	19 (16–22)	0.2% [12]	3.5% (2.9–4.0%)
Alcohol abuse	3.3 (2.1–5.2)	13.5% [13]	23.7% (12.9–36.2%)
Undernourishment	3.2 (3.1–3.3)	11.5% [14]	20.2% (19.5–20.9%)
Smoking	1.6 (1.2–2.1)	24.8% [15]	13.0% (4.7–21.4%)
Diabetes Mellitus	1.5 (1.3–1.8)	8.6% [16]	4.1% (2.5–6.4%)
Indoor Air Pollution	2.0 (1.2–3.2)	38.6% [17]	27.8% (7.2–45.9%)

* Source: Global TB report 2019 [6]); ** these are approximates and vary widely across countries; *** PAF indicates the proportion of all cases of a particular disease in a population that is attributable to a specific exposure and is estimated based on the relative risk and the prevalence of the risk factor in the population [18].

Box 1. Factors influencing the "exposure-infection-disease-adverse outcome" spectrum of TB.

The essential factor for TB infection and TB disease
• Close contact with a person with infectious TB disease
Major health-related risk factors (factors that increase the chances of infection, disease, adverse TB treatment outcomes)
• Age, sex, tobacco use, alcohol abuse, malnutrition, HIV infection, diabetes mellitus, exposure to indoor air pollution, silicosis, intake of immunosuppressive drugs/medications (e.g., tumor necrosis factor-alpha (TNF) antagonists, corticosteroids)
Major underlying determinants
• Poverty, socio-economic and gender inequality, overcrowding, food and job insecurity, weak health systems

4.1. Relationship between Various Health-Related Risk factors and Major Underlying Socio-Economic Determinants of TB

In the past, the trends in TB incidence rates in high-income countries clearly show that efforts towards improving the socio-economic status, living conditions and nutritional status (as was seen before and soon after the world wars) resulted in the rapid decline in the TB burden, and, deterioration in these conditions (during times of war) increased the TB incidence rates. Both in high and low-income countries, TB predominantly affects people of lower socio-economic status [19,20].

Most of the risk factors for TB are associated with poverty, socio-economic and gender inequalities, and living conditions [21]. Malnutrition, poor housing/living conditions, and overcrowding are direct markers of poverty [22]. People from lower socio-economic groups are more likely to live and/or work in overcrowded settings, experience greater food insecurity, have lower levels of awareness about healthy behavior, and are less likely to have access to quality health care services [23]. They are also more likely to come into contact with people with active TB disease. The prevalence of tobacco use, alcohol use, HIV, and diabetes mellitus is relatively higher in people of low socio-economic status groups in various settings [24–28].

The Multisectoral Accountability Framework to accelerate progress to end TB (MAF-TB) by 2035 developed by the WHO in 2019 [29] urges governments to address a wide range of socio-economic determinants through collaborations and partnerships. Although the primary responsibility to pursue public health in all policies rests with different ministries within governments, the national TB programs, as champions and implementers of the TB care and prevention services in the countries, should take the lead in developing partnerships and support the implementation of the multisectoral accountability framework, both through advocacy and by helping to address the social conditions of patients and their families.

4.2. Need for Action on Risk Factors and Major Determinants of TB

TB (as described earlier) is a multifactorial disease, and the achievement of the End TB Strategy milestones requires universal access to quality-assured diagnosis, treatment, and prevention services promptly. For this, it is necessary to strengthen the national TB programs, by ensuring adequate resources for deploying latest WHO-endorsed rapid TB diagnostics and drug susceptibility testing (DST) facilities, the provision of appropriate treatment services for drug-susceptible and drug-resistant TB, preventive treatment for high risk individuals (people living with HIV and household and other close contacts of TB patients), and the implementation of infection control measures in all health facilities. While these are necessary, it is being increasingly recognized that End TB targets are ambitious and unlikely to be achieved by these measures alone [10,11,30]. Massive efforts are needed to mitigate the prevalence of health-related risk factors, preferably through broader actions on the determinants of the "exposure-infection-disease-adverse outcome" spectrum, such as health system strengthening, poverty alleviation, addressing socio-economic and gender inequality, limiting job loss and food insecurity, improving housing quality and reducing overcrowding. An increase in the health-related risk factors of TB or the worsening of the determinants of TB (as is currently happening due to the socio-economic consequences of the SARS-CoV-2 pandemic [31]) can harm the global progress made towards ending TB.

5. Framework for Action on Social Determinants of Tuberculosis: Sustainable Development Goals

The sustainable development goals (SDGs) [32] are a list of 17 global goals, which outline the vision, principles, and commitments of all United Nations member countries to a fairer and more sustainable world, now and in the future. The SDGs, launched in 2015 by the United Nations General Assembly, and intended to be achieved by the year 2030, are part of UN Resolution 70/1, the 2030 Agenda. The 17 SDGs are mentioned in Box 2.

Box 2. The Sustainable Development Goals (2015 to 2030) *.

1.	**No Poverty**
2.	**Zero Hunger**
3.	**Good Health and Well-being**
4.	**Quality Education**
5.	**Gender Equality**
6.	**Clean Water and Sanitation**
7.	**Affordable and Clean Energy**
8.	**Decent Work and Economic Growth**
9.	Industry, Innovation, and Infrastructure
10.	**Reducing Inequality**
11.	**Sustainable Cities and Communities**
12.	Responsible Consumption and Production
13.	**Climate Action**
14.	Life Below Water
15.	Life on Land
16.	Peace, Justice, and Strong Institutions
17.	Partnerships for the Goals

The seventeen SDGs each have a list of targets that are measured with indicators [33]. These goals necessitate collaboration and the alignment of all actions to secure a fair, healthy, and prosperous future for everyone on this planet—Earth. These SDGs provide a framework for action on the determinants of TB disease. Action on the determinants of TB through the SDGs framework will also mean endorsing the socio-ecological model of health which outlines that disease prevention and its mitigation may require action at five levels: individual, interpersonal, organisational, community and public policy [34] and addressing every TB determinant may require actions at these five levels.

5.1. Sustainable Development Goals that Are Likely to Have a Significant Impact on the Burden of TB

5.1.1. SDG Goal 1: No Poverty

As discussed above, poverty is a significant determinant of several aspects of health including TB [22,35]. Globally, more than 90% of TB cases and deaths occur in low and middle income countries [36]. There is an inverse correlation between a country's gross domestic product (GDP) per capita and TB incidence rates [21]. Therefore, efforts to reduce poverty will have a substantial impact on the TB burden. Despite great progress made globally in reducing poverty levels, some countries in the WHO South-East Asia and Western Pacific Regions, such as India (~21%) and Papua New Guinea (38%), have high reported levels of people living below the international poverty line (SDG Indicator 1.1.1 in Table (SDG Indicator 2.1.1 in Table 4).

5.1.2. SDG Goal 2: Zero Hunger

Hunger leads to undernutrition, which is one of the significant determinants of TB [37]. It is estimated that in India (the highest TB burden country in the world), where the prevalence of undernutrition is high, nearly 50% of TB cases are attributable to undernutrition [38,39]. Undernutrition is also ubiquitous in all high TB burden countries in Asia and the Pacific region (SDG Indicator 2.1.1 in Table 4). Therefore, ending hunger and improving the nutritional status of populations can dramatically reduce the burden of TB.

5.1.3. SDG Goal 3: Good Health and Well Being

One of the key targets of this goal (Target 8) is to achieve universal health coverage (UHC) by 2030 [40]. UHC means that everyone can access and receive sufficient and quality health services that they need without suffering financial hardship. There are two key indicators to monitor progress. They are: a) UHC service coverage index (SCI)—SDG Indicator 3.8.1 (Table 5), and b) the percentage of the population experiencing expenditures on health care that are relatively large in relation to the household expenditures or income—SDG Indicator 3.8.2 (Table 5). The achievement of UHC and improved patient-centered TB care will have a direct effect on the reach and delivery of quality TB services and on catastrophic costs incurred by TB patients and their families [40]. Apart from this, the SDG goal also has indicators for dramatically reducing the prevalence of HIV, tobacco and alcohol use, and diabetes mellitus, all of which will have a considerable impact on reducing the TB burden.

5.1.4. SDG Goal 4: Quality Education

Quality education typically leads to better and secure jobs, more money and higher purchasing power, resulting in better access to quality health care (including for TB) [41]. Higher earnings also allow people to afford homes in safer neighbor hoods, as well as consume healthier diets. Incorporating health within the ambit of 'quality education' builds knowledge, skills, and positive attitudes about health and all other determinants of health, which can directly or indirectly have a considerable impact on efforts to End TB [42]. Education also improves the ability to identify the symptoms suggestive of TB and seek timely care for diagnosis and treatment of TB [43], thus, limiting the delays in the diagnosis of TB and the community spread of the disease.

5.1.5. SDG Goal 5: Gender Equality

TB can affect either gender. In almost all countries, the notification rates of TB are higher in males than in females. Although more men than women develop TB disease and die from it, TB is nevertheless a leading infectious cause of death among women. Higher tuberculosis notification rates in men partly reflect epidemiological and biological differences in exposure, risk of infection, and progression from infection to disease [44]. Despite this, in several countries, gender inequality, socio-economic, and cultural factors act as barriers to accessing health care among women. These may lead to the under-detection and under-notification of TB in women. The stigma and discrimination associated with TB and certain co-morbidities, such as HIV infection, adversely affect women more than men, often leaving them in a more vulnerable position [45,46]. It is also widely believed that the medical care-seeking behavior of men and women with TB is mostly determined by how they and those around them perceive the symptoms, regard the diagnosis, accept the treatment, and complete it. Gender may influence each of these components and affect the early detection of the disease and its outcome [47]. Studies that have assessed gender differences have shown that, on average, women are either undiagnosed, or diagnosed late in the course of TB disease when compared to men [48,49]. Promoting gender equality in all spheres of life helps to mitigate some of these issues and contribute towards ending TB.

5.1.6. SDG Goal 6: Clean Water and Sanitation

Access to clean water and sanitation is essential to reduce illness, malnutrition, poor physical and cognitive development, and death due to water-borne diseases [50]. In countries of the Asia-Pacific region, the proportion with access to clean water ranges from 16.7% in rural Cambodia to 92.3% in urban China. The proportion with access to safe sanitation ranges from 5.1% in rural Democratic People's Republic of Korea to 83.7% in urban China. The provision of clean water and sanitation can affect the TB burden by reducing infections and improving nutritional status.

5.1.7. SDG Goal 7: Affordable and Clean Energy

There is evidence of an association between indoor air pollution (such as that caused by the burning of solid fuels for cooking at homes), outdoor ambient air pollution and TB infection and TB disease [51–54]. Depending on the prevalence of indoor air pollution, the fraction of TB cases attributable to indoor air pollution varies across countries. The proportion of the population using clean fuels in the South-East Asia and Western Pacific regions ranges from 11% in DPR Korea to 74% in Thailand (Table 4; indicator 7.1.2). Interventions such as clean cook stoves to reduce the adverse effects of indoor air pollution merit rigorous evaluation [50], particularly in high TB burden countries in Asia and the Pacific, where the prevalence of both indoor air pollution and TB is high. Clean energy is also expected to reduce outdoor air pollution and improve ambient air quality, which can reduce the risk of TB [55].

5.1.8. SDG Goal 8: Decent Work and Economic Growth

TB predominantly affects people in the economically productive age-groups [56]. Apart from providing stable and regular job opportunities for the economically productive age groups, provision for early diagnosis and treatment of TB at workplaces, making workplaces safe by reducing the chances of airborne transmission of infections, adopting favorable policies towards social/job security in case of diseases and reducing occupational diseases like silicosis, will help in reducing the TB burden and improving the economic productivity of the workforce [57]. Stable/formal employment also increases access to employer-sponsored social health insurance programs and paid sick leaves, both of which are known to be associated with the reduced risk of occupational diseases and all-cause mortality [58–60].

5.1.9. SDG Goal 10: Reduced Inequalities

Empowering and promoting social, economic and political inclusion of all, irrespective of age, sex, sexual orientation, disability, race, ethnicity, origin, religion or economic or another status will help in mitigating the effects of socio-economic disparities—disparities that are key drivers of all the risk factors of TB [61].

5.1.10. SDG Goal 11: Sustainable Cities and Communities

Rapid industrialization, urbanization, and migration—dominant occurrences in most developing countries in the Asia Pacific region—can create ideal conditions for infectious diseases (including TB) to flourish [62,63], unless accompanied by proper urban planning, social reforms, environmental protection, adequate housing, transportation, and a well-coordinated and robust health system.

5.1.11. SDG Goal 13: Climate Action

Climate change that manifests itself in the form of higher variations in temperatures and rainfall is known to have a substantial effect on several aspects of human health and behaviour (such as crowding, migration, changes in food habits), either directly or through several intermediaries, resulting in an increase in the burden of infectious diseases including TB [64,65].

The linkages between the various SDGs and TB are pictorially depicted in Figure 1.

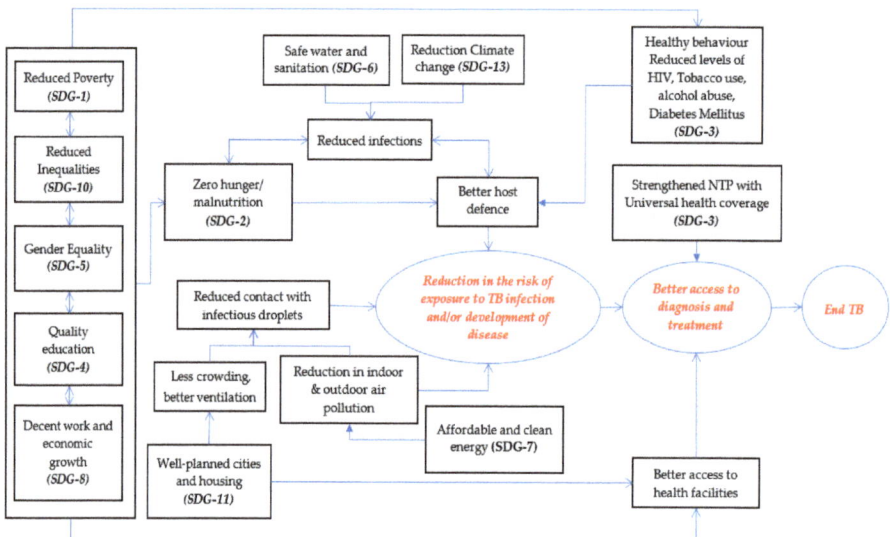

Figure 1. The possible direct and indirect linkages between SGDs 1, 2, 3, 4, 5, 6, 7, 8, 10, 11, 13 and reduction in tuberculosis burden. The arrows indicate the probable direction of action, with the bi-directional arrow indicating that effects in both the directions are possible. The relationships/pathways shown in this figure are 'indicative' only and not 'definitive'. The size of the square boxes in the figure have been arrived at using the best fit function, and therefore the varying sizes or shapes of the text boxes/circles in the figure do not carry any special significance. SDGs 1, 4, 5, 8, 10 are grouped together, to indicate the author's view that they are interdependent and can act alone or in a combined manner to influence the other aspects in the pathway.

Table 4. Current levels of TB relevant SDG 1, 2, 7, 8, 10, 11 indicators in high TB burden countries in the WHO South-East Asia and Western Pacific Regions (in 2018).

Country	1.1.1 Proportion of the Population Living below the International Poverty Line	1.3.1 Proportion of the Population Covered by Social Protection Floors or Systems	2.1.1 Prevalence of Undernourishment	7.1.2 Proportion of the Population with Primary Reliance on Clean Fuels and Technology	8.1.1 Gross Domestic Product (GDP) Per Capita, PPP (Constant 2011 International Dollars)	10.1.1 Gini Index for Income Inequality *	11.1.1 Proportion of the Urban Population Living in Slums
Bangladesh	15%	18%	15%	18%	3500	32	55%
Cambodia	NA	3.1%	18%	18%	3700	NA	55%
China	0.7%	63%	8.7%	59%	15,300	39	25%
DPR Korea	NA	NA	43%	11%	NA	NA	NA
India	21%	30%	15%	41%	6500	36	24%
Indonesia	5.7%	57%	7.7%	58%	11,200	38	22%
Myanmar	6.4%	2.3%	10%	18%	5600	38	41%
Papua New Guinea	38%	4.2%	NA	13%	3800	48	NA
Philippines	NA	41%	14%	43%	7600	40	38%
Thailand	0%	79%	9%	74%	16,300	36	25%
Vietnam	2%	35%	11%	67%	6200	35	27%

PPP = Purchasing Power Parity; NA = Not available; Source of data: [66–68]; * Gini index = measure of income distribution across income percentiles in a population. It ranges from 0% to 100%, with 0% representing perfect equality and 100% representing perfect inequality.

Table 5. Estimated prevalence of TB relevant SDG-3 indicators in high TB burden countries in the WHO South-East Asia and Western Pacific Regions (in 2018).

Country	3.8.1 Coverage of Essential Health Services (UHC) Measure with an UHC Index Based Essential Health Services and Ranges between 0 and 100	3.8.2 Proportion of the Population with Large Household Expenditures on Health as a Share of Total Household Expenditure or Income	3.c.1 Current Health Expenditure Per Capita in Current International Dollars	3.3.1 Prevalence of HIV	3.a.1 Prevalence of Smoking		3.4.1 Prevalence of Diabetes		3.5.2 Prevalence of Alcohol Use Disorder	
					Male	Female	Male	Female	Male	Female
Bangladesh	48	25%	91	0.1%	45%	1%	10%	9.3%	1.4%	0.3%
Cambodia	60	15%	229	0.5%	34%	2%	7.4%	6.9%	8.7%	1.8%
China	79	20%	761	NA	48%	1.9%	9.9%	7.6%	8.4%	0.2%
DPR Korea	71	NA	NA	NA	NA	NA	5.8%	5.9%	6.2%	1.0%
India	55	17%	241	0.2%	21%	1.9%	9.1%	8.3%	9.1%	0.5%
Indonesia	57	2.7%	363	0.4%	76%	2.8%	7.6%	8.0%	1.4%	0.3%
Myanmar	61	14%	291	0.7%	35%	6.3%	6.9%	7.9%	3.2%	0.6%
Papua New Guinea	40	NA	92	0.9%	49%	24%	15%	14%	8.8%	1.8%
Philippines	61	6.3%	342	0.1%	41%	7.8%	7.1%	7.3%	8.8%	1.8%
Thailand	80	2.2%	635	1.1%	39%	1.9%	8.3%	8.8%	10%	0.9%
Vietnam	75	9.4%	356	0.3%	46%	1.0%	5.5%	5.1%	9.8%	1.2%

NA = Not available; Source of data: [66–68].

6. Role of National TB Programs in Accelerating the Progress towards Achieving SDGs

Together, TB and poverty form a vicious cycle: TB decreases people's capacity to work and adds to treatment expenses. This, in turn, exacerbates their poverty. Poor people also go hungry and live in close, unhygienic quarters, where TB and its risk factors flourish. Progress in ending TB will accelerate the progress on SDG goal 1, and through it, progress on other related SDGs [36].

According to the WHO's "A Multisectoral Accountability Framework to accelerate progress to end Tuberculosis by 2030 (MAF-TB)" [29], the following are recommended actions for national TB programs:

- Development of national (and local) strategic and operational plans to end (or eliminate) TB, with a multisectoral perspective involving government and partners, consistent with the End TB Strategy.
- Development and use of a national MAF-TB.
- Establishment, strengthening or maintenance of a national multisectoral mechanism (e.g., inter-ministerial commission), tasked with providing oversight, coordination and a periodic review of the national tuberculosis response.
- Implementation of multisectoral actions on the social determinants of tuberculosis.
- Revisions to plans and policies, and associated activities, based on monitoring, reporting, and recommendations from reviews.

WHO has identified the following fourteen SDG indicators as relevant to TB. These include

A. Seven indicators relevant to TB under SDG 1, 2, 7, 8, 10 and 11 and seven indicators within SDG-3.

   (1) SDG 1 (No poverty)—Indicator 1.1.1: Proportion of the population living below the international poverty line
   (2) SDG 1 (No poverty)—Indicator 1.3.1: Proportion of the population covered by social protection floors or systems
   (3) SDG 2 (Zero hunger)—Indicator 2.1.1: Prevalence of undernourishment
   (4) SDG 7 (Affordable and clean energy)—Indicator 7.1.2: Proportion of the population with primary reliance on clean fuels and technology
   (5) SDG 8 (Decent work and economic growth)—Indicator: 8.1.1: Gross domestic product (GDP) per capita
   (6) SDG 10 (Reduced inequalities)—Indicator: 10.1.1: Gini index for income inequality
   (7) SDG 11 (Sustainable Cities and Communities)—Indicator: 11.1.1: Proportion of the urban population living in slums

The levels of these seven indicators under SDG 1, 2, 7, 8, 10 and 11 at the end of 2018 in the 11 high TB burden countries in WHO South-East Asia and Western Pacific Regions are given in Table 4.

B. Seven indicators relevant to TB within SDG 3 are as follows:

   (1) SDG Indicator 3.8.1: Coverage of essential health services (UHC) measure with an UHC index based essential health services and ranges between 0 and 100
   (2) SDG Indicator 3.8.2: Proportion of the population with large household expenditures on health, as a share of total household expenditure or income
   (3) SDG Indicator 3.c.1: Current health expenditure per capita in current international dollars
   (4) SDG Indicator 3.3.1: Prevalence of HIV
   (5) SDG Indicator 3.a.1: Prevalence of smoking
   (6) SDG Indicator 3.4.1: Prevalence of diabetes
   (7) SDG Indicator 3.5.2: Prevalence of alcohol use disorder

The levels of these seven within SDG-3 indicators at the end of 2018 is in the 11 high TB burden countries in WHO South-East Asia, and Western Pacific Regions is given in Table 5.

National TB programs, Ministries of Health and Governments in the 11 high TB burden countries must realize that interventions beyond diagnosis and treatment of TB and LTBI are needed to reduce the risk factors and determinants of TB. TB programs must take a lead and list the stakeholders in their countries who are working on the other SDGs and equip themselves with resources and the necessary skillsets to engage with them. Since TB is not homogenously distributed within the country, there will be geographical areas/communities with high TB burdens. As a first step, TB programs should share details/information of high TB burden geographical areas, assess the socio-economic determinants that are locally relevant/prevalent, and facilitate concentrated action on those socio-economic determinants as a priority in these areas wherever possible. The list of sample interventions that can be undertaken to reduce the prevalence of the socio-economic determinants of TB (based on needs assessment) are given in Table 6. (In this table, using India as an example, we have highlighted public programs [69–82] that can be galvanized to address the determinants at the local level.)

The stakeholders/partners who can be involved in carrying out the interventions could be respective government departments (who have the mandate and jurisdiction to perform the intervention), non-governmental/community based organizations, private sector, developmental partners etc., who may share the common vision of improving the lives of the people. Identifying suitable partners will help the national TB programs, in facilitating their interventions in such geographic high TB burden areas. This holistic approach may contribute towards ending TB in such communities or geographic areas in a sustainable manner. Demonstration projects on how to operationalize intersectoral coordination and build partnerships (at the local level) are urgently needed to generate evidence and to show that the impact of such initiatives goes beyond the simple sum of its immediate returns. Research—to find out the optimal mechanisms for collaboration and to measure the impact of such collaborations—must also be undertaken, so that the lessons learnt are disseminated widely. Apart from this, national TB programs must also find themselves represented in all in-country developmental committees and agendas of the government, so that ending TB is seen, not just as a responsibility of the health sector, but seen as a necessity for human development in all spheres of life. International technical and funding agencies/organizations, like WHO, the Global Fund, etc., should advocate for progress on broader SDGs and provide technical and financial assistance on this aspect to TB programs.

Table 6. Sample policies/interventions that can be implemented at the community level in high TB burden geographical areas within a country by the National TB program and its partners to address determinants of tuberculosis.

Determinant of TB	Sample Community Level Policies/Interventions to Address the Determinant	Example: Public Programs in India that Can Be Galvanized to Address the Determinant at the Local Level
To reduce poverty (SDG-1)	• Skills building programs • Providing access to credit/microfinance and markets • Generating employment opportunities	• Pradhan Mantri Kaushal Vikas Yojana (PMKVY)—A skill development scheme [69] • Mahatma Gandhi National Rural Employment Guarantee Act (MGNREGA) 2005 (India)—Aims to enhance livelihood security in rural areas [70]
To reduce hunger (SDG-2)	• Nutrition education • Food subsidy interventions/ Cash transfers • Targeted Supplemental nutrition assistance programs • Finding ways to increase agricultural production and cost of food crops	• National Food for Work Program (India) • School mid-day meals program [75]
Improve the quality of education (SDG-4)	• Improving physical infrastructure of schools (including sanitation facilities), providing teaching and learning materials, and training and hiring extra teachers. • Enhancing community ownership and engagement in education • Adult literacy, numeracy and education programs and special education programs to children and youth with disabilities and learning difficulties • Compulsory and free education programs for children and youth	• National Education Mission (Samagra Shiksha Abhiyan) [76]
Gender equality (SDG-5)	• Awareness-raising and sensitization programs to reduce gender inequality, raise awareness about different gender identities and reduce gender-based violence • Engagement with political leaders, religious leaders, community leaders to address practices that impair the rights of women and girls • Empowering young girls and women by creating employment and education opportunities for their holistic growth and development • Provide legal and psychosocial support services to address gender discrimination and human rights violations	• Beti Bachao Beti Padhao Scheme (To provide education to girls' and their welfare. To prevent the violation in the interest of girls. To celebrate the birth of a girl child.) [77] • Support to Training and Employment Program for Women (STEP) [78] • Mahila E-Haat (To help women to make financial and economic choices which will enable them to be a part of 'Make in India' and 'Stand Up India' initiatives) [79]
Clean water and sanitation (SDG-6)	• Construction of toilets and latrines in all households and public spaces that flush into a sewer or safe enclosure. • Information, Education and Communication to promote good hygiene habits (e.g., hand washing). • Rainwater harvesting to collect and store rainwater for drinking or recharging underground aquifers. • Provide low cost home water-treatment capability through the use of filters, chlorine tablets, plastic bottles for solar disinfection, or flocculants, to make drinking water safe. • Invest in public piped water supply systems that provide good quality and potable water particularly for the poor.	• Swachh Bharat Abhiyan–gramin (to eliminate open defecation and improve solid waste management in rural areas) [80] • National Water Supply and Sanitation Program in India [81] • National Rural Drinking Water Program (to provide safe and adequate water for drinking, cooking and other domestic needs to every rural person on a sustainable basis) [82]

Table 6. *Cont.*

Determinant of TB	Sample Community Level Policies/Interventions to Address the Determinant	Example: Public Programs in India that Can Be Galvanized to Address the Determinant at the Local Level
Affordable and clean energy (SDG-7)	• Provision of improved cookstoves, cleaner and drier fuels which aim to burn fuel more efficiently and therefore produce fewer harmful combustion products; • Improving natural and artificial ventilation, to avoid air pollution inside the household; • Changing cooking behavior and patterns, to reduce the amount of time an individual spends in proximity to a fire or stove; • Altering regulatory or financial policies, with intent to improve access to advanced cookstoves or fuels and provide incentives for changes within communities or towards community development. • Strict industrial regulations to control environmental air pollution	• Pradhan Mantri Ujjwala Yojana (to distribute LPG gas connections to women of below poverty line families) [71]
Decent work and economic growth (SDG-8)	• Encouragement for locally available micro, small, and medium sized enterprises through access to necessary financial services • Generate employment opportunities • Trainings/mentorship support for entrepreneurship • Low interest loan schemes	• Entrepreneurship Development Program (EDP) [72] • Mahatma Gandhi National Rural Employment Guarantee Act (MGNREGA) 2005 (India) [70]
Reduced inequalities (SDG-10)	• Local programs aimed at financial inclusion and social security or linkages to existing social security schemes	• Jan Dhan-Aadhaar-Mobile programs (For Financial Inclusion to ensure access to financial services, namely banking savings and deposit accounts, remittance, credit, insurance and pension in an affordable manner and to prevent leakage of government subsidies) [73]
Sustainable cities and communities (SDG-11)	• Local implementation of slum development schemes/ slums upgrading programs which includes improvements in housing conditions, water supply and sanitation, roads, ground stabilization, storm water drainage etc.,	• Jawaharlal Nehru National Urban Renewal Mission (a city-modernization scheme) [74]
Climate action (SDG-13)	• Efforts to reduce carbon emissions through increased generation of power using renewable sources of energy • Increase additional forest and tree cover	• National Solar mission [83] • National Afforestation Program [84]

7. Conclusions

Achieving End TB targets with the current pace of progress is highly challenging and un-realistic if the thrust is mainly medical and focusing only on 'diagnosis and treatment' of TB and LTBI, without addressing the underlying determinants of TB. While the strengthening of national TB programs under the framework of universal health coverage is quintessential for accelerating the progress towards End TB targets, the SDG framework provides an excellent opportunity for acting on several determinants and risk factors of TB. All stakeholders, be it government ministries, non-governmental organizations or private sectors involved in achieving SDGs and the End TB targets must recognize that most of their goals are strongly interlinked. Failure to acknowledge this fact may result in ineffective and inappropriate actions and a delay in the achievement of both SDG goals and End TB targets.

Author Contributions: S.S. and P.T. wrote the first draft which was critically reviewed by A.M.V.K., Y.L., R.A.D., M.K., R.Z. and A.D.H. All authors contributed to subsequent drafts and agreed upon and approved the final version. All authors have read and agreed to the published version of the manuscript.

Funding: The research received no external funding.

Conflicts of Interest: The authors declare no conflict of interest.

Disclaimer: The views expressed in this document are those of the authors and may not necessarily reflect those of their affiliated institutions.

References

1. World Health Organisation. The Top 10 Causes of Death. Available online: https://www.who.int/en/news-room/fact-sheets/detail/the-top-10-causes-of-death (accessed on 19 March 2020).
2. Pai, M.; Behr, M.A.; Dowdy, D.; Dheda, K.; Divangahi, M.; Boehme, C.C.; Ginsberg, A.; Swaminathan, S.; Spigelman, M.; Getahun, H.; et al. Tuberculosis. *Nat. Rev. Dis. Prim.* **2016**, *2*, 16076. [CrossRef] [PubMed]
3. Behr, M.A.; Edelstein, P.H.; Ramakrishnan, L. Revisiting the timetable of tuberculosis. *BMJ* **2018**, *362*, k2738. [CrossRef] [PubMed]
4. Behr, M.A.; Edelstein, P.H.; Ramakrishnan, L. Is *Mycobacterium tuberculosis* infection life long? *BMJ* **2019**, *367*, l5770. [CrossRef] [PubMed]
5. Houben, R.M.G.J.; Dodd, P.J. The global burden of latent tuberculosis infection: A re-estimation using mathematical modelling. *PLoS Med.* **2016**, *13*, e1002152. [CrossRef]
6. Global Tuberculosis Report 2019. Available online: https://www.who.int/tb/publications/global_report/en/ (accessed on 19 March 2020).
7. Trauer, J.M.; Dodd, P.J.; Gomes, M.G.M.; Gomez, G.B.; Houben, R.M.G.J.; McBryde, E.S.; Melsew, Y.A.; Menzies, N.A.; Arinaminpathy, N.; Shrestha, S. The Importance of Heterogeneity to the Epidemiology of Tuberculosis. *Clin. Infect. Dis.* **2019**, *69*, 159–166. [CrossRef]
8. The End TB Strategy. Available online: https://www.who.int/tb/post2015_strategy/en/ (accessed on 13 June 2020).
9. Cadena, A.M.; Fortune, S.M.; Flynn, J.L. Heterogeneity in tuberculosis. *Nat. Rev. Immunol.* **2017**, *17*, 691–702. [CrossRef] [PubMed]
10. Lönnroth, K.; Jaramillo, E.; Williams, B.G.; Dye, C.; Raviglione, M. Drivers of tuberculosis epidemics: The role of risk factors and social determinants. *Soc. Sci. Med.* **2009**, *68*, 2240–2246. [CrossRef] [PubMed]
11. Pedrazzoli, D.; Boccia, D.; Dodd, P.J.; Lönnroth, K.; Dowdy, D.W.; Siroka, A.; Kimerling, M.E.; White, R.G.; Houben, R.M.G.J. Modelling the social and structural determinants of tuberculosis: Opportunities and challenges. *Int. J. Tuberc. Lung Dis.* **2017**, *21*, 957–964. [CrossRef]
12. Avert. HIV and AIDS in the Asia and the Pacific Regional Overview. Available online: https://www.avert.org/professionals/hiv-around-world/asia-pacific/overview (accessed on 11 May 2020).
13. Epidemiology of Alcohol Use in the WHO South-East Asia Region. Available online: https://apps.who.int/iris/handle/10665/259831 (accessed on 13 June 2020).
14. Hunger Notes. Asia Hunger facts. Available online: https://www.worldhunger.org/asia-hunger-facts-2018/ (accessed on 11 May 2020).

15. World Health Statistics Data Visualisation Dashboard: Prevalance of Tobacco Smoking. Available online: https://apps.who.int/gho/data/node.sdg.3-a-viz?lang=en (accessed on 13 June 2020).
16. Global Report on Diabetes. Available online: https://apps.who.int/iris/bitstream/handle/10665/204874/WHO_NMH_NVI_16.3_eng.pdf;jsessionid=244DC978B0833D7128BD508B32D46E9A?sequence=1 (accessed on 16 June 2020).
17. Lin, H.-H.; Ezzati, M.; Murray, M. Tobacco Smoke, Indoor air pollution and tuberculosis: A systematic review and meta-analysis. *PLoS Med.* **2007**, *4*, e20. [CrossRef]
18. Mansournia, M.A.; Altman, D.G. Population attributable fraction. *BMJ* **2018**, *360*, k757. [CrossRef]
19. Murray, J.F. A Century of Tuberculosis. *Am. J. Respir. Crit. Care Med.* **2004**, *169*, 1181–1186. [CrossRef] [PubMed]
20. Murray, J.F. Tuberculosis and World War I. *Am. J. Respir. Crit. Care Med.* **2015**, *192*, 411–414. [CrossRef] [PubMed]
21. Janssens, J.P.; Rieder, H.L. An ecological analysis of incidence of tuberculosis and per capita gross domestic product. *Eur. Respir. J.* **2008**, *32*, 1415–1416. [CrossRef] [PubMed]
22. Carter, D.J.; Glaziou, P.; Lönnroth, K.; Siroka, A.; Floyd, K.; Weil, D.; Raviglione, M.; Houben, R.M.G.J.; Boccia, D. The impact of social protection and poverty elimination on global tuberculosis incidence: A statistical modelling analysis of Sustainable Development Goal 1. *Lancet Glob. Heal.* **2018**, *6*, e514–e522. [CrossRef]
23. Adler, N.E.; Newman, K. Socioeconomic disparities in health: Pathways and policies. *Health Aff.* **2002**, *21*, 60–76. [CrossRef] [PubMed]
24. Tobacco and Poverty: A Vicious Circle. Available online: https://apps.who.int/iris/handle/10665/68704 (accessed on 16 June 2020).
25. Karriker-Jaffe, K.J.; Roberts, S.C.M.; Bond, J. Income inequality, alcohol use, and alcohol-related problems. *Am. J. Public Health* **2013**, *103*, 649–656. [CrossRef]
26. Killewo, J. Poverty, TB, and HIV infection: A vicious cycle. *J. Health. Popul. Nutr.* **2002**, *20*, 281–284.
27. Gaskin, D.J.; Thorpe, R.J.; McGinty, E.E.; Bower, K.; Rohde, C.; Young, J.H.; LaVeist, T.A.; Dubay, L.; Dubay, L. Disparities in diabetes: The nexus of race, poverty, and place. *Am. J. Public Health* **2014**, *104*, 2147–2155. [CrossRef]
28. Agardh, E.; Allebeck, P.; Hallqvist, J.; Moradi, T.; Sidorchuk, A. Type 2 diabetes incidence and socio-economic position: A systematic review and meta-analysis. *Int. J. Epidemiol.* **2011**, *40*, 804–818. [CrossRef]
29. *Multisectoral Accountability Framework to Accelerate Progress to End Tuberculosis by 2030*; World Health Organisation: Geneva, Switzerland, 3 August 2019.
30. MacNeil, A.; Glaziou, P.; Sismanidis, C.; Date, A.; Maloney, S.; Floyd, K. Global Epidemiology of Tuberculosis and Progress Toward Meeting Global Targets—Worldwide, 2018. *MMWR. Morb. Mortal. Wkly. Rep.* **2020**, *69*, 281–285. [CrossRef]
31. Nicola, M.; Alsafi, Z.; Sohrabi, C.; Kerwan, A.; Al-Jabir, A.; Iosifidis, C.; Agha, M.; Agha, R. The Socio-Economic Implications of the Coronavirus and COVID-19 Pandemic: A Review. *Int. J. Surg.* **2020**, *78*, 185–193. [CrossRef]
32. United Nations. Sustainable Development Goals. Available online: https://sustainabledevelopment.un.org/?menu=1300 (accessed on 13 June 2020).
33. United Nations. Global indicator framework for the Sustainable Development Goals and targets of the 2030 Agenda for Sustainable Development. Available online: https://unstats.un.org/sdgs/indicators/GlobalIndicatorFrameworkafter2020review_Eng.pdf (accessed on 26 March 2020).
34. Golden, S.D.; Earp, J.A.L. Social ecological approaches to individuals and their contexts: Twenty years of health education & behavior health promotion interventions. *Health Educ. Behav.* **2012**, *39*, 364–372. [PubMed]
35. Oxlade, O.; Murray, M. Tuberculosis and poverty: Why are the poor at greater risk in India? *PLoS One* **2012**, *7*, e47533. [CrossRef]
36. Stop TB Partnership. What is the Relation between TB and Poverty? Available online: http://www.stoptb.org/assets/documents/events/world_tb_day/2002/1Therelationship.pdf (accessed on 27 March 2020).

37. Gupta, K.B.; Gupta, R.; Atreja, A.; Verma, M.; Vishvkarma, S. Tuberculosis and nutrition. *Lung India* **2009**, *26*, 9–16. [CrossRef]
38. Bhargava, A.; Benedetti, A.; Oxlade, O.; Pai, M.; Menzies, D. Undernutrition and the incidence of tuberculosis in India: National and subnational estimates of the population-attributable fraction related to undernutrition. *Natl. Med. J. India* **2014**, *27*, 128–133.
39. Padmapriyadarsini, C.; Shobana, M.; Lakshmi, M.; Beena, T.; Swaminathan, S. Undernutrition & tuberculosis in India: Situation analysis & the way forward. *Indian J. Med. Res.* **2016**, *144*, 11–20. [PubMed]
40. Reid, M.J.A.; Arinaminpathy, N.; Bloom, A.; Bloom, B.R.; Boehme, C.; Chaisson, R.; Chin, D.P.; Churchyard, G.; Cox, H.; Ditiu, L.; et al. Building a tuberculosis-free world: The lancet commission on tuberculosis. *Lancet* **2019**, *393*, 1331–1384. [CrossRef]
41. Hahn, R.A.; Truman, B.I. Education improves public health and promotes health equity. *Int. J. Health Serv.* **2015**, *45*, 657–678. [CrossRef] [PubMed]
42. Cutler, D.M.; Lleras-Muney, A. Understanding differences in health behaviors by education. *J. Health Econ.* **2010**, *29*, 1–28. [CrossRef]
43. Samal, J. Health Seeking Behaviour among Tuberculosis Patients in India: A Systematic Review. *J. Clin. Diagn. Res.* **2016**, *10*, LE01. [CrossRef]
44. Nhamoyebonde, S.; Leslie, A. Biological differences between the sexes and susceptibility to tuberculosis. *J. Infect. Dis.* **2014**, *209*, S100–S106. [CrossRef] [PubMed]
45. Holmes, C.B.; Hausler, H.; Nunn, P. A review of sex differences in the epidemiology of tuberculosis. *Int. J. Tuberc. Lung Dis.* **1998**, *2*, 96–104. [PubMed]
46. Connolly, M.; Nunn, P. Women and tuberculosis. *World Health Stat. Q.* **1996**, *49*, 115–119. [PubMed]
47. Krishnan, L.; Akande, T.; Shankar, A.V.; McIntire, K.N.; Gounder, C.R.; Gupta, A.; Yang, W.-T. Gender-Related Barriers and Delays in Accessing Tuberculosis Diagnostic and Treatment Services: A Systematic Review of Qualitative Studies. *Tuberc. Res. Treat.* **2014**, *2014*, 1–14. [CrossRef] [PubMed]
48. Horton, K.C.; MacPherson, P.; Houben, R.M.G.J.; White, R.G.; Corbett, E.L. Sex Differences in Tuberculosis Burden and Notifications in Low- and Middle-Income Countries: A Systematic Review and Meta-analysis. *PLoS Med.* **2016**. [CrossRef]
49. Yang, W.-T.; Gounder, C.R.; Akande, T.; De Neve, J.-W.; McIntire, K.N.; Chandrasekhar, A.; de Lima Pereira, A.; Gummadi, N.; Samanta, S.; Gupta, A. Barriers and Delays in Tuberculosis Diagnosis and Treatment Services: Does Gender Matter? *Tuberc. Res. Treat.* **2014**, *2014*, 1–15. [CrossRef]
50. Quansah, R.; Semple, S.; Ochieng, C.A.; Juvekar, S.; Armah, F.A.; Luginaah, I.; Emina, J. Effectiveness of interventions to reduce household air pollution and/or improve health in homes using solid fuel in low-and-middle income countries: A systematic review and meta-analysis. *Environ. Int.* **2017**, *103*, 73–90. [CrossRef]
51. Jafta, N.; Jeena, P.M.; Barregard, L.; Naidoo, R.N. Childhood tuberculosis and exposure to indoor air pollution: A systematic review and meta-analysis. *Int. J. Tuberc. Lung Dis.* **2015**, *19*, 596–602. [CrossRef]
52. Sumpter, C.; Chandramohan, D. Systematic review and meta-analysis of the associations between indoor air pollution and tuberculosis. *Trop. Med. Int. Heal.* **2013**, *18*, 101–108. [CrossRef]
53. Lin, H.-H.; Suk, C.-W.; Lo, H.-L.; Huang, R.-Y.; Enarson, D.A.; Chiang, C.-Y. Indoor air pollution from solid fuel and tuberculosis: A systematic review and meta-analysis. *Int. J. Tuberc. Lung Dis.* **2014**, *18*, 613–621. [CrossRef]
54. Lai, T.C.; Chiang, C.-Y.; Wu, C.-F.; Yang, S.-L.; Liu, D.-P.; Chan, C.-C.; Lin, H.-H. Ambient air pollution and risk of tuberculosis: A cohort study. *Occup. Environ. Med.* **2016**, *73*, 56–61. [CrossRef]
55. Lin, Y.J.; Lin, H.-C.; Yang, Y.-F.; Chen, C.-Y.; Ling, M.-P.; Chen, S.-C.; Chen, W.-Y.; You, S.-H.; Lu, T.-H.; Liao, C.-M. Association between ambient air pollution and elevated risk of tuberculosis development. *Infect. Drug Resist.* **2019**, *12*, 3835–3847. [CrossRef] [PubMed]
56. Donald, P.R.; Marais, B.J.; Barry, C.E. Age and the epidemiology and pathogenesis of tuberculosis. *Lancet* **2010**, *375*, 1852–1854. [CrossRef]
57. Maher, D.; Boldrini, F.; Alli, B.O.; Gabriel, P.; Kisting, S.; Norval, P.-Y. Guidelines for workplace TB control activities the contribution of workplace TB control activities to TB control in the community. Available online: http://www.stoptb.org/assets/documents/resources/publications/technical/workplace_guidelines.pdf (accessed on 27 March 2020).

58. Heymann, J.; Rho, H.J.; Schmitt, J.; Earle, A. Ensuring a healthy and productive workforce: Comparing the generosity of paid sick day and sick leave policies in 22 countries. *Int. J. Health Serv.* **2010**, *40*, 1–22. [CrossRef]
59. Asfaw, A.; Pana-Cryan, R.; Rosa, R. Paid sick leave and nonfatal occupational injuries. *Am. J. Public Health* **2012**, *102*, e59–e64. [CrossRef] [PubMed]
60. Kim, D. Paid Sick Leave and Risks of All-Cause and Cause-Specific Mortality among Adult Workers in the USA. *Int. J. Environ. Res. Public Health* **2017**, *14*, 1247. [CrossRef]
61. Duarte, R.; Lönnroth, K.; Carvalho, C.; Lima, F.; Carvalho, A.C.C.; Muñoz-Torrico, M.; Centis, R. Tuberculosis, social determinants and co-morbidities (including HIV). *Pulmonology* **2018**, *24*, 115–119. [CrossRef]
62. Reyes, R.; Ahn, R.; Thurber, K.; Burke, T.F. Urbanization and Infectious Diseases: General Principles, Historical Perspectives, and Contemporary Challenges. In *Challenges in Infectious Diseases*; Springer New York: New York, NY, USA, 2013; pp. 123–146.
63. Prasad, A.; Ross, A.; Rosenberg, P.; Dye, C. A world of cities and the end of TB. *Trans. R. Soc. Trop. Med. Hyg.* **2016**, *110*, 151–152. [CrossRef]
64. Nardell, E.; Lederer, P.; Mishra, H.; Nathavitharana, R.; Theron, G. Cool but dangerous: How climate change is increasing the risk of airborne infections. *Indoor Air* **2020**, *30*, 195–197. [CrossRef]
65. Harries, A.D. Chronic kidney disease, tuberculosis and climate change. *Int. J. Tuberc. Lung Dis.* **2020**, *24*, 132–133. [CrossRef]
66. WHO Global TB Report App launched. Available online: https://www.who.int/tb/features_archive/TB-report-App/en/ (accessed on 11 June 2020).
67. Tuberculosis Country Profiles. Available online: https://www.who.int/tb/country/data/profiles/en/ (accessed on 11 June 2020).
68. Measuring progress towards the Sustainable Development Goals - SDG Tracker. Available online: https://sdg-tracker.org/ (accessed on 27 March 2020).
69. Pradhan Mantri Kaushal Vikas Yojana (PMKVY). Available online: https://pmkvyofficial.org/ (accessed on 11 May 2020).
70. Mahatma Gandhi National Rural Employment Gurantee Act. Available online: https://nrega.nic.in/netnrega/home.aspx (accessed on 11 May 2020).
71. Pradhan Mantri Ujjwala Yojana. Available online: https://pmuy.gov.in/ (accessed on 11 May 2020).
72. Ministry of Skill Development and Entrepreneurship. Available online: https://www.msde.gov.in/proposed-scheme.html (accessed on 11 May 2020).
73. Pradhan Mantri Jan-Dhan Yojana, Ministry of Finance, Government of India. Available online: https://www.pmjdy.gov.in/scheme (accessed on 11 May 2020).
74. Jawaharlal Nehru National Urban Renewal Mission: Ministry of Housing and Urban Affairs, Goverment of India. Available online: http://mohua.gov.in/cms/jawaharlal-nehru-national-urban-renewal-mission.php (accessed on 11 May 2020).
75. School Education, Government of India, Ministry of Human Resource Development. Available online: https://mhrd.gov.in/mid-day-meal (accessed on 11 May 2020).
76. Samagra Shiksha. Available online: http://samagra.mhrd.gov.in/ (accessed on 11 May 2020).
77. Beti Bachao Beti Padhao, Ministry of Women & Child Development, Government of India. Available online: https://wcd.nic.in/bbbp-schemes (accessed on 11 May 2020).
78. Governement of India. Ministry of Women and Child Development, Revised Guidelines and Application Format on Support to Training and Employment Programmer for Women (STEP) 2009. Available online: https://wcd.nic.in/sites/default/files/RevisedschemeofSTEP_0.pdf (accessed on 11 May 2020).
79. Ministry of Women & Child Development. Available online: http://mahilaehaat-rmk.gov.in/en/ (accessed on 11 May 2020).
80. Swachh Bharat Mission-Gramin. Available online: https://sbm.gov.in/sbmReport/home.aspx (accessed on 11 May 2020).
81. National Water and Sanitation Programmer, Ministry of Environment & Forest, Govt. of India. Available online: http://www.sulabhenvis.nic.in/Database/NationalWater_176.aspx (accessed on 11 May 2020).
82. National Rural Drinking Water Programmer. Available online: https://www.prsindia.org/content/national-rural-drinking-water-programme-22 (accessed on 16 May 2020).

83. Jawaharlal Nehru National Solar Mission. Available online: https://vikaspedia.in/energy/policy-support/renewable-energy-1/solar-energy/jawaharlal-nehru-national-solar-mission (accessed on 1 June 2020).
84. National Afforestation Programmer, Ministry of Environment and Forests, Government of India. Available online: http://www.naeb.nic.in/documents/NAP_intro.htm (accessed on 31 May 2020).

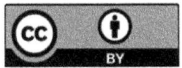

© 2020 by the authors. Licensee MDPI, Basel, Switzerland. This article is an open access article distributed under the terms and conditions of the Creative Commons Attribution (CC BY) license (http://creativecommons.org/licenses/by/4.0/).

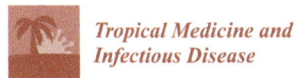

Article

Yield of Systematic Longitudinal Screening of Household Contacts of Pre-Extensively Drug Resistant (PreXDR) and Extensively Drug Resistant (XDR) Tuberculosis Patients in Mumbai, India

Roma Haresh Paryani [1], Vivek Gupta [2], Pramila Singh [1], Madhur Verma [3], Sabira Sheikh [1], Reeta Yadav [1], Homa Mansoor [1], Stobdan Kalon [1], Sriram Selvaraju [4], Mrinalini Das [1,*], Chinmay Laxmeshwar [1], Gabriella Ferlazzo [5] and Petros Isaakidis [5]

1. Médecins Sans Frontières (MSF)/Doctors Without Borders, Mumbai 400088, India; MSFOCB-Mumbai-OS@brussels.msf.org (R.H.P.); msfocb-mumbai2@brussels.msf.org (P.S.); sabirayasin74@gmail.com (S.S.); reeta242015@gmail.com (R.Y.); msfocb-delhi-med@brussels.msf.org (H.M.); Msfocb-India-ops-strategic-advisor@brussels.msf.org (S.K.); chinmay2210@gmail.com (C.L.)
2. Dr RP Centre for Ophthalmic Sciences, All India Institute of Medical Sciences (AIIMS), New Delhi 110029, India; vgupta@aiims.edu
3. Department of Community & Family Medicine, All India Institute of Medical Sciences (AIIMS), Bathinda, Punjab 151001, India; drmadhurverma@gmail.com
4. National Institute for Research in Tuberculosis, Chennai 600031, India; sriram.s@nirt.res.in
5. Southern Africa Medical Unit (SAMU), Médecins Sans Frontières, Cape Town 7925, South Africa; Gabriella.FERLAZZO@joburg.msf.org (G.F.); Petros.Isaakidis@joburg.msf.org (P.I.)
* Correspondence: msfocb-delhi-epi@brussels.msf.org; Tel.: +91-8010261984

Received: 13 April 2020; Accepted: 6 May 2020; Published: 15 May 2020

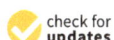

Abstract: While risk of tuberculosis (TB) is high among household contacts (HHCs) of pre-extensively drug resistant (pre-XDR) TB and XDR-TB, data on yield of systematic longitudinal screening are lacking. We aim to describe the yield of systematic longitudinal TB contact tracing among HHCs of patients with pre-XDR-TB and XDR-TB. At the Médecins Sans Frontières (MSF) clinic, Mumbai, India a cohort comprising 518 HHCs of 109 pre-XDR and XDR index cases was enrolled between January 2016 and June 2018. Regular HHC follow-ups were done till one year post treatment of index cases. Of 518 HHCs, 23 had TB (21 on TB treatment and two newly diagnosed) at the time of first visit. Of the rest, 19% HHCs had no follow-ups. Fourteen (3.5%) TB cases were identified among 400 HHCs; incidence rate: 2072/100,000 person-years (95% CI: 1227–3499). The overall yield of household contact tracing was 3% (16/518). Of 14 who were diagnosed with TB during follow-up, six had drug susceptible TB (DSTB); six had pre-XDR-TB and one had XDR-TB. Five of fourteen cases had resistance patterns concordant with their index case. In view of the high incidence of TB among HHCs of pre-XDR and XDR-TB cases, follow-up of HHCs for at least the duration of index cases' treatment should be considered.

Keywords: incidence; tuberculosis; household contacts tracing; operational research

1. Introduction

Tuberculosis (TB) is a long-standing global health issue, disproportionately affecting low- and middle-income countries. India is a country with a high TB burden [1]. Drug-resistant tuberculosis (DR-TB) is also reported to have an increasing trend in the country. Pre-extensively drug resistant (pre-XDR-TB) is the presence of resistance to rifampicin and isoniazid along with resistance to either one of the fluoroquinolones (ofloxacin, levofloxacin or moxifloxacin) or second-line injectables (amikacin, capreomycin or kanamycin). In case the TB bacilli have resistance to both fluoroquinolones and second-line injectables, along with rifampicin and isoniazid, they are classified as extensively drug resistant (XDR). In India, the estimated incidence of TB in India was 2,700,000 [2]. According to the drug-resistance survey report, in India, 28% patients with TB have resistance to any anti-tubercular drugs and 6.2% have multi-drug resistant TB (MDR-TB); among MDR-TB, 21.8% have pre-XDR-TB and 1.3% have XDR-TB [3]. Some studies from the country have reported a higher prevalence of XDR-TB [4–6].

Systematic reviews suggest that contact investigations are an important intervention in early identification of active TB cases, thus minimizing TB transmission [7–9]. Fox and colleagues have reported active TB among 3.4% contacts of patients with multi-drug-resistant or extensively drug-resistant TB in low-and middle-income settings [9]. In Pakistan, baseline contact investigation of index cases with MDR-TB identified MDR-TB in 17.4% and DS-TB in 4.2% of close contacts [10]. A longitudinal study of household contact (HHC) among newly diagnosed TB patients in Vietnam reported incident TB in 0.5% of contacts at 12-month follow-up and in 0.3% of contacts at 24-month follow-up, while the prevalence at baseline evaluation was 0.5% [11]. In China, four-year follow-up of close contacts of bacteria-positive TB index cases reported a high risk of incident TB (333/100,000 person years) [12].

To add to the evidence around longitudinal contact tracing in addition to baseline contact tracing among drug-resistant TB cases, the present study aimed to determine the yield of systematic longitudinal household contact tracing among patients with pre-XDR-TB and XDR-TB initiated on treatment at Médecins Sans Frontières (MSF) Clinic, Mumbai. Secondary objectives included (1) assessment of profile of index cases and HHCs developing TB and (2) drug resistance patterns in TB diagnosed among HHCs.

2. Materials and Methods

2.1. Study Design

This was a retrospective cohort study using routine program data.

2.2. Setting

The study was done in Mumbai, which is among the most populous cities of India. Located in the western part of India in the state of Maharashtra, it has a population density of 21,000/km^2. The city has high rates of migration and is home to a large slum population. Nearly 9895 patients with DR-TB were diagnosed in Maharashtra, and TB case notifications were nearly 209,642 in 2018 [2,12–14].

The MSF clinic in Mumbai started offering treatment to patients with pre-XDR and XDR-TB in 2012 [15]. Eligibility criteria for enrollment are based on resistance profile and treatment history. Individualized treatment is offered on an outpatient basis based on drug sensitivity patterns. Bedaquiline and Delamanid are provided to patients who require it. All patients receive free-of-charge services, which include counseling, diagnosis, treatment, social enabler (dry ration), travel support and medical reimbursement for co-morbid conditions as per need. Treatment is provided using an ambulatory model of care described elsewhere [15].

2.2.1. Household Contact (HHC) Investigation

Since 2013, the clinic has been performing investigation of HHCs of registered pre-XDR and XDR-TB patients. HHCs of DR-TB cases were members of the household regularly living with the patients registered for care in the MSF Clinic (hereafter mentioned as index cases). At enrollment of a new index case, a trained nurse visited their homes, a list of HHCs was prepared, and details were noted in a standardized form. All the HHCs are examined for signs and symptoms of TB and following risk factors: pregnancy, diabetes mellitus, HIV, alcohol use disorder, drug use, previous history of TB, age >55 years and immune-suppressive therapy.

Adults and adolescents HHCs over 15 years of age with risk factors and all pediatric (aged <15 years) HHCs are invited to visit the MSF clinic for a detailed screening. Those who visit the clinic are assessed using chest X-ray (CXR) and physical examination. If they have symptoms suggestive of TB or CXR abnormality, sputum examination or gastric lavage for smear, cartridge based nucleic acid amplification test (CBNAAT)/GeneXpert and culture and drug susceptibility testing (C-DST) are done. HHCs that are diagnosed with active TB are initiated on treatment as per their TB drug susceptibility pattern.

2.2.2. Follow-Up of HHCs

HHCs aged >15 years and not having any high-risk factors are followed every six months in their homes. Those who have risk factors are followed at three-monthly intervals during the first year and then six-monthly at home. All children <15 years are followed up three-monthly at the MSF clinic. At each follow-up visit, screening of contacts is done for presumptive TB, defined as any of the symptoms/signs: (a) cough >2 weeks, (b) fever >2 weeks, (c) significant weight loss, (d) any abnormality in chest radiograph. Contacts with presumptive TB undergo detailed clinical, radiological and laboratory evaluations. All laboratory investigations are done in an accredited private laboratory contracted by MSF. In case a contact does not report for follow-up at the clinic, they are contacted telephonically and encouraged to visit the clinic. The follow-up continues for the entire duration of TB treatment of the index case and one year after treatment completion. In case of the death of the index case, follow-up of HHCs is still offered for the next one year.

2.3. Study Population and Participants

For the present analysis, we included all HHCs of index cases with pre-XDR and XDR-TB registered for treatment between January 2016 and June 2018. Index cases who did not have bacteriologically confirmed pre-XDR or XDR-TB, and those who refused treatment, were excluded.

2.4. Data Variables and Sources, Data Analysis

Data for each index case and HHCs is maintained in EMR software (Bahmni™), individual care record files, and in Microsoft Excel™ spreadsheets. Data for this study were extracted from these sources. Data was analyzed using EpiData Analysis (version 2.2.2.178 EpiData Association, Odense, Denmark) and Stata version 15.1 (StataCorp, College Station, TX). The numbers of HHCs assessed at each stage of follow-up were noted to understand the contact investigation cascade. Survival analysis was used to analyze the incidence rate of incident TB overall, by age, sex and time from follow-up initiation. HHCs were censored in case of loss to follow-up (LTFU), completion of follow-up period, or on 30th April 2019, whichever was earlier. The date of last visit was taken as the date of censoring. Per-capita floor area of the house was calculated, and overcrowding was considered present in case the per-capita area was less than 50 square feet. In all analyses, $p < 0.05$ was considered statistically significant. Wherever appropriate, 95% confidence intervals (95% CI) are being reported.

2.5. Operational Definitions

(1) Index case: patients with pre-XDR or XDR-TB registered for treatment in MSF Clinic.
(2) Incident TB: any HHC diagnosed as suffering from TB after one month of baseline contact evaluation.
(3) Lost to follow-up (LTFU): HHCs not evaluated during a scheduled visit and any time during the subsequent 6-month period.

2.6. Ethics

Ethics approval was obtained from the Ethics Advisory Group of the International Union Against Tuberculosis and Lung Disease, Paris, France (EAG No. 96/18). The study met the criteria for a posteriori analysis of routinely collected clinical data and did not require MSF Ethics Review Board full review. It was conducted with permission of the medical director, Operational Centre Brussels, MSF.

3. Results

The clinic enrolled 129 cases of pre-XDR and XDR-TB during the study period; among these, we excluded 11, and nine refused treatment later, yielding 109 eligible index cases (Figure 1). There were 58 (53.4%) cases with XDR-TB; nine (8.3%) were under 15 years of age, and 60 (55.1%) were female (Table 1). Two index cases were from the same household. These 109 index cases had 530 HHCs, among whom 518 (97.7%) underwent baseline evaluation. Among 518 HHCs, 23 were reported to have TB at the time of first visit (21 already on treatment, two newly diagnosed). The rest of the 495 HHCs were eligible for follow-up.

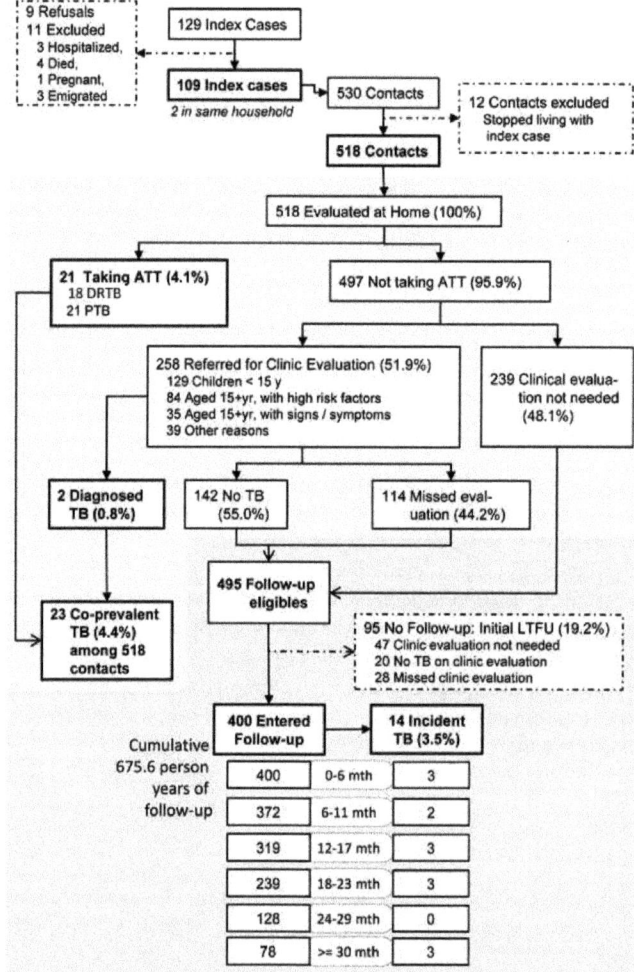

Figure 1. Assembly and follow-up of cohort comprising household contacts of index cases with pre-XDR and XDR tuberculosis registered at the MSF Clinic, Mumbai between Jan 2016 and June 2018. TB = Tuberculosis; DSTB = Drug-sensitive TB; DRTB = Drug-resistant TB; pre-XDR = Pre-extensively drug-resistant; XDR-TB = Extensively drug-resistant tuberculosis; PTB = Pulmonary TB; ATT = Anti-tubercular therapy; LTFU = Loss to follow-up. While 114 HHCs missed clinic evaluation, we considered them as eligible for follow-up since they were at risk of incident tuberculosis.

Table 1. Characteristics of index cases with pre-XDR and XDR tuberculosis registered at the MSF clinic, Mumbai, India, January 2016 to June 2018 (N = 109). IQR: Inter-quartile range.

Characteristics	Groups	Index Cases N	%
Type of TB drug resistance	Pre-Extensive Drug Resistance (pre-XDR)	51	(47)
	Extensive Drug Resistance (XDR)	58	(53)
Age at enrolment (years)	0–14	9	(8)
	15 and above	100	(92)
Sex	Male	49	(45)
	Female	60	(55)
Previous TB treatment	No treatment	6	(6)
	History of previous TB treatment	103	(94)
Site of TB in Index Case	Extra-pulmonary (EPTB)	15	(14)
	Pulmonary (PTB)	94	(86)
X-ray results (n = 105)	Abnormal	92	(88)
	Normal	13	(12)
Sputum conversion (in months) [Median (IQR)] (n = 76)		2 (1–4)	
Human Immunodeficiency Virus (HIV) co-infection		5	(5)
Diabetes mellitus co-morbidity		10	(9)
Overcrowding (area per person <= 50 square feet)		60	(55)
Staying in rented house		33	(30)

3.1. TB Diagnosis among HHCs

Among the 495 HHCs eligible for follow-up, 95 (19.2%) did not complete the first follow-up visit (at 3 or 6 months, based on age and risk profile) and were early LTFUs. For the remaining 400 HHCs, median follow-up of 18.9 months [Interquartile range (IQR): 14.0–25.8] and cumulative follow-up of 675 person-years (py) was achieved. During the follow-up period, we identified 14 (3.5%) new TB cases (Figure 1). The median time to TB diagnosis among HHCs was 18 months (IQR: 6–21 months). The incidence rate of TB was 2072 (95% CI: 1227–3499) per 100,000 person-years over the entire follow-up period.

Of 14 HHCs with incident TB, ten (69.2%) incident cases were 15 years of age or older, and eight (61.5%) were female (Table 2). Six cases occurred in siblings of index cases and three in children. None of the index cases or HHC characteristics were associated with incident disease in univariate analysis.

Table 2. Profile and factors associated with incident TB among household contacts of patients with pre-XDR and XDR tuberculosis in Mumbai, India, January 2016–June 2018 (N = 400). * Column percentage; ** Row percentage; N(%) were compared using the Chi-square test or Fisher's exact test; †: Median (Inter-quartile range), compared using the Wilcoxon rank-sum test; Pre-XDR TB: Pre-extensive drug resistant TB; XDR-TB: Extensive drug-resistant TB; PTB = Pulmonary TB; EPTB = Extra-Pulmonary Tuberculosis; AFB = Acid fast bacilli.

Variable		Household Contacts (n = 400) *	Household Contacts with Incident TB(n = 14) **	p-Value
Index Case Characteristics		n (%)	n (%)	
Type of index case	Pre-XDR	166 (41)	7 (4)	0.51
	XDR	234 (59)	7 (3)	
Age (Median(IQR), years) †		24 (19–30)	24 (18–26)	0.43
Sex	Male	156 (39)	6 (4)	0.76
	Female	244 (61)	8 (3)	
Prior TB treatment	No treatment	23 (6)	2 (9)	0.43
	TB treatment	377 (94)	12 (3)	
HIV in index case	No	384 (96)	12 (3)	0.10
	Yes	16 (4)	2 (13)	
AFB result	Negative	183 (47)	8 (4)	0.59
	Scanty	42 (11)	2 (5)	
	Positive	162 (42)	4 (3)	
Site of TB	EPTB	51 (13)	0 (0)	
	PTB	349 (87)	14 (4)	
X-ray results	Abnormal	344 (88)	14 (4)	
	Normal	47 (12)	0 (0)	
Number of household contacts †		6 (4–8)	6 (5–10)	0.21
Household Contact Characteristics				
Age group	0–14 years	94 (23)	4 (4)	0.75
	15 years or more	306 (97)	10 (3)	
Sex	Male	205 (51)	6 (3)	0.52
	Female	195 (49)	8 (4)	
Relationship with index case	Child	68 (17)	3 (4)	0.37
	Parent	120 (30)	4 (3)	
	Sibling	97 (24)	6 (6)	
	Spouse	22 (6)	0 (0)	
	Other	93 (23)	1 (1)	
Area < 50 sq/feet/capita	No	226 (59)	10 (4)	0.32
	Yes	159 (41)	4 (3)	
Past history of TB	No	358 (90)	11 (3)	0.17
	Yes	42 (10)	3 (7)	

3.2. Overall Yield of TB in HHCs

The overall yield among 518 identified HHCs was 3%. A total of 16 patients were diagnosed with TB, which included two patients who were diagnosed with TB on first day of screening and 14 who were identified during follow-up.

3.3. Drug Resistance Patterns

Among 37 identified TB cases among HHCs, the TB resistance profiles of 23 patients who were reported with TB on the first day of screening (including 21 on TB treatment and two newly diagnosed) were as follows: three had DSTB, seven had MDR TB, five had pre-XDR, and eight had XDR-TB, respectively. Among 14 cases found during follow-up, six had DSTB, six had pre-XDR-TB, one had XDR-TB and a TB resistance profile could not be ascertained for one. Five (38.5%) of these 14 cases were concordant with index case (4 Pre-XDR-TB and 1 XDR-TB).

4. Discussion

The overall yield was 3% during the longitudinal household contact tracing for TB in patients diagnosed with pre-XDR and XDR-TB receiving care in MSF Clinic in Mumbai, India. Through systematic longitudinal evaluation of HHCs, the study reported a higher incidence of TB disease than the previously reported study from India [2].

The yield of TB reported in our study is comparable to findings of systematic reviews [6–8]. However, the systematic review by Morrison et al. [6] also included studies where TB index cases were bacteriologically and clinically confirmed patients, while our study included only biologically confirmed cases as index cases.

Our findings are in line with those of Leung and colleagues, who conducted follow-up of HHCs of MDR-TB and reported that presence of XDR-TB significantly increased the odds of identifying a prevalent TB as well as hazard of incident case by almost five times after 18 months [16]. However, they did not have pre-XDR cases in their cohort. The observed incidence is higher than in China, Gambia and Peru [17–19], though it matches results from a Vietnam active case finding setting [10].

We observed discordant TB resistance profiled in HHCs compared to index cases; about half of the cases were DSTB, while the index cases were either pre-XDR-TB or XDR-TB [7]. These may hint towards community transmission of DSTB in a high burden setting.

4.1. Limitations

The study could not differentiate whether incident cases were the result of infection within the household or community acquired, since we did not conduct molecular fingerprinting. Molecular fingerprinting would have assisted in identifying the transmission pathways. We also did not evaluate for latent TB infection. Given the high incidence of TB in the program setting, it is likely that transmission would have occurred outside households, as is suggested by recent literature [20]. We observed that 44.2% of HHCs did not come for baseline clinic evaluation and 19.2% of HHCs had initial LTFU. A commonly reported reason for this was family members moving away from the index case. The index cases were largely slum-dwellers staying in rented accommodation, and the family members moving away could be a result of stigma, or a reaction to protect the health of family members. Finally, our findings may be representative of an urban Mumbai slum context and not directly applicable in other settings.

4.2. Implications for Policy and Practice

Under the Programmatic Management of Drug Resistant TB (PMDT) in India, it has been recommended that all close contacts of DR-TB cases be identified through contact tracing and evaluated for active TB disease. If the contact is found to be suffering from TB disease, irrespective of bacteriological confirmation, s/he should be identified as "presumptive DR-TB" and therapy be initiated based on their history of previous anti-TB treatment or TB resistance profile of index TB case. Simultaneously, two sputum samples should be transported for culture and DST. No definitive guidelines have been provided for prophylaxis among contacts with no active disease, and follow-up duration and close monitoring is suggested as the recommended action [21]. Our results suggest the need for follow-up of HHCs of patients with DR-TB after baseline evaluation for at least the duration of the index case's treatment.

4.3. Implications for Future Research

Cost-effectiveness analyses have shown the utility of active case finding among HHCs [22]. Since we are proposing a longitudinal follow-up of contacts of pre-XDR and XDR cases, future research should focus on establishing the cost effectiveness of this approach. An assessment of latent TB infection among contacts of pre-XDR and XDR cases is also recommended in view of the high incidence rates of active infection. Molecular fingerprinting and linkage analyses will clarify the epidemiology of transmission. Longer follow-up of more pre-XDR and XDR contacts is also recommended in research settings along with analyses of implementation effects of various screening preventive and infection control strategies so that their relationship with incident disease may be better understood.

5. Conclusions

We observed a high incidence of TB among HHCs of pre-XDR and XDR-TB in Mumbai, India. Systematic longitudinal TB screening of HHCs in cases with pre-XDR and XDR-TB must be strengthened, as they are at a high risk of incident disease.

Author Contributions: Conceptualization and protocol writing: R.H.P., V.G., M.V., C.L., M.D., P.S., S.S. (Sriram Selvaraju), P.I., G.F.; Data collection: R.H.P., S.S. (Sabira Sheikh), R.Y.; Data analysis: R.H.P., V.G.; Drafting the paper: R.H.P., V.G., C.L., M.D., M.V., S.S. (Sabira Sheikh); Critical review and approval for submission: R.H.P., V.G., P.S., M.V., S.S. (Sriram Selvaraju), H.M., S.K., M.D., C.L., G.F., P.I. All authors have read and agreed to the published version of the manuscript.

Funding: This research received no external funding.

Acknowledgments: This research was conducted through the Structured Operational Research and Training Initiative (SORT IT), a global partnership led by the Special Programme for Research and Training in Tropical Diseases at the World Health Organization (WHO/TDR). The model is based on a course developed jointly by the International Union Against Tuberculosis and Lung Disease (The Union) and Medécins sans Frontières (MSF/Doctors Without Borders). The specific SORT IT programme which resulted in this publication was jointly developed and implemented by: The Union South-East Asia Office, New Delhi, India; the Centre for Operational Research, The Union, Paris, France; Department of Preventive and Social Medicine, Jawaharlal Institute of Postgraduate Medical Education and Research, Puducherry, India; Department of Community Medicine and School of Public Health, Postgraduate Institute of Medical Education and Research, Chandigarh, India; Department of Community Medicine, All India Institute of Medical Sciences, Nagpur, India; Rajendra Prasad Centre for Ophthalmic Sciences, All India Institute of Medical Sciences, New Delhi, India; Department of Community Medicine, Pondicherry Institute of Medical Science, Puducherry, India; Department of Community Medicine, Kalpana Chawla Medical College, Karnal, India; National Centre of Excellence and Advance Research on Anemia Control, All India Institute of Medical Sciences, New Delhi, India; Department of Community Medicine, Sri Manakula Vinayagar Medical College and Hospital, Puducherry, India; Department of Community Medicine, Velammal Medical College Hospital and Research Institute, Madurai, India; Department of Community Medicine, Yenepoya Medical College, Mangalore, India; Karuna Trust, Bangalore, India and National Institute for Research in Tuberculosis, Chennai, India. The authors are grateful for the contribution of healthcare workers from the MSF clinic as well as the patients living with TB and their families.

Conflicts of Interest: The authors declare no conflict of interest.

References

1. World Health Organization. *Global Tuberculosis Report 2017*; World Health Organization: Geneva, Switzerland, 2017.
2. Central TB Division. *India TB Report 2019: Revised National Tuberculosis Control Program—Annual Status Report*; Directorate General of Health Services, Ministry of Health and Family Welfare, Government of India: New Delhi, India, 2019.
3. *Report of the First National Anti-Tuberculosis Drug Resistance Survey India 2014–2016 [Internet]*; Ministry of Health and Family Welfare, Government of India: New Delhi, India, 2018.
4. Shah, I.; Shah, F. Changing prevalence and resistance patterns in children with drug-resistant tuberculosis in Mumbai. *Paediatr. Int. Child Health* **2017**, *37*, 135–138. [CrossRef] [PubMed]
5. Goyal, V.; Kadam, V.; Narang, P.; Singh, V. Prevalence of drug-resistant pulmonary tuberculosis in India: Systematic review and meta-analysis. *BMC Public Health* **2017**, *17*, 817. [CrossRef] [PubMed]
6. Dalal, A.; Pawaskar, A.; Das, M.; Desai, R.; Prabhudesai, P.; Chhajed, P.; Rajan, S.; Reddy, D.; Babu, S.; Jayalakshmi, T.K.; et al. Resistance patterns among multidrug-resistant tuberculosis patients in greater metropolitan Mumbai: Trends over time. *PLoS ONE* **2015**, *10*, e0116798. [CrossRef] [PubMed]
7. Morrison, J.; Pai, M.; Hopewell, P.C. Review Tuberculosis and latent tuberculosis infection in close contacts of people with pulmonary tuberculosis in low-income and middle-income countries: A systematic review and meta-analysis. *Lancet Infect. Dis.* **2008**, *8*, 359–368. [CrossRef]

8. Shah, N.S.; Yuen, C.M.; Heo, M.; Tolman, A.W.; Becerra, M.C. Yield of Contact Investigations in Households of Patients with Drug-Resistant Tuberculosis: Systematic Review and Meta-Analysis. *Clin. Infect. Dis.* **2014**, *58*, 381–391. [CrossRef] [PubMed]
9. Fox, G.J.; Barry, S.E.; Britton, W.J.; Marks, G.B. Contact investigation for tuberculosis: A systematic review and meta-analysis. *Eur. Respir. J.* **2013**, *41*, 140–156. [CrossRef]
10. Javaid, A.; Khan, M.A.M.A.; Khan, M.A.M.A.; Mehreen, S.; Basit, A.; Khan, R.A.; Ihtesham, M.; Ullah, I.; Khan, A.; Ullah, U. Screening outcomes of household contacts of multidrug-resistant tuberculosis patients in Peshawar, Pakistan. *Asian Pac. J. Trop. Med.* **2016**, *9*, 909–912. [CrossRef] [PubMed]
11. Fox, G.J.; Nhung, N.V.; Sy, D.N.; Hoa, N.L.P.; Anh, L.T.N.; Anh, N.T.; Hoa, N.B.; Dung, N.H.; Buu, T.N.; Loi, N.T.; et al. Household-Contact Investigation for Detection of Tuberculosis in Vietnam. *N. Engl. J. Med.* **2018**, *378*, 221–229. [CrossRef] [PubMed]
12. Jiang, Q.; Lu, L.; Wu, J.; Yang, C.; Prakash, R.; Zuo, T.; Liu, Q.; Hong, J.; Guo, X.; Gao, Q. Assessment of tuberculosis contact investigation in Shanghai, China: An 8-year cohort study. *Tuberculosis* **2018**, *108*, 10–15. [CrossRef] [PubMed]
13. Mumbai (Greater Mumbai) City Population Census 2011 | Maharashtra [Internet]. Available online: https://www.census2011.co.in/census/city/365-mumbai.html (accessed on 28 November 2019).
14. Registrar General and Census Commissioner-India. *Census of India 2011: Provisional Population Totals-India Data Sheet*; Office of the Registrar General and Census Commissioner: Delhi, India, 2011.
15. Isaakidis, P.; Cox, H.S.; Varghese, B.; Montaldo, C.; Silva, E.D.; Mansoor, H.; Ladomirska, J.; Sotgiu, G.; Migliori, G.B.; Pontali, E.; et al. Ambulatory multi-drug resistant tuberculosis treatment outcomes in a cohort of HIV-infected patients in a slum setting in Mumbai, India. *PLoS ONE* **2011**, *6*, e28066. [CrossRef] [PubMed]
16. Leung, E.C.C.; Leung, C.C.; Kam, K.M.; Yew, W.W.; Chang, K.C.; Leung, W.M.; Tam, C.M. Transmission of multidrug-resistant and extensively drug-resistant tuberculosis in a metropolitan city. *Eur. Respir. J.* **2013**, *41*, 901–908. [CrossRef] [PubMed]
17. Guo, J.; Yang, M.; Wu, Z.; Shen, X.; Wang, Y.; Zhao, G. High incidence and low case detection rate among contacts of tuberculosis cases in Shanghai, China. *BMC Infect. Dis.* **2019**, *19*, 320. [CrossRef] [PubMed]
18. Hill, P.C.; Jackson-Sillah, D.J.; Fox, A.; Brookes, R.H.; de Jong, B.C.; Lugos, M.D.; Adetifa, I.M.; Donkor, S.A.; Aiken, A.M.; Howie, S.R.; et al. Incidence of Tuberculosis and the Predictive Value of ELISPOT and Mantoux Tests in Gambian Case Contacts. *PLoS ONE* **2008**, *3*, e1379. [CrossRef] [PubMed]
19. Saunders, M.J.; Tovar, M.A.; Collier, D.; Baldwin, M.R.; Montoya, R.; Valencia, T.R.; Gilman, R.H.; Evans, C.A. Active and passive case-finding in tuberculosis-affected households in Peru: A 10-year prospective cohort study. *Lancet Infect. Dis.* **2019**, *19*, 519–528. [CrossRef]
20. Cudahy, P.G.T.; Andrews, J.R.; Bilinski, A.; Dowdy, D.W.; Mathema, B.; Menzies, N.A.; Salomon, J.A.; Shrestha, S.; Cohen, T. Spatially targeted screening to reduce tuberculosis transmission in high-incidence settings. *Lancet Infect. Dis.* **2019**, *19*, e89–e95. [CrossRef]
21. *National Strategic Plan for Tuberculosis Elimination 2017–2025 [Internet]*; Central TB Division, Directorate General of Health Services, Ministry of Health and Family Welfare, Government of India: New Delhi, India, 2017. Available online: https://tbcindia.gov.in/WriteReadData/NSP%20Draft%2020.02.2017%201.pdf (accessed on 25 June 2019).
22. Lung, T.; Marks, G.B.; Nhung, N.V.; Anh, N.T.; Hoa, N.L.P.; Anh, L.T.N.; Hoa, N.B.; Britton, W.J.; Bestrashniy, J.; Jan, S.; et al. Household contact investigation for the detection of tuberculosis in Vietnam: Economic evaluation of a cluster-randomised trial. *Lancet Glob. Health* **2019**, *7*, E376–E384. [CrossRef]

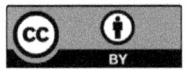

© 2020 by the authors. Licensee MDPI, Basel, Switzerland. This article is an open access article distributed under the terms and conditions of the Creative Commons Attribution (CC BY) license (http://creativecommons.org/licenses/by/4.0/).

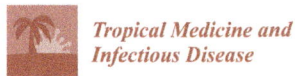

Perspective

The Growing Importance of Tuberculosis Preventive Therapy and How Research and Innovation Can Enhance Its Implementation on the Ground

Anthony D. Harries [1,2,*], Ajay M.V. Kumar [1,3,4], Srinath Satyanarayana [1,3], Pruthu Thekkur [1,3], Yan Lin [1,5], Riitta A. Dlodlo [1], Mohammed Khogali [6] and Rony Zachariah [6]

1. International Union Against Tuberculosis and Lung Disease, 68 Boulevard Saint Michel, 75006 Paris, France; akumar@theunion.org (A.M.V.K.); SSrinath@theunion.org (S.S.); Pruthu.TK@theunion.org (P.T.); ylin@theunion.org (Y.L.); rdlodlo@theunion.org (R.A.D.)
2. London School of Hygiene and Tropical Medicine, Keppel Street, London WC1E 7HT, UK
3. International Union Against Tuberculosis and Lung Disease, South-East Asia Office, C-6 Qutub Institutional Area, New Delhi 110016, India
4. Yenepoya Medical College, Yenepoya (Deemed to be University), University Road, Deralakatte, Mangalore 575018, India
5. International Union Against Tuberculosis and Lung Disease, No.1 Xindong Road, Beijing 100600, China
6. Special Programme for Research and Training in Tropical Disease (TDR), World Health Organization, Avenue Appia 20, 1211 Geneva 27, Switzerland; khogalim@who.int (M.K.); zachariahr@who.int (R.Z.)
* Correspondence: adharries@theunion.org; Tel.: +44-(0)-1962-714-297

Received: 24 March 2020; Accepted: 14 April 2020; Published: 16 April 2020

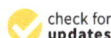

Abstract: Ending the tuberculosis (TB) epidemic by 2030 requires two key actions: rapid diagnosis and effective treatment of active TB and identification and treatment of latent TB infection to prevent progression to active disease. We introduce this perspective by documenting the growing importance of TB preventive therapy on the international agenda coupled with global data showing poor implementation of preventive activities in programmatic settings. We follow this with two principal objectives. The first is to examine implementation challenges around diagnosis and treatment of active TB. Within this, we include recent evidence about the continued morbidity and heightened mortality that persists after TB treatment is successfully completed, thus elevating the importance of TB preventive therapy. The second objective is to outline how current TB preventive therapy activities have been shaped and are managed and propose how these can be improved through research and innovation. This includes expanding and giving higher priority to certain high-risk groups including those with fibrotic lung lesions on chest X-ray, showcasing the need to develop and deploy new biomarkers to more accurately predict risk of disease and making shorter treatment regimens, especially with rifapentine-isoniazid, more user-friendly and widely available. Ending the TB epidemic requires not only cure of the disease but preventing it before it even begins.

Keywords: tuberculosis; post-tuberculosis morbidity and mortality; TB preventive therapy; latent TB infection; Asia Pacific; rifapentine-isoniazid

1. Introduction

The international community has pledged to end the tuberculosis (TB) epidemic by 2030. The principal targets for meeting this ambitious goal include a 90% reduction in TB deaths and an 80% reduction in TB incidence rate by 2030 compared with 2015 [1]. On the ground, there are two key actions that need to take place if this goal is to be realised. First, every individual who develops active TB (estimated at about 10 million each year) must be rapidly diagnosed and effectively treated.

This benefits not only the individual with active TB but also reduces the risk of further transmission of *Mycobacterium tuberculosis* (*MTB*) within the family, other close contacts and the community. Second, of the 1.7 billion individuals estimated globally to have latent infection with *MTB* [2], those at risk of progressing to active disease need to be identified and treated.

While the prevention of TB makes intuitive public health sense, this has been a relatively neglected component of TB control efforts. However, recent years have begun to see a change. The World Health Organization's (WHO) End TB Strategy, adopted by the World Health Assembly in 2014, emphasises preventive therapy in persons at high risk of TB under its first pillar of patient-centred care and prevention [1]. During the United Nations High Level Meeting (UNHLM) on the fight against TB in September 2018, world leaders committed to provide preventive therapy to at least 30 million people between 2018 and 2022. This included 4 million children aged <5 years, 20 million other household contacts of people diagnosed and treated for TB and 6 million people living with HIV (PLHIV) [3]. This translates to giving TB preventive therapy globally to 800,000 children aged <5 years per year, 4 million other household contacts per year and 1.2 million PLHIV per year.

In 2018, the proportions of children aged <5 years (who were household contacts of people with bacteriologically confirmed TB) and PLHIV (newly enrolled in care) who were placed on TB preventive therapy were well below target at the global level and in the WHO South-East Asia and Western Pacific Regions (which comprise the Asia Pacific) (Table 1) [4]. Moreover, at the global level, only 79,000 other household contacts aged ≥ 5 years (2% of annual target) were given TB preventive therapy. Clearly a lot more work is needed to raise performance and get anywhere near the UNHLM preventive therapy targets.

Table 1. Tuberculosis (TB) preventive treatment in 2018.

WHO Region	PLHIV Newly Enrolled in Care Who Were Given TB Preventive Treatment [a] %	Household Children (aged < 5) Contacts of Bacteriologically Confirmed TB Patients Who Were Given TB Preventive Treatment %
Africa	60	29
Americas	9	55
Eastern Mediterranean	13	23
European	69	>100
South-East Asia	15	26
Western Pacific	39	12
Global	49	27

WHO = World Health Organization; PLHIV = persons living with HIV. [a] Calculations exclude countries with missing numerators or denominators. Asia Pacific comprises South-East Asia and the Western Pacific Adapted from [4].

There are two main objectives of this perspective. The first is to outline the implementation challenges around the diagnosis and treatment of TB. This includes highlighting the morbidity, disability and heightened mortality that persist after successful treatment completion, in order for readers to appreciate the importance of TB preventive therapy in the overall context of ending the TB epidemic and ensuring healthy lives. The second objective is to describe how current TB preventive therapy activities have been shaped and are managed. We further assess some of the implementation challenges of TB preventive therapy and propose how activities can be improved and enhanced through research and innovation.

2. Challenges with the Diagnosis and Treatment of Active TB

2.1. Screening and Diagnosis

There are two components to the efficient screening and diagnosis of TB. People with symptoms suggestive of TB must recognise that they are ill and seek appropriate and timely care, and the health services must respond quickly and efficiently. Unfortunately, symptomatic individuals can take on average 3 months or more to present to the health sector and the health system can take a further 1 month to diagnose TB [5,6]. Substantial delays from first symptoms to diagnosis are therefore often the norm. Large numbers of symptomatic individuals presenting to health facilities may also fail to be properly screened or investigated with appropriate microbiological or radiological tests and the diagnosis of TB therefore can be completely missed [7,8]. These problems of so-called "passive case finding" have plagued TB Control Programmes for decades and programmes frequently overlook the proportion of patients who suffer the fate of pre-diagnostic loss to follow-up.

Active case finding, in which people who do not actively seek health care are proactively sought out and screened for TB regardless of symptoms, has the potential to overcome some of these limitations. Some pilot projects have shown that community-wide screening for active TB can reduce TB prevalence and TB infection, as shown recently in Vietnam [9]. However, an evaluation of several active case finding projects in 16 countries showed no impact on national case notifications mainly because the projects had not been taken to scale due to costs and shortages of human resources [10]. Other active case finding projects have found low detection yields of TB [11], and at the programmatic level are beset with challenges of inadequate health care worker training, staff shortages, community distrust, illiteracy and lack of community awareness about TB [12]. Much more investment and commitment are needed to take active case finding to scale and overcome multiple implementation challenges.

Finally, an overview of 21 national TB prevalence surveys in Asia between 1990 and 2012 showed that between 40% and 79% of patients with bacteriologically-positive TB did not report TB symptoms and were only detected due to chest X-ray screening of all survey participants [13]. Such high proportions of asymptomatic TB patients present important challenges for standard screening and diagnostic algorithms and bring up the question about whether community use of chest X-ray should be expanded in the routine setting.

2.2. Initiating Anti-TB Treatment

While it should be straightforward to initiate treatment in all those diagnosed with TB, in practice this is far more difficult than it seems. In low- and middle-income countries in Africa, Asia and the Western Pacific between 4% and 38% of patients with laboratory-detected sputum smear-positive or culture-positive TB fail to start treatment [14]. This pre-treatment loss to follow-up appears to be no better with the use of rapid molecular technology [15–17]. For those who do get treated, turn-around times between confirmed diagnosis and treatment initiation can also be lengthy, compromising individual care and increasing the risk of *MTB* transmission within families and communities.

2.3. Providing Effective Treatment

TB is a treatable and curable infectious disease. The duration of treatment for drug-susceptible TB is 6 months, with previous attempts to shorten this to 4 months with third generation fluoroquinolones and/or rifapentine being unsuccessful [18–20]. In contrast, there has been relatively good progress in shortening the treatment of multidrug-resistant TB (MDR-TB, resistant to isoniazid and rifampicin) from 24 months down to 9 or 12 months [21,22]. Trials are in progress to assess whether even shorter regimens of 6 months are effective and whether fully oral treatment with new or repurposed second-line drugs can be used [23].

Despite this progress with TB treatment regimens, treatment outcomes at the global level and in the Asia Pacific remain substandard (Table 2). Globally, treatment success for new and previously treated TB patients is below 85%, and this is even lower for patients with HIV-positive TB and drug-resistant TB [4]. In patients with new/previously treated TB, death, lost to follow-up and not evaluated are the main adverse outcomes while treatment failure, death and lost to follow-up are the main adverse outcomes in drug-resistant TB. Many of these outcomes are potentially correctable. For example, late detection of HIV-associated TB and delays in starting antiretroviral therapy (ART) and TB treatment account for most HIV-related TB deaths [4]. On the other hand, enabling local staff to make sense of their TB data has been associated with reduced losses to follow-up and better treatment success [24].

Table 2. Treatment success in cohorts of TB patients registered for treatment.

2A: Global		
Cohorts of TB patients registered for treatment	Registered in cohort N	Treatment Success %
New/previously treated patients registered in 2017 [a]	6,381,295	84
HIV-positive TB patients registered in 2017	445,922	75
MDR/RR-TB patients started on SLD in 2016	126,089	56
XDR-TB patients started on SLD in 2016	9258	39
2B: South-East Asia Region		
Cohorts of TB patients registered for treatment	Registered in cohort N	Treatment Success %
New/previously treated patients registered in 2017 [a]	2,746,023	82
HIV-positive TB patients registered in 2017	56,872	71
MDR/RR-TB patients started on SLD in 2016	40,725	52
XDR-TB patients started on SLD in 2016	2567	31
2C: Western Pacific Region		
Cohorts of TB patients registered for treatment	Registered in cohort N	Treatment Success %
New/previously treated patients registered in 2017 [a]	1,360,505	91
HIV-positive TB patients registered in 2017	12,170	79
MDR/RR-TB patients started on SLD in 2016	14,602	59
XDR-TB patients started on SLD in 2016	88	58

[a] Some countries reported on new patients only. Treatment success = cured and treatment completed; MDR-TB = multidrug-resistant TB; RR-TB = rifampicin-resistant TB; XDR-TB = extensively drug-resistant TB; SLD = second-line anti-TB drugs. Asia Pacific comprises South-East Asia and the Western Pacific. Adapted from [4].

2.4. Taking Account of Post-Tuberculosis Morbidity and Mortality

It is widely thought that the outcome of "treatment success" signifies the end of TB treatment and a return to active healthy life. Indeed, most TB disease burden analyses, using disability-adjusted life-years (DALYs), assume that survivors return to full health post-tuberculosis [25]. However, a growing body of evidence shows that this is far from the truth.

Many individuals who successfully complete TB treatment continue to be burdened with chronic pulmonary impairment from obstructive and restrictive lung disease that either pre-existed or developed as a result of TB [26]. Other morbidities such as permanent hearing loss from second-line injectable anti-TB drugs [27] and mental health disorders [28,29] compound these serious and long-term post-TB sequelae. Not surprisingly, a recent systematic review and meta-analysis found that all-cause mortality was nearly three times higher in individuals post-tuberculosis compared with age- and sex-matched controls [30]. A study using conservative estimates of post-TB morbidity and mortality from chronic obstructive lung disease only showed that the burden of TB in India would increase by 6.1 million DALYs—a 54% increase on the current estimates that assume a full return to health at the end of anti-TB treatment [31]. This burden would increase further if other post-TB conditions such as restrictive lung disease or permanent hearing loss from second-line injectable drugs were included.

2.5. Implications of Shortfalls in Diagnosis, Treatment and Cure of TB

In summary, in 2018 only 7 million out of an estimated 10 million new patients with TB were notified. The rest, referred to as the 'missing millions', were not notified due to underdiagnosis and/or underreporting of detected patients [4]. Of the 7 million notified TB patients, about 5.8 million successfully completed treatment [4]. Good quality targeted operational research should lead to better programmatic implementation of proven interventions around diagnosis and treatment and therefore potentially better outcomes [32]. Prevention of TB, when coupled with improved diagnosis and treatment, would have an added and synergistic effect on TB control. With a considerable number of patients also continuing to experience significant morbidity and heightened mortality in the post-TB period, preventive therapy becomes even more important due to the greater DALYs averted per TB episode prevented.

3. Current Status and Management of TB Preventive Therapy

The WHO provides guidelines for the programmatic management of latent TB infection (LTBI) and TB preventive therapy. The most recent published version was released in 2018 [33] and forthcoming changes are due to appear later in 2020 [34]. The key components of TB preventive therapy are briefly outlined below.

3.1. Identifying High Risk Groups for TB Preventive Therapy

Among those with LTBI, there are various populations at much higher risk of TB compared with the general population [35]. These high-risk groups need to be identified for testing and/or treatment of LTBI providing active TB is ruled out. The two highest priority groups are PLHIV and household contacts of people with bacteriologically confirmed TB. For PLHIV, while it is not necessary to systematically screen for LTBI because benefits of preventive therapy for all affected people outweigh any risks, those with positive results to tuberculin skin testing (TST) and interferon-gamma release assays (IGRAs) appear to benefit more from TB preventive therapy [33]. Similarly, for household contacts there is a higher ratio of benefit to risk from preventive therapy, and systematic screening for LTBI is only recommended for HIV-negative adults, adolescents and children ≥ 5 years if they are from a low TB incidence country (<100 patients per 100,000 population).

Other HIV-negative high-risk groups are listed in Table 3. For those in Categories 1–3, systematic testing for LTBI is recommended if TB preventive therapy is to be considered, and those who test positive can be offered treatment. For those in Category 4, systematic testing for LTBI is generally not recommended but treatment can be offered on an individual basis if testing is done and is positive.

3.2. Diagnosis of LTBI

There are no perfect ways of testing for and diagnosing LTBI. The two main tests in use (TST and IGRAs) both measure the immunological response to *MTB* antigens. TST is inexpensive but logistically challenging for patients and health care staff, different results may be obtained depending on which purified protein derivative products are used [37] and there continue to be widespread shortages of quality-assured tuberculin in many low- and middle-income countries [38]. IGRAs are more specific than TST and only one clinic visit is required by the patient for a venous blood sample. However, they are costly, there is a need for specialised laboratory equipment and there are issues related to reproducibility of results. The validity of both tests has recently been questioned with evidence to suggest that only 10% of persons showing immunoreactivity to TST or IGRAs harbour viable *MTB* organisms capable of causing disease [39].

Table 3. Testing and treatment of latent TB infection (LTBI) in HIV-negative high-risk groups who are not household contacts.

Category	Type of Person	Need for Systematic Testing of LTBI	Treatment of LTBI
1	• Patient with Silicosis	Yes	Recommended if LTBI test is positive
2	• Patients in end-stage renal failure receiving dialysis • Patients who have received haematological or organ transplants • Patients receiving tumour necrosis factor α-neutralising agents for Crohn's disease or rheumatoid arthritis • Patients using oral or inhaled corticosteroids	Yes for all Category 2	Recommended if LTBI test is positive for all Category 2
3	In countries with low TB incidence: • Prisoners • Homeless people • People who inject drugs • Health care workers • Immigrants from countries with a high TB burden	Yes for all Category 3	Recommended if LTBI test is positive for all Category 3
4	• Persons with diabetes mellitus • Persons with harmful alcohol consumption • People who smoke tobacco • People who are underweight	No for all Category 4	Recommended if LTBI testing is done on individual basis and LTBI test is found to be positive

TB = tuberculosis; LTBI = latent tuberculosis infection. Adapted from [33] and [36].

3.3. TB Preventive Therapy Regimens

For many years, isoniazid preventive therapy (IPT), self-administered for 6–12 months, has been the mainstay of treatment for HIV-infected and HIV-uninfected persons and household contacts. Six-months IPT is highly effective in high-risk groups, it adds to the already considerable TB preventive benefits of ART in PLHIV and is recommended by WHO [33,36]. Amongst PLHIV in high TB exposure areas, for example in Southern Africa, continuous IPT for 36 months or longer provides more durable and robust TB prevention and is therefore recommended [40]. The likely reason for this effect is that isoniazid treats existing LTBI and also prevents new *MTB* infections from taking hold and progressing to active TB.

Alternative and shorter regimens for treating LTBI are available (Table 4). In clinical trials these regimens appear to have the same efficacy as IPT but have higher rates of completion, improved medication adherence and better safety profiles [33,36]. The 3- or 4-month regimen of daily rifampicin and isoniazid (RH) is popular with children because of child friendly, dispersible, paediatric fixed-dose formulations. The 3- or 4-month regimen of rifampicin alone is not so widely used because of possible irrational use of the drug (which has broad spectrum antibacterial activity) to treat many non-TB conditions which could lead to widespread rifampicin resistance [36].

Table 4. Alternative shorter TB preventive therapy regimens.

Treatment Regimen	Duration	Dosage Frequency	Common Abbreviation
Rifampicin	3–4 months	Daily	3R/4R
Rifampicin and isoniazid	3–4 months	Daily	3RH/4RH
Rifapentine and isoniazid	3 months	Weekly	3HP
Rifapentine and isoniazid	4 weeks	Daily	1HP

The 3-month weekly rifapentine and isoniazid (3HP) regimen, 12 doses in total, is rapidly becoming an attractive option and there is growing experience with this regimen from clinical studies and implementation in the field [33,41]. A recently completed trial of 4-weeks daily rifapentine and isoniazid (1HP) in adults or adolescents with HIV showed non-inferiority in preventing TB compared with 9-months IPT along with significantly better rates of treatment completion [42]. One of the important concerns with rifapentine has been the high cost. However, in 2018 the Global Drug Facility and the pharmaceutical company that manufactures the drug, Sanofi, reached agreement to offer rifapentine for USD$45 per patient course of 3HP, and activist pressure is being applied to produce generic patient-friendly formulations for as little as USD$10–USD$15 per patient course [43].

For household contacts of patients with MDR-TB or XDR-TB (MDR-TB with added resistance to fluoroquinolones and second-line injectable agents) there are only observational studies to guide recommendations [44–47]. The drugs used for MDR-TB contacts have been mainly fluoroquinolones with or without other drugs such as ethambutol or ethionamide. As about a quarter of the TB patients amongst households exposed to MDR-TB do not have drug-resistant disease [48], TB preventive treatment has to be individualised with selected drugs based on the drug susceptibility profile of the index patient. For XDR-TB contacts there is no specific guidance and currently close observation and follow-up is advised.

4. Research and Innovation to Improve Delivery and Uptake of TB Preventive Therapy

4.1. Expanding the High-Risk Groups for TB Preventive Therapy

Currently, it is recommended that PLHIV newly enrolled in care and treatment receive TB preventive therapy [33]. The number of PLHIV newly enrolled in care is considered as the denominator against which WHO reports the percentage receiving TB preventive therapy on an annual basis [4]. However, giving TB preventive therapy to all PLHIV, regardless of how long they have been on ART, is likely to be beneficial and should be considered. Laboratory studies have shown that long-term recovery of TB specific immune function is incomplete on ART [49], and clinical studies have shown that length of time on therapy and ART-induced immune recovery still do not fully protect against TB in high exposure environments [50].

Household contacts of patients with bacteriologically confirmed TB are high priority for TB preventive therapy. There are several research questions that need to be answered around the index patient and the household contacts if practice is to be refined and improved (Table 5). The accepted definition of a household contact is "a person who shared the same enclosed living space for one or more nights or for frequent or extended periods during the day with the index case during the 3 months before commencement of the current treatment episode" [51]. This is an arbitrary definition and in the local context it needs to be tested out through operational research and adapted as necessary. For example, the amount of exposure to *MTB* will vary from sharing the same bed to living somewhere else within the same household complex and the actual duration of infectiousness may be longer or shorter than 3 months.

Currently, only patients with end-stage renal disease are recommended for systematic testing and treatment of LTBI [33]. However, a well-conducted cohort study in Taiwan showed that there is an increased risk of TB in early stage chronic kidney disease (CKD) [52], and it has been suggested that TB prevention efforts be targeted to all people with this condition. This recommendation needs further study because over the last 25 years, the global all-age prevalence of CKD has increased by 29% with nearly 700 million patients of all-stage CKD recorded in 2017 [53].

In high TB burden countries, prisoners, people who inject drugs and health care workers are all at high risk of TB [35,36]. Operational research should be conducted to assess whether in the local context and based on available resources it is cost-effective to systematically enrol such groups into TB preventive therapy services. Finding ways to ensure adherence in prisoners and people who inject drugs will need operational research.

Currently, WHO does not recommend that persons with diabetes mellitus (DM) be systematically screened and treated for LTBI [33]. This needs to be revisited especially in the Asia Pacific Region. Persons with DM have an overall three-times higher risk of TB compared with the general population [54,55]. A systematic review and meta-analysis estimated that the pooled prevalence of DM amongst TB patients between 1986 and 2017 was 15%, with the Asia Pacific in particular having a higher prevalence than other regions at 19% [56]. In Indonesia, TB incidence was found to be significantly higher in persons with DM with established LTBI (1.7 per 100 person-years) compared with those without LTBI (0.5 per 100 person-years) [57]. In Singapore, TB incidence was higher in persons with DM compared with the normal population and increased significantly in persons with DM as their body mass index dropped, being highest in those who were underweight [58]. Further research is needed to determine whether persons with DM should be targeted for systematic LTBI testing and TB preventive therapy. In this regard, a prospective randomised controlled study is approved and about to start in Tanzania and Uganda using 3HP (European Union–EDTCP2 programme and grant number RIA2018CO-2514-PROTID). If TB preventive therapy is found to be cost-effective and taken up by WHO, this would considerably expand the pool of people potentially eligible for LTBI testing and TB preventive therapy. In 2019, there were 463 million people living with DM (54% living in the Asia Pacific) and this is predicted to rise to 578 million by 2030 [59].

Finally, there is no mention in the WHO Guidelines about what to do with HIV-uninfected persons who have fibrotic lung lesions on chest X-ray. A trial in Eastern Europe 40 years ago found a high incidence of TB in this population group with TB preventive therapy using isoniazid significantly reducing this risk [60]. In this regard, the expanded use of chest X-ray should be further considered, and those with fibrotic lung lesions consistent with inactive TB could be assessed for LTBI testing and treatment.

Table 5. Research and innovation on the index patient and their household contacts.

Research questions around index patient	• Determine the value in assessing the index patient's drug susceptibility status in order to better prescribe the type of TB preventive therapy for household contacts
	• Assess whether the index patient should be systematically screened for risk factors such as HIV, DM, smoking, alcohol abuse and malnutrition
Research questions around household contacts	• Clarify the definition of household contact for the local context
	• Assess whether household contact screening should be done just for index patients with bacteriologically confirmed pulmonary TB or include index patients with clinically diagnosed pulmonary TB
	• Explore whether household contacts should be systematically screened for risk factors such as HIV, DM, smoking, alcohol abuse and malnutrition irrespective of whether the index patient has these risk factors
	• In countries that still insist on LTBI testing of household contacts, assess in the local context whether this is needed or whether all household contacts can just be treated

TB = tuberculosis; HIV = human immunodeficiency virus; DM = diabetes mellitus.

4.2. Better Tests for LTBI

There is an urgent need to develop and then deploy sensitive and specific biomarkers that can distinguish infection with *MTB* from immunological memory of past infection (which is essentially what TST and IGRAs do) and predict who will progress from LTBI to active TB disease. It is becoming clear that LTBI is not a single entity but rather represents a broad spectrum of asymptomatic TB infection where different degrees of inflammation, bacterial replication and host immunity determine whether disease will develop or not [61]. An exciting development in this direction has been the use of a whole blood transcriptomic messenger RNA expression signature that in Cape Town, South Africa, predicted progression from LTBI to active TB disease with 66% sensitivity and 81% specificity [62]. Further research is continuing in this direction [61], but currently there are no clinically useful or affordable tests for use in the field.

4.3. Ruling Out Active TB

A "sine qua non" of TB preventive therapy is ensuring that no person with active TB starts mono- or dual therapy. Screening adults and children for suggestive symptoms of TB is recommended by WHO [33]. Those with symptoms are investigated and if TB is not diagnosed, TB preventive therapy can be considered. While molecular technology, particularly with Xpert MTB/RIF or Xpert MTB/RIF Ultra, has greatly improved the sensitivity and specificity of diagnosing active TB [63], diagnostic certainty cannot be guaranteed. For this reason, symptomatic persons are often not offered TB preventive therapy.

The big question is whether absence of symptoms in adults or children is sufficient for ruling out active disease or whether chest X-ray should also be performed. The systematic use of chest X-ray is not considered mandatory in resource-limited settings [33], although WHO states that the combination of absence of any chest X-ray abnormality plus the absence of TB-related symptoms has the highest negative predictive value for ruling out TB [64]. Mobile vans equipped with a digital chest X-ray machine are increasingly being piloted and used in resource-limited settings. A study in Zimbabwe using a mobile van and digital chest X-ray showed that nearly 10% of asymptomatic persons with chest x-rays suggestive of pulmonary TB were diagnosed and treated for TB, with 13% of them found to have bacteriologically confirmed disease [65]. A similar study in India confirmed the value of chest X-ray in asymptomatic persons both in operational and economic terms [66]. Currently, digital chest X-rays are read by medical officers or other trained personnel. Accuracy of TB diagnosis can be improved using artificial intelligence to read the chest X-ray [67]: the automated technology is available and this should be considered and further researched and assessed by TB programmes where human resources are constrained.

4.4. Expanding and Refining the Use of 3HP

A growing number of countries are using 3HP although there are several issues that require further research (Table 6). Caution is currently required before 3HP can be given safely to children < 2 years, pregnant women, injecting drug users on opioid substitution therapies (OST) and women using oral or injectable contraceptives. There is no published data on the use of 3HP in children < 2 years although a study is underway to assess safety and optimal dosing in this age group [43]. While 3HP was given to 125 pregnant women and showed rates of abortion and birth defects similar to those in the general population [68], this area needs further research in light of a randomised controlled trial on isoniazid preventive therapy showing a higher incidence of adverse pregnancy outcomes (stillbirth, low-birthweight, congenital anomalies) in HIV-infected women receiving isoniazid [69]. The risk of using 3HP in injecting drug users on Opioid Substitution Therapy (OST) is that the rifamycin component may lead to an "opiate withdrawal syndrome" due to decreased serum concentrations of the drugs [43]: this needs further study.

All rifamycin-containing regimens have potential drug–drug interactions with ARV drugs, although in general rifapentine has less interaction than rifampicin. Dolutegravir (DTG) is now recommended as a preferred drug in first-line ARV regimens in PLHIV [70], and it has been established that 3HP can safely be used with this regimen without the need to adjust DTG doses [43].

In the 3HP regimen for adults, 900 mg rifapentine (6 × 150 mg tablets) is taken with 900 mg isoniazid (3 × 300 mg tablets) along with pyridoxine: 10 tablets on one day per week [43]. Lowering the pill burden (by offering rifapentine as a 300 mg tablet in a fixed-dose combination together with isoniazid 300 mg) would make 3HP more acceptable for people to take and would simplify procurement, distribution and storage issues at peripheral health facilities. These concerns are being taken up by generic drug manufacturers.

Systematic monitoring is needed for common and important side effects. The most serious side effect of any isoniazid-containing regimen is drug-induced hepatitis [36], which if unrecognised can lead to acute liver failure and death. 3HP is associated with less hepatotoxicity than 9-months IPT [71]. Nevertheless, programmes need to think about systematically excluding those at high risk of drug-induced hepatitis (for example, with pre-existing liver disease or chronic hepatitis C infection) and monitor this aspect closely. Given the absence of laboratory monitoring in most resource-constrained countries, those taking 3HP and health workers must be educated about the symptoms and signs of hepatitis and the need to stop the drug and immediately report to a health facility if these occur.

3HP is said to be more cost-effective when given by clinic-based direct observation (DOT) [72]. However, in the USA, self-administered 3HP with monthly monitoring with or without weekly text messaging was non-inferior to 3HP by DOT in terms of safety and treatment completion [73]. Video observed therapy (VOT) has also emerged recently as a method to mimic in-person visits, especially in the smartphone era with internet data connections. VOT was associated with higher treatment completion in persons taking 3HP compared with DOT in New York [74], and in South India VOT was preferred over DOT in terms of support during care and treatment of TB [75]. This is an important research topic in low- and middle-income countries where local information on demographics and smartphone ownership is crucial to understand who might and might not benefit from this digital technology.

TB preventive therapy reduces but does not completely prevent TB, and all individuals must be monitored for the development of active TB during treatment, and, if possible, after treatment as well. This requires education of those initiated on preventive therapy as well as their attending health care workers, with clear instructions to attend health facilities for screening and investigation if suggestive TB symptoms arise. For PLHIV living in high TB exposure environments, there is a need to determine whether repeat courses of 3HP are required to maintain TB preventive effects.

Table 6. Research and innovation on the 3-month weekly rifapentine and isoniazid (3HP) treatment regimen.

Issues Around 3HP	Category	Research and Evidence Needed
Caution and safety	Children < 2 years	Acceptability of water-dispersible formulations: one trial underway
	Pregnant women	Frequency of maternal adverse events and pregnancy adverse outcomes
	PWID on OST	Frequency of opiate withdrawal syndrome and measures needed to avoid it
	Women on oral or injectable contraceptives	Interactions with contraceptives and possible dosage adjustments
	Drug-drug interactions in PLHIV	3HP interactions with nevirapine, efavirenz and protease inhibitors
Acceptable formulations	Pill burden: 10 pills once a week: 6 pills of rifapentine 3 pills of isoniazid 1 pill of pyridoxine	Simpler fixed-dose combination—e.g., three tablets combined rifapentine (300 mg) and isoniazid (300 mg) once a week
Monitoring for adverse events	Drug-induced hepatitis and acute liver failure	How to monitor without laboratory infrastructure and how to educate people and health care workers about hepatitis and acute liver failure
Administration of medication	Clinic-based DOT or self-administered treatment or VOT through smartphones	Locally based operational research on how best to administer 3HP in terms of medication adherence, safety and treatment completion
Number of courses of 3HP	PLHIV living in high TB exposure environments	The need, if any, of repeat courses of 3HP to further reduce risk of TB and the frequency of these repeat courses

3HP = 3 months of weekly isoniazid and rifapentine; PWID = people who inject drugs: OST = opioid substitution therapies; PLHIV = people living with HIV; DOT = directly observed therapy; VOT = video-observed therapy.

4.5. Recording and Reporting

Keeping track of who is eligible, who initiates, who completes TB preventive therapy and who is free of TB 12 months after completing therapy is essential for (i) monitoring each individual's journey, (ii) assessing the TB preventive therapy cascade, (iii) charting the progress made against indicators (such as rates of coverage, completion or failure) at subnational, national and international level and (iv) drug forecasting so that procurement and distribution match demand. Drug shortages and interrupted supplies were the most common reasons for discontinuing IPT in children in an Ethiopian community-based LTBI treatment study [76].

In PLHIV, National HIV/AIDS Programmes take responsibility for recording and reporting on who is screened for TB, diagnosed with TB and given TB preventive therapy. These data, collated annually for countries and at global level, are usually presented in the Global TB Reports [4].

For household contacts of index TB patients and for all other high-risk groups, the National TB Programme generally takes responsibility. Done properly, this is an enormous task requiring adequate human, financial and technical resources. To fully comprehend how all the steps of preventive therapy work at the programme level, a sufficient amount of detail must initially be collected. Table 7 outlines the key indicators for which data should be collected in household contacts of index patients with TB. This should identify bottlenecks or problem areas where operational research or further work might be required to close gaps in the TB preventive therapy cascade and better streamline activities. If the index patient is HIV-positive or has DM, further testing of household contacts with respect to these parameters would be indicated.

Table 7. TB Preventive therapy master card for household contacts of index patients with TB. Index Patient Details: Name; registration number: type and category of TB; age; sex; cigarette smoker; consumes alcohol; HIV status; diabetes mellitus status. Line List of Household contacts with details of TPT.

Name	Age	Sex	Relationship to index patient	Symptom Screen	CXR	Active TB diagnosis	Eligible for TPT	Reason for non-eligibility	TPT started	TPT completed	TB status at 12 months after TPT completion
				Positive Negative Not done	Positive Negative Not done	Yes No	Yes No	a	Yes (Date) No	Yes (Date) No	No TB (Date) TB (Date)

a Reasons = known alcohol abuse; acute hepatitis; chronic liver disease; infection with hepatitis B or C; other TB = tuberculosis; CXR = chest X-ray; TPT = TB preventive therapy; Note: if index patient is HIV-positive then screen household contacts for HIV: stratify the numbers below for HIV.

Number of household contacts < 5 years: Number of other household contacts:
Number diagnosed with TB: Number diagnosed with TB:
Number given TPT: Number given TPT:
Number finished TPT: Number finished TPT:

4.6. Consideration of Other TB Prevention Activities

TB preventive therapy is an important part of a larger effort to prevent TB. The development and widespread use of an effective vaccine would have an enormous impact. BCG vaccine protects children from severe disease such as disseminated TB and meningitis, but it does not afford long term protection against pulmonary disease. However, a novel candidate vaccine, $M72/AS01_E$, provided 50% protection over three years against progression to pulmonary TB in adults with LTBI enrolled in Kenya, South Africa and Zambia [77]. While more work on this vaccine is needed in different populations and age-groups as well as people with no evidence of LTBI, this is an exciting and promising development.

Intervening on socioeconomic and other determinants of TB can yield valuable preventive dividends. For example, ART is an excellent TB prevention tool in PLHIV [78], and in South Korea the use of metformin in elderly people with DM significantly reduced their risk of TB [79]. On a much larger scale, poverty reduction at the country level predictably reduces TB incidence [80], and targeted socioeconomic poverty reduction interventions such as cash transfers can also reduce TB risk [81]. Good infection control policies and practices in health care facilities and congregate settings such as refugee camps and prisons can reduce *MTB* transmission and lower TB incidence.

5. Conclusions

The Lancet Commission on TB outlined two main strategies for better progress towards ending the TB epidemic [82], and they both apply to TB preventive therapy. First, we need to improve the implementation of proven interventions and ensure efficient and rapid scale-up as described earlier in this perspective. This applies to finding high risk-groups, considering the expanded use of chest X-ray, properly assessing who is eligible for preventive therapy, initiating appropriate and acceptable treatment and ensuring that a course of treatment is completed with due attention to safety and medication adherence. It is also important to see how TB preventive services can be integrated with those that are already established for diagnosis and treatment. Second, we need to invest in and deploy new products, the most important of which would be an affordable, reliable and easy-to-use biomarker to predict who is at risk of progressing to active disease. More effort is also needed to embrace digital technology, not only for diagnostic tools and monitoring treatment adherence, but for data services, recording and reporting and health service management [83].

For years, the diagnosis and treatment of TB has been the cornerstone of TB control efforts. Given the inefficiencies of this process, the ensuing morbidity and mortality that accompany the treatment period and the recognition of disability and enhanced mortality after treatment is completed, prevention has to be better embraced, properly implemented and scaled up. As Benjamin Franklin famously stated almost 300 years ago "an ounce of prevention is worth a pound of cure".

Author Contributions: A.D.H. wrote the first draft which was critically reviewed by A.M.V.K., S.S., P.T., Y.L., R.A.D., M.K. and R.Z. All authors contributed to subsequent drafts, and agreed upon and approved the final version. All authors have read and agreed to the published version of the manuscript.

Funding: The research received no external funding.

Conflicts of Interest: The authors declare no conflicts of interest.

Disclaimer: The views expressed in this document are those of the authors and may not necessarily reflect those of their affiliated institutions.

References

1. World Health Organization. The End TB Strategy. Available online: https://www.who.int/tb/End_TB_brochure.pdf?ua=1 (accessed on 20 March 2020).
2. Houben, R.M.G.J.; Dodd, P.J. The Global Burden of Latent Tuberculosis Infection: A Re-estimation Using Mathematical Modelling. *PLoS Med.* **2016**, *13*, e1002152. [CrossRef] [PubMed]
3. *Political Declaration on the Fight Against Tuberculosis. Co-facilitators' Revised Text*; United Nations: New York, NY, USA, 2018.
4. World Health Organization. *Global Tuberculosis Report 2019*; World Health Organization: Geneva, Switzerland, 2019.
5. Getnet, F.; Demissie, M.; Assefa, N.; Mengistie, B.; Worku, A. Delay in diagnosis of pulmonary tuberculosis in low-and middle-income settings: Systematic review and meta-analysis. *BMC Pulm. Med.* **2017**, *17*, 202. [CrossRef] [PubMed]
6. Bello, S.; Afolabi, R.F.; Ajayi, D.T.; Sharma, T.; Owoeye, D.O.; Oduyoye, O.; Jasanya, J. Empirical evidence of delays in diagnosis and treatment of pulmonary tuberculosis: Systematic review and meta-regression analysis. *BMC Public Health* **2019**, *19*, 820. [CrossRef] [PubMed]
7. Kweza, P.F.; Van Schalkwyk, C.; Abraham, N.; Uys, M.; Claassens, M.M.; Medina-Marino, A. Estimating the magnitude of missed pulmonary TB patients by primary health care clinics, South Africa. *Int. J. Tuberc. Lung Dis.* **2017**, *22*, 264–272. [CrossRef] [PubMed]
8. Murongazvombo, A.S.; Dlodlo, R.A.; Shewade, H.D.; Robertson, V.; Hirao, S.; Pikira, E.; Zhanero, C.; Taruvinga, R.K.; Andifasi, P.; Tshuma, C. Where, when, and how many tuberculosis patients are lost from presumption until treatment initiation? A step by step assessment in a rural district in Zimbabwe. *Int. J. Infect. Dis.* **2019**, *78*, 113–120. [CrossRef]
9. Marks, G.B.; Nguyen, N.V.; Nguyen, P.T.B.; Nguyen, T.-A.; Nguyen, H.B.; Tran, K.H.; Nguyen, S.V.; Luu, K.B.; Tran, D.T.T.; Vo, Q.T.N.; et al. Community-wide Screening for Tuberculosis in a High-Prevalence Setting. *N. Engl. J. Med.* **2019**, *381*, 1347–1357. [CrossRef]
10. Koura, K.G.; Trébucq, A.; Schwoebel, V. Do active case-finding projects increase the number of tuberculosis cases notified at national level? *Int. J. Tuberc. Lung Dis.* **2017**, *21*, 73–78. [CrossRef]
11. Dey, A.; Thekkur, P.; Ghosh, A.; Dasgupta, T.; Bandopadhyay, S.; Lahiri, A.; Sanju, S.V.C.; Dinda, M.K.; Sharma, V.; Dimari, N.; et al. Active Case Finding for Tuberculosis through TOUCH Agents in Selected High TB Burden Wards of Kolkata, India: A Mixed Methods Study on Outcomes and Implementation Challenges. *Trop. Med. Infect. Dis.* **2019**, *4*, 134. [CrossRef]

12. Shamanewadi, A.N.; Naik, P.R.; Thekkur, P.; Madhukumar, S.; Nirgude, A.S.; Pavithra, M.B.; Poojar, B.; Sharma, V.; Urs, A.P.; Nisarga, B.V.; et al. Enablers and Challenges in the Implementation of Active Case Findings in a Selected District of Karnataka, South India: A Qualitative Study. *Tuberc. Res. Treat.* **2020**, *2020*, 9746329. [CrossRef]
13. Onozaki, I.; Law, I.; Sismanidis, C.; Zignol, M.; Glaziou, P.; Floyd, K. National tuberculosis prevalence surveys in Asia, 1990–2012: An overview of results and lessons learned. *Trop. Med. Int. Health* **2015**, *20*, 1128–1145. [CrossRef]
14. MacPherson, P.; Houben, R.M.G.J.; Glynn, J.R.; Corbett, E.L.; Kranzer, K. Pre-treatment loss to follow-up in tuberculosis patients in low- and lower-middle-income countries and high-burden countries: A systematic review and meta-analysis. *Bull. World Health Organ.* **2014**, *92*, 126–138. [CrossRef] [PubMed]
15. Cox, H.; Dickson-Hall, L.; Ndjeka, N.; van't Hoog, A.; Grant, A.; Cobelens, F.; Stevens, W.; Nicol, M. Delays and loss to follow-up before treatment of drug-resistant tuberculosis following implementation of Xpert MTB/RIF in South Africa: A retrospective cohort study. *PLoS Med.* **2017**, *14*, e1002238. [CrossRef] [PubMed]
16. Onyoh, E.F.; Kuaban, C.; Lin, H.H. Pre-Treatment loss to follow-up of pulmonary tuberculosis patients in two regions of Cameroon. *Int. J. Tuberc. Lung Dis.* **2018**, *22*, 378–384. [CrossRef] [PubMed]
17. Htet, K.K.K.; Soe, K.T.; Kumar, A.M.V.; Saw, S.; Maung, H.M.W.; Myint, Z.; Khine, T.M.M.; Aung, S.T. Rifampicin-resistant tuberculosis patients in Myanmar in 2016: How many are lost on the path to treatment? *Int. J. Tuberc. Lung Dis.* **2018**, *22*, 385–392. [CrossRef]
18. Gillespie, S.H.; Crook, A.M.; McHugh, T.D.; Mendel, C.M.; Meredith, S.K.; Murray, S.R.; Pappas, F.; Phillips, P.P.J.; Nunn, A.J. Four-Month Moxifloxacin-Based Regimens for Drug-Sensitive Tuberculosis. *N. Engl. J. Med.* **2014**, *371*, 1577–1587. [CrossRef]
19. Merle, C.S.; Fielding, K.; Sow, O.B.; Gninafon, M.; Lo, M.B.; Mthiyane, T.; Odhiambo, J.; Amukoye, E.; Bah, B.; Kassa, F.; et al. A four-month gatifloxacin-containing regimen for treating tuberculosis. *N. Engl. J. Med.* **2014**, *371*, 1588–1598. [CrossRef]
20. Jindani, A.; Harrison, T.S.; Nunn, A.J.; Phillips, P.P.J.; Churchyard, G.J.; Charalambous, S.; Hatherill, M.; Geldenhuys, H.; McIlleron, H.M.; Zvada, S.P.; et al. High-Dose Rifapentine with Moxifloxacin for Pulmonary Tuberculosis. *N. Engl. J. Med.* **2014**, *371*, 1599–1608. [CrossRef]
21. Nunn, A.J.; Phillips, P.P.J.; Meredith, S.K.; Chiang, C.-Y.; Conradie, F.; Dalai, D.; van Deun, A.; Dat, P.-T.; Lan, N.; Master, I.; et al. A Trial of a Shorter Regimen for Rifampin-Resistant Tuberculosis. *N. Engl. J. Med.* **2019**, *380*, 1201–1213. [CrossRef]
22. Trebucq, A.; Schwoebel, V.; Kashongwe, Z.; Bakayoko, A.; Kuaban, C.; Noeske, J.; Hassane, S.; Souleymane, B.; Piubello, A.; Ciza, F.; et al. Treatment outcome with a short multidrug-resistant tuberculosis regimen in nine African countries. *Int. J. Tuberc. Lung Dis.* **2018**, *22*, 17–25. [CrossRef] [PubMed]
23. Furin, J.; Cox, H.; Pai, M. Tuberculosis. *Lancet* **2019**, *393*, 1642–1656. [CrossRef]
24. Heldal, E.; Dlodlo, R.A.; Mlilo, N.; Nyathi, B.B.; Zishiri, C.; Ncube, R.T.; Siziba, N.; Sandy, C. Local staff making sense of their tuberculosis data: Key to quality care and ending tuberculosis. *Int. J. Tuberc. Lung Dis.* **2019**, *23*, 612–618. [CrossRef]
25. Menzies, N.A.; Gomez, G.B.; Bozzani, F.; Chatterjee, S.; Foster, N.; Baena, I.G.; Laurence, Y.V.; Qiang, S.; Siroka, A.; Sweeney, S.; et al. Cost-effectiveness and resource implications of aggressive action on tuberculosis in China, India, and South Africa: A combined analysis of nine models. *Lancet Glob. Health* **2016**, *4*, e816–e826. [CrossRef]
26. Harries, A.D.; Dlodlo, R.A.; Brigden, G.; Mortimer, K.; Jensen, P.; Fujiwara, P.I.; Castro, J.L.; Chakaya, J.M. Should we consider a 'fourth 90' for tuberculosis? *Int. J. Tuberc. Lung Dis.* **2019**, *23*, 1253–1256. [CrossRef]
27. Reuter, A.; Tisile, P.; Von Delft, D.; Cox, H.; Cox, V.; Ditiu, L.; Garcia-Prats, A.; Koenig, S.; Lessem, E.; Nathavitharana, R.; et al. The devil we know: Is the use of injectable agents for the treatment of MDR-TB justified? *Int. J. Tuberc. Lung Dis.* **2017**, *21*, 1114–1126. [CrossRef] [PubMed]
28. Mason, P.H.; Sweetland, A.C.; Fox, G.J.; Halovic, S.; Nguyen, T.A.; Marks, G.B. Tuberculosis and mental health in the Asia-Pacific. *Australas. Psychiatry* **2016**, *24*, 553–555. [CrossRef] [PubMed]
29. Alene, K.A.; Clements, A.C.A.; McBryde, E.S.; Jaramillo, E.; Lönnroth, K.; Shaweno, D.; Gulliver, A.; Viney, K. Mental health disorders, social stressors, and health-related quality of life in patients with multidrug-resistant tuberculosis: A systematic review and meta-analysis. *J. Infect.* **2018**, *77*, 357–367. [CrossRef] [PubMed]

30. Romanowski, K.; Baumann, B.; Basham, C.A.; Ahmad Khan, F.; Fox, G.J.; Johnston, J.C. Long-term all-cause mortality in people treated for tuberculosis: A systematic review and meta-analysis. *Lancet Infect. Dis.* **2019**, *19*, 1129–1137. [CrossRef]
31. Quaife, M.; Houben, R.M.G.J.; Allwood, B.; Cohen, T.; Coussens, A.K.; Harries, A.D.; van Kampen, S.; Marx, F.M.; Sweeney, S.; Wallis, R.S.; et al. Post-tuberculosis mortality and morbidity: Valuing the hidden epidemic. *Lancet Respir. Med.* **2020**, *8*, 332–333. [CrossRef]
32. Harries, A.D.; Kumar, A.M.V.; Satyanarayana, S.; Thekkur, P.; Lin, Y.; Dlodlo, R.A.; Zachariah, R. How Can Operational Research Help to Eliminate Tuberculosis in the Asia Pacific Region? *Trop. Med. Infect. Dis.* **2019**, *4*, 47. [CrossRef]
33. *Latent Tuberculosis Infection. Updated and Consolidated Guidelines for Programmatic Management. 2018*; World Health Organization: Geneva, Switzerland, 2018.
34. World Health Organization. Rapid Communication on Forthcoming Changes to the Programmatic Management of Tuberculosis Preventive Treatment. Available online: http://apps.who.int/bookorders. (accessed on 21 March 2020).
35. Campbell, J.; Winters, N.; Menzies, D. Absolute risk of tuberculosis among untreated populations with a positive tuberculin skin test or interferon-gamma release assay result: Systematic review and meta-analysis. *BMJ* **2020**, *368*, m549. [CrossRef]
36. Harries, A.D.; Kumar, A.M.V.; Satyanarayana, S.; Takarinda, K.C.; Timire, C.; Dlodlo, R.A. Treatment for latent tuberculosis infection in low- and middle-income countries: Progress and challenges with implementation and scale-up. *Expert Rev. Respir. Med.* **2020**, *14*, 195–208. [CrossRef] [PubMed]
37. Chandrasekaran, P.; Mave, V.; Thiruvengadam, K.; Gupte, N.; Yogendra Shivakumar, S.V.B.; Hanna, L.E.; Kulkarni, V.; Kadam, D.; Dhanasekaran, K.; Paradkar, M.; et al. Tuberculin skin test and QuantiFERON-Gold In Tube assay for diagnosis of latent TB infection among household contacts of pulmonary TB patients in high TB burden setting. *PLoS ONE* **2018**, *13*, e0199360. [CrossRef]
38. Getahun, H.; Matteelli, A.; Chaisson, R.E.; Raviglione, M. Latent Mycobacterium tuberculosis infection. *N. Engl. J. Med.* **2015**, *372*, 2127–2135. [CrossRef] [PubMed]
39. Behr, M.A.; Edelstein, P.H.; Ramakrishnan, L. Is Mycobacterium tuberculosis infection life long? *BMJ* **2019**, *367*, l5770. [CrossRef] [PubMed]
40. Den Boon, S.; Matteelli, A.; Ford, N.; Getahun, H. Continuous isoniazid for the treatment of latent tuberculosis infection in people living with HIV. *AIDS* **2016**, *30*, 797–801. [CrossRef]
41. Hamada, Y.; Ford, N.; Schenkel, K.; Getahun, H. Three-month weekly rifapentine plus isoniazid for tuberculosis preventive treatment: A systematic review. *Int. J. Tuberc. Lung Dis.* **2018**, *22*, 1422–1428. [CrossRef] [PubMed]
42. Swindells, S.; Ramchandani, R.; Gupta, A.; Benson, C.A.; Leon-Cruz, J.; Mwelase, N.; Jean Juste, M.A.; Lama, J.R.; Valencia, J.; Omoz-Oarhe, A.; et al. One month of rifapentine plus isoniazid to prevent HIV-related Tuberculosis. *N. Engl. J. Med.* **2019**, *380*, 1001–1011. [CrossRef]
43. Treatment Action Group. An Activist's Guide to Rifapentine for the Treatment of TB Infection—Treatment Action Group. Available online: https://www.treatmentactiongroup.org/publication/an-activists-guide-to-rifapentine-for-the-treatment-of-tb-infection/ (accessed on 21 March 2020).
44. Simon Schaaf, H.; Gie, R.P.; Kennedy, M.; Beyers, N.; Hesseling, P.B.; Donald, P.R. Evaluation of young children in contact with adult multidrug-resistant pulmonary tuberculosis: A 30-month follow-up. *Pediatrics* **2002**, *109*, 765–771. [CrossRef]
45. Garcia-Prats, A.J.; Zimri, K.; Mramba, Z.; Schaaf, H.S.; Hesseling, A.C. Children exposed to multidrug-resistant tuberculosis at a homebased day care centre: A contact investigation. *Int. J. Tuberc. Lung Dis.* **2014**, *18*, 1292–1298. [CrossRef]
46. Bamrah, S.; Brostrom, R.; Dorina, F.; Setik, L.; Song, R.; Kawamura, L.M.; Heetderks, A.; Mase, S. Treatment for LTBI in contacts of MDR-TB patients, Federated States of Micronesia, 2009–2012. *Int. J. Tuberc. Lung Dis.* **2014**, *18*, 912–918. [CrossRef]
47. Trieu, L.; Proops, D.C.; Ahuja, S.D. Moxifoxacin prophylaxis against MDR TB, NEW YORK, NEW YORK, USA. *Emerg. Infect. Dis.* **2015**, *21*, 500–503. [CrossRef]
48. Fox, G.J.; Schaaf, H.S.; Mandalakas, A.; Chiappini, E.; Zumla, A.; Marais, B.J. Preventing the spread of multidrug-resistant tuberculosis and protecting contacts of infectious cases. *Clin. Microbiol. Infect.* **2017**, *23*, 147–153. [CrossRef] [PubMed]

49. Lawn, S.D.; Bekker, L.G.; Wood, R. How effectively does HAART restore immune responses to Mycobacterium tuberculosis? Implications for tuberculosis control. *AIDS* **2005**, *19*, 1113–1124. [CrossRef] [PubMed]
50. Gupta, A.; Wood, R.; Kaplan, R.; Bekker, L.-G.; Lawn, S.D. Tuberculosis Incidence Rates during 8 Years of Follow-Up of an Antiretroviral Treatment Cohort in South Africa: Comparison with Rates in the Community. *PLoS ONE* **2012**, *7*, e34156. [CrossRef] [PubMed]
51. World Health Organization. *Recommendations for Investigating Contacts of Persons with Infectious Tuberculosis in Low-and Middle-Income Countries*; WHO: Geneva, Switzerland, 2012; ISBN 9789241504492.
52. Cho, P.J.Y.; Wu, C.Y.; Johnston, J.; Wu, M.Y.; Shu, C.C.; Lin, H.H. Progression of chronic kidney disease and the risk of tuberculosis: An observational cohort study. *Int. J. Tuberc. Lung Dis.* **2019**, *23*, 555–562. [CrossRef]
53. GBD Chronic Kidney Disease Collaboration. Global, regional, and national burden of chronic kidney disease, 1990–2017: A systematic analysis for the Global Burden of Disease Study 2017. *Lancet* **2020**, *395*, 709–733. [CrossRef]
54. Stevenson, C.R.; Critchley, J.A.; Forouhi, N.G.; Roglic, G.; Williams, B.G.; Dye, C.; Unwin, N.C. Diabetes and the risk of tuberculosis: A neglected threat to public health? *Chronic Illn.* **2007**, *3*, 228–245. [CrossRef]
55. Jeon, C.Y.; Murray, M.B. Diabetes mellitus increases the risk of active tuberculosis: A systematic review of 13 observational studies. *PLoS Med.* **2008**, *5*, e152.
56. Noubiap, J.J.; Nansseu, J.R.; Nyaga, U.F.; Nkeck, J.R.; Endomba, F.T.; Kaze, A.D.; Agbor, V.N.; Bigna, J.J. Global prevalence of diabetes in active tuberculosis: A systematic review and meta-analysis of data from 2·3 million patients with tuberculosis. *Lancet Glob. Health* **2019**, *7*, e448–e460. [CrossRef]
57. McAllister, S.M.; Koesoemadinata, R.C.; Santoso, P.; Soetedjo, N.N.M.; Kamil, A.; Permana, H.; Ruslami, R.; Critchley, J.A.; van Crevel, R.; Hill, P.C.; et al. High tuberculosis incidence among people living with diabetes in Indonesia. *Trans. R. Soc. Trop. Med. Hyg.* **2020**, *114*, 79–85. [CrossRef]
58. Soh, A.Z.; Chee, C.B.E.; Wang, Y.T.; Yuan, J.M.; Koh, W.P. Diabetes and body mass index in relation to risk of active tuberculosis: A prospective population-based cohort. *Int. J. Tuberc. Lung Dis.* **2019**, *23*, 1277–1282. [CrossRef] [PubMed]
59. International Diabetes Federation. *IDF Diabetes Atlas*, 9th ed.; International Diabetes Federation, 2019; Available online: https://diabetesatlas.org/upload/resources/2019/IDF_Atlas_9th_Edition_2019.pdf (accessed on 21 March 2020).
60. International Union against Tuberculosis Committee on Prophylaxis. Efficacy of various durations of isoniazid preventive therapy for tuberculosis: Five years of follow-up in the IUAT trial. International union against tuberculosis committee on prophylaxis. *Bull. World Health Organ.* **1982**, *60*, 555–564.
61. Goletti, D.; Lee, M.R.; Wang, J.Y.; Walter, N.; Ottenhoff, T.H.M. Update on tuberculosis biomarkers: From correlates of risk, to correlates of active disease and of cure from disease. *Respirology* **2018**, *23*, 455–466. [CrossRef]
62. Zak, D.E.; Penn-Nicholson, A.; Scriba, T.J.; Thompson, E.; Suliman, S.; Amon, L.M.; Mahomed, H.; Erasmus, M.; Whatney, W.; Hussey, G.D.; et al. A blood RNA signature for tuberculosis disease risk: A prospective cohort study. *Lancet* **2016**, *387*, 2312–2322. [CrossRef]
63. Harries, A.D.; Kumar, A.M.V. Challenges and Progress with Diagnosing Pulmonary Tuberculosis in Low- and Middle-Income Countries. *Diagnostics* **2018**, *8*, 78. [CrossRef]
64. World Health Organization. *Chest Radiography in Tuberculosis Detection*; WHO, Ed.; WHO: Geneva, Switzerland, 2016; ISBN 9789241511506.
65. Sengai, T.; Timire, C.; Harries, A.D.; Tweya, H.; Kavenga, F.; Shumba, G.; Tavengerwei, J.; Ncube, R.; Zishiri, C.; Mapfurira, M.J.; et al. Mobile targeted screening for tuberculosis in Zimbabwe: Diagnosis, linkage to care and treatment outcomes. *Public Health Action* **2019**, *9*, 159–165. [CrossRef] [PubMed]
66. Datta, B.; Prakash, A.K.; Ford, D.; Tanwar, P.K.; Goyal, P.; Chatterjee, P.; Vipin, S.; Jaiswal, A.; Trehan, N.; Ayyagiri, K. Comparison of clinical and cost-effectiveness of two strategies using mobile digital x-ray to detect pulmonary tuberculosis in rural India. *BMC Public Health* **2019**, *19*, 99. [CrossRef] [PubMed]
67. Qin, Z.Z.; Sander, M.S.; Rai, B.; Titahong, C.N.; Sudrungrot, S.; Laah, S.N.; Adhikari, L.M.; Carter, E.J.; Puri, L.; Codlin, A.J.; et al. Using artificial intelligence to read chest radiographs for tuberculosis detection: A multi-site evaluation of the diagnostic accuracy of three deep learning systems. *Sci. Rep.* **2019**, *9*, 15000. [CrossRef]

68. Moro, R.N.; Scott, N.A.; Vernon, A.; Tepper, N.K.; Goldberg, S.V.; Schwartzman, K.; Leung, C.C.; Schluger, N.W.; Belknap, R.W.; Chaisson, R.E.; et al. Exposure to latent tuberculosis treatment during pregnancy the PREVENT TB and the iadhere trials. *Ann. Am. Thorac. Soc.* **2018**, *15*, 570–580. [CrossRef]
69. Gupta, A.; Montepiedra, G.; Aaron, L.; Theron, G.; McCarthy, K.; Bradford, S.; Chipato, T.; Vhembo, T.; Stranix-Chibanda, L.; Onyango-Makumbi, C.; et al. Isoniazid preventive therapy in HIV-infected pregnant and postpartum women. *N. Engl. J. Med.* **2019**, *381*, 1333–1346. [CrossRef]
70. World Health Organization. *Updated Recommendations on First-Line and Second-Line Antiretroviral Regimens and Post-Exposure Prophylaxis and Recommendations on Early Infant Diagnosis of HIV*; WHO, Ed.; WHO: Geneva, Switzerland, 2018.
71. Bliven-Sizemore, E.E.; Sterling, T.R.; Shang, N.; Benator, D.; Schwartzman, K.; Reves, R.; Drobeniuc, J.; Bock, N.; Villarino, M.E. Three months of weekly rifapentine plus isoniazid is less hepatotoxic than nine months of daily isoniazid for LTBI. *Int. J. Tuberc. Lung Dis.* **2015**, *19*, 1039–1044. [CrossRef]
72. Doan, T.N.; Fox, G.J.; Meehan, M.T.; Scott, N.; Ragonnet, R.; Viney, K.; Trauer, J.M.; McBryde, E.S. Cost-effectiveness of 3 months of weekly rifapentine and isoniazid compared with other standard treatment regimens for latent tuberculosis infection: A decision analysis study. *J. Antimicrob. Chemother.* **2019**, *74*, 218–227. [CrossRef] [PubMed]
73. Belknap, R.; Holland, D.; Feng, P.J.; Millet, J.P.; Cayla, J.A.; Martinson, N.A.; Wright, A.; Chen, M.P.; Moro, R.N.; Scott, N.A.; et al. Self-administered versus directly observed once-weekly isoniazid and rifapentine treatment of latent tuberculosis infection. *Ann. Intern. Med.* **2017**, *167*, 689–697. [CrossRef] [PubMed]
74. Lam, C.K.; Pilote, K.M.G.; Haque, A.; Burzynski, J.; Chuck, C.; Macaraig, M. Using video technology to increase treatment completion for patients with latent tuberculosis infection on 3-month isoniazid and rifapentine: An implementation study. *J. Med. Internet Res.* **2018**, *20*, e287. [CrossRef] [PubMed]
75. Kumar, A.A.; De Costa, A.D.; Das, A.; Srinivasa, G.A.; D'Souza, G.; Rodrigues, R. Mobile health for tuberculosis management in south India: Is video-based directly observed treatment an acceptable alternative? *J. Med. Internet Res.* **2019**, *7*, e11687. [CrossRef]
76. Datiko, D.G.; Yassin, M.A.; Theobald, S.J.; Cuevas, L.E. A community-based isoniazid preventive therapy for the prevention of childhood tuberculosis in Ethiopia. *Int. J. Tuberc. Lung Dis.* **2017**, *21*, 1002–1007. [CrossRef]
77. Tait, D.R.; Hatherill, M.; Van Der Meeren, O.; Ginsberg, A.M.; Van Brakel, E.; Salaun, B.; Scriba, T.J.; Akite, E.J.; Ayles, H.M.; Bollaerts, A.; et al. Final Analysis of a Trial of M72/AS01E Vaccine to Prevent Tuberculosis. *N. Engl. J. Med.* **2019**, *381*, 2429–2439. [CrossRef]
78. Suthar, A.B.; Lawn, S.D.; del Amo, J.; Getahun, H.; Dye, C.; Sculier, D.; Sterling, T.R.; Chaisson, R.E.; Williams, B.G.; Harries, A.D.; et al. Antiretroviral therapy for prevention of tuberculosis in adults with hiv: A systematic review and meta-analysis. *PLoS Med.* **2012**, *9*, e1001270. [CrossRef]
79. Park, S.; Yang, B.R.; Song, H.J.; Jang, S.H.; Kang, D.Y.; Park, B.J. Metformin and tuberculosis risk in elderly patients with diabetes mellitus. *Int. J. Tuberc. Lung Dis.* **2019**, *23*, 924–930. [CrossRef]
80. Dye, C.; Lönnroth, K.; Jaramillo, E.; Williams, B.G.; Raviglione, M. Trends in tuberculosis incidence and their determinants in 134 countries. *Bull. World Health Organ.* **2009**, *87*, 683–691. [CrossRef]
81. Siroka, A.; Ponce, N.A.; Lönnroth, K. Association between spending on social protection and tuberculosis burden: A global analysis. *Lancet Infect. Dis.* **2016**, *16*, 473–479. [CrossRef]
82. Reid, M.J.A.; Arinaminpathy, N.; Bloom, A.; Bloom, B.R.; Boehme, C.; Chaisson, R.; Chin, D.P.; Churchyard, G.; Cox, H.; Ditiu, L.; et al. Building a tuberculosis-free world: The Lancet Commission on tuberculosis. *Lancet* **2019**, *393*, 1331–1384. [CrossRef]
83. Lee, Y.; Raviglione, M.C.; Flahault, A. Use of Digital Technology to Enhance Tuberculosis Control: Scoping Review. *J. Med. Internet Res.* **2020**, *22*, e15727. [CrossRef] [PubMed]

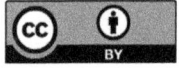

© 2020 by the authors. Licensee MDPI, Basel, Switzerland. This article is an open access article distributed under the terms and conditions of the Creative Commons Attribution (CC BY) license (http://creativecommons.org/licenses/by/4.0/).

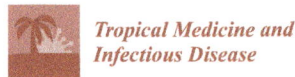

Article

High Levels of Treatment Success and Zero Relapse in Multidrug-Resistant Tuberculosis Patients Receiving a Levofloxacin-Based Shorter Treatment Regimen in Vietnam

Le T. N. Anh [1,*], Ajay M. V. Kumar [2,3,4], Gomathi Ramaswamy [5], Thurain Htun [6], Thuy Thanh Hoang Thi [7], Giang Hoai Nguyen [8], Mamel Quelapio [9], Agnes Gebhard [9], Hoa Binh Nguyen [1,3] and Nhung Viet Nguyen [1]

1. Vietnam Integrated Center for TB and Respirology Research, National Lung Hospital, Ha Noi 100000, Vietnam; nguyenbinhhoatb@yahoo.com (H.B.N.); vietnhung@yahoo.com (N.V.N.)
2. International Union Against Tuberculosis and Lung Disease, South East Asia Office, New Delhi 110016, India; akumar@theunion.org
3. International Union Against Tuberculosis and Lung Disease, 75006 Paris, France
4. Yenepoya Medical College, Yenepoya (Deemed to be University), Mangaluru 575018, India
5. National Centre of Excellence and Advanced Research on Anemia Control, Centre for Community Medicine, All India Institute of Medical Sciences, New Delhi 110029, India; gmthramaswamy@gmail.com
6. International Union Against Tuberculosis and Lung Disease, Mandalay 05021, Myanmar; drthurain07@gmail.com
7. Programmatic Management of Drug Resistant Tuberculosis Unit, National Lung Hospital, Ha Noi 100000, Vietnam; hoangthanht@gmail.com
8. Interactive Research and Development, Ho Chi Minh 700000, Vietnam; nhgiang@gmail.com
9. KNCV Tuberculosis Foundation, 2596 BC The Hague, The Netherlands; mameldquelapio@gmail.com (M.Q.); agnes.gebhard@kncvtbc.org (A.G.)
* Correspondence: ngocanhntp2015@gmail.com; Tel.: +84-94705610

Received: 17 November 2019; Accepted: 7 January 2020; Published: 10 March 2020

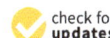

Abstract: Vietnam has been using a levofloxacin-based shorter treatment regimen (STR) for rifampicin resistant/multidrug-resistant tuberculosis (RR/MDR-TB) patients since 2016 on a pilot basis. This regimen lasts for 9–11 months and is provided to RR/MDR-TB patients without second-line drug resistance. We report the treatment outcomes and factors associated with unsuccessful outcomes. We conducted a cohort study involving secondary analysis of data extracted from electronic patient records maintained by the national TB program (NTP). Of the 302 patients enrolled from April 2016 to June 2018, 259 (85.8%) patients were successfully treated (246 cured and 13 'treatment completed'). Unsuccessful outcomes included: treatment failure (16, 5.3%), loss to follow-up (14, 4.6%) and death (13, 4.3%). HIV-positive TB patients, those aged ≥65 years and patients culture-positive at baseline had a higher risk of unsuccessful outcomes. In a sub-group of patients enrolled in 2016 (n = 99) and assessed at 12 months after treatment completion, no cases of relapse were identified. These findings vindicate the decision of the Vietnam NTP to use a levofloxacin-based STR in RR/MDR-TB patients without second-line drug resistance. This regimen may be considered for nationwide scale-up after a detailed assessment of adverse drug events.

Keywords: STR; Bangladesh regimen; operational research; SORT IT

1. Introduction

Multidrug-resistant tuberculosis (MDR-TB), defined as TB resistant to both isoniazid and rifampicin, is a global public health challenge. In 2018, an estimated 484,000 people developed TB that was resistant to rifampicin (RR-TB), and of these, 78% had MDR-TB [1]. Treatment coverage and treatment success rates among MDR-TB patients have been poor. Globally, only 32% of estimated RR/MDR-TB patients were treated in 2018, and only 56% of them were successfully treated [1], mostly because of challenges related to the long duration of the treatment and toxic drugs.

There has been great progress in the development and availability of new diagnostic tools, new drugs and new treatment regimens for MDR-TB. The new diagnostic tools include Xpert® MTB/RIF assay (including the Ultra [2] and Omni versions [3] and a new assay under development to diagnose resistance to second-line drugs [4]) and line probe assay (LPA) to diagnose resistance to the most important first-line and second-line drugs (SLD) [5]. On the treatment front, there are two new drugs in the armamentarium against TB—Bedaquiline and Delamanid—and some of the existing drugs are being repurposed for use in MDR-TB treatment [6–8]. Further, the duration of treatment has been shortened. Owing to a large body of evidence accumulated over the past few years, WHO recommends use of standardized shorter treatment regimen (STR) for patients with MDR-TB (in whom SLD resistance has been excluded) [9–15].

There has been a debate about the choice of fluoroquinolone to be used in the STRs. While the initial studies in Bangladesh, Niger and Cameron used Gatifloxacin [10–12], later studies in nine African countries and the STREAM trial used Moxifloxacin [14,16], owing to concerns about dysglycaemia (low or high blood sugar) caused by Gatifloxacin and the subsequent withdrawal of the drug from the market [17]. Experts have argued that these concerns about safety of Gatifloxacin have to be balanced against those of Moxifloxacin [18,19], which is not immune to causing dysglycemia [20]. In addition, Moxifloxacin causes QT interval prolongation (a measure of delayed ventricular repolarization as measured on electrocardiogram) leading to cardiac arrhythmias and sudden death [21].

Owing to these concerns, there has been interest in the use of Levofloxacin in STRs [22] because it does not significantly prolong the mean QT interval [23] and the initial data support its effectiveness [24]. There has been limited evidence about the effectiveness of Levofloxacin-based STRs among MDR-TB patients, barring a sub-group analysis from Bangladesh showing high treatment success [25]. Vietnam is one of the unique settings, which has always used a Levofloxacin-based STR. A systematic assessment of the treatment outcomes in Vietnam has the potential to contribute to the global evidence base on this issue.

So, we conducted an operational research with the following objectives: (i) to describe the demographic and clinical profile of MDR-TB patients who received the Levofloxacin-based STR from April 2016 to June 2018 under the national tuberculosis program (NTP) of Vietnam (ii) to assess their treatment outcomes, including 12 months' recurrence in a sub-group of patients and (iii) to determine the factors associated with unsuccessful treatment outcomes.

2. Materials and Methods

2.1. Study Design

This was a cohort study involving secondary analysis of routinely collected program data.

2.2. Setting

Vietnam is a lower-middle income country situated in East Asia with a population of 92 million. The country has 63 provinces, 673 districts and 10,925 communes. Vietnam is considered as one of the 30 high-burden countries in the world, with a MDR-TB prevalence of 3.6% and 17% among new and previously treated TB patients respectively [1]. Vietnam started the programmatic management of drug resistant TB (PMDT) in 2009 using the conventional regimen (20–24 months), which was scaled-up nationwide in 2016. The latest available outcome data indicates a relatively high treatment success of 68% among a cohort of MDR-TB patients enrolled in 2016, which is substantially higher than the global average [1].

The NTP network follows the hierarchy of the health system. The National Lung Hospital in Hanoi is the national referral hospital. There are three sub-national TB referral hospitals: Pham Ngoc Thach hospital in Ho Chi Minh City, TB and Lung Hospital in Da Nang Province and TB and Lung hospital in Can Tho province. There are 63 provincial TB hospitals or TB units as part of the provincial preventive medicine department. Each of the districts has a TB coordinator and each commune has a commune health worker responsible for TB. The commune health workers educate the community on TB, refer people with symptoms suggestive for TB and provide treatment support.

2.2.1. Diagnosis and Treatment of MDR-TB

Under the PMDT program, all TB patients are screened for rifampicin resistance using Xpert® MTB/RIF assay. Patients diagnosed with rifampicin resistance are then tested for evidence of second-line drug resistance (fluoroquinolone, second-line injectables) using LPA (Genotype® MTBDRsl assay, Hain Lifescience, Nehren, Germany) and/or phenotypic culture (either in liquid media using BACTEC MGIT 960 instrument or solid Lowenstein–Jensen media) and drug susceptibility test (DST using proportion method) at the sub-national reference laboratories. All the laboratories are quality-assured and under the supervision of supranational reference laboratory at Adelaide, Australia.

While waiting for the results of SLD resistance, patients are referred to the provincial hospital for conducting baseline tests which include testing for HIV, diabetes, hepatic and renal function, audiometry and routine biochemistry and assessing if they are eligible for STR. Accordingly, a decision is made by a committee to start STR. All the patients are hospitalized for a period of two to four weeks at the time of starting treatment. This is followed by ambulatory treatment delivered under direct observation of the health workers at either district or commune levels. If the results of the initial LPA or DST show that there is resistance to SLDs, the treatment is stopped and the patient is shifted to an individualized regimen based on the drug resistance pattern.

For all patients, a family (or friend) is designated as treatment supporter whose role is to remind the patient to consume the medicines regularly and visit the health facility for follow-up. Psychosocial support is provided by the community-based organizations (Women's Union, Farmers' Union, Youth Union, and the Red Cross) which run the 'TB patient clubs'. In addition, food allowance, hospitalization costs during intensive phase and transport costs incurred during follow-up visits are reimbursed by the NTP.

2.2.2. The Treatment Regimen

The STR is provided for 9–11 months and consists of two phases: intensive phase for 4–6 months and continuation phase for a fixed duration of 5 months (Table 1). The intensive phase consists of the following drugs: Levofloxacin, Kanamycin, Clofazimine, Prothionamide, Ethambutol, high-dose Isoniazid, and Pyrazinamide, given daily. The continuation phase consists of Levofloxacin, Clofazimine, Ethambutol and Pyrazinamide, given daily.

2.2.3. Follow-Up Schedule during the Treatment

The treatment response is monitored using clinical examination, follow-up sputum smear microscopy and culture, done monthly. If the sputum smear is positive at four months of treatment, the intensive phase is extended for a month or two. During the extended intensive phase, kanamycin is provided intermittently (thrice a week) to reduce toxicity. Patients are switched to continuation phase once two consecutive culture results taken at least 30 days apart in intensive phase are negative. If the person remains culture positive at the end of the 4th month or later, or reverts after conversion, DST (for second-line drugs) is done for every positive culture and the patient is shifted to an individualized regimen based on the susceptibility pattern. A treatment outcome is assigned for each person. The operational definitions of treatment outcomes and other outcome indicators are detailed in Table 2 [26].

Patients who experience adverse drug events are followed-up until clinical recovery is complete and laboratory results have returned to normal, or until the event has stabilized. All the treatment related details are recorded in the TB treatment card by the health care providers and electronically captured in the e-TB manager system as per national guidelines.

Table 1. Weight-based drug dosages used among MDR-TB patients treated with shorter treatment regimen in Vietnam, 2016–2018.

Drug	Months	Drug Doses by Weight Group			
		<33 kg	33–50 kg	>50–70 kg	>70 kg
Kanamycin *(Km)	1–4 (6)	0.5 g	0.75 g	0.75 g	1 g
Levofloxacin (Lx)	1–9	500 mg	750 mg	750 mg	1000 mg
Clofazimine (Cfz)	1–9	50 mg	100 mg	100 mg	100 mg
Ethambutol (E)	1–9	600 mg	800 mg	1000 mg	1200 mg
Pyrazinamide (Z)	1–9	750 mg	1500 mg	2000 mg	2000 mg
Isoniazid (H)	1–4	300 mg	400 mg	600 mg	600 mg
Prothionamide (Pto)	1–4	500 mg	500 mg	750 mg	1000 mg

* with a maximum of 0.75 g for people over 45 years of age, mg = milligram, g = gram.

2.2.4. Follow-Up Schedule Post-Treatment

Patient whose treatment outcome is either cured or completed are invited to come back to the provincial hospital for post-treatment follow-up every six months till 24 months after treatment completion. TB symptom screening and chest radiography are done at each follow-up visit. If the patient has TB symptoms (cough ≥ 2 weeks, hemoptysis) or abnormalities on chest X-ray, s/he is asked to produce a sputum sample which is tested using Xpert MTB/RIF and culture and drug susceptibility test. If patient does not return for follow-up as scheduled, health staffs at the provincial hospital follow-up over phone or conduct a home visit for screening.

2.3. Study Population

All the RR/MDR-TB patients who received the levofloxacin-based STR under NTP in Vietnam between April 2016 and June 2018 were included in the study. All the patients had a confirmed rifampicin resistance result by a genotypic (Xpert MTB/RIF assay) or a phenotypic test (culture and DST). STR was implemented on a pilot basis in the seven sites of the country which include Ha Noi, Ho Chi Minh, Can Tho, Da Nang, Nam Dinh, Soc Trang and Khanh Hoa. The number of patients enrolled depended on the number of treatment courses available with the NTP Vietnam. Patients with known resistance to second-line drugs, children aged <15 years, pregnant or breastfeeding women, those who received SLDs for more than a month, patients with hypersensitivity to any of the drugs used were excluded from receiving the STR.

2.4. Data Variables, Sources of Data and Data Collection

The data were extracted from the e-TB manager and reviewed. The data of each MDR-TB patient in the e-TB system was validated by referring to the original paper-based source (treatment card) for completeness and consistency. If there was any inconsistency between data in e-TB system and treatment card, we considered the treatment card as final and updated information into the e-TB system, before extracting for final analysis.

Table 2. Treatment outcome and adherence to follow up definitions among MDR-TB patients started on shorter treatment regimen in Vietnam, 2016–2018.

Term	Definitions
Cured	Treatment completed without evidence of failure and two consecutive negative cultures taken at least 30 days apart in the continuation phase
Treatment completed	Treatment completed without evidence of failure but there is no record of two consecutive negative cultures taken at least 30 days apart in the continuation phase.
Died	A patient who dies for any reason during the course of treatment
Failure	A patient who has a positive culture after ≥6 months of treatment (except for an isolated positive culture, which is a culture preceded by ≥1 and followed ≥2 negative cultures) OR A patient who after an initial conversion, has a reversion after ≥6 months of treatment with two consecutive positive cultures taken at-least 30 days apart OR evidence of additional acquired resistance to fluoroquinolones or second-line injectables OR treatment terminated or need for permanent change of at least two of anti-TB drugs due to adverse drug reactions
Lost to follow-up (LTFU)	A patient whose treatment was interrupted for ≥2 consecutive months
Not evaluated	A patient for whom no treatment outcome is assigned (this includes patients "transferred out" to another treatment unit and whose treatment outcome is unknown)
Treatment success	The sum of cured and treatment completed
Unsuccessful treatment outcomes	The sum of death, lost to follow-up, failure and not evaluated
Relapse	Patient after completing a course of STR and declared "cured" or "treatment completed", is diagnosed with another episode of confirmed RR-TB (based on Xpert MTB/RIF assay or culture) during a follow-up period of one year post-treatment
Adherence to follow-up	Number who had a follow-up smear or culture divided by number eligible for follow-up for a given month. Number eligible will be calculated by subtracting the number dead and lost to follow-up before the scheduled follow-up time.
Bacteriological effectiveness	This is calculated by dividing the number successfully treated by the number of patients who had a bacteriological outcome (excluding death, LTFU and not evaluated)

2.5. Analysis and Statistics

Data was analyzed using Stata (v14.1, Statacorp, College Station, TX, USA). We described the demographic and clinical profile of patients using mean (and standard deviation), or median (and interquartile range) or frequency (and proportions) as appropriate to the type of variable and the normality of distribution. Adherence to follow-up examination was summarized using frequencies and percentages (for each month of follow-up). We initially planned to use a Cox proportional hazards model, but the proportionality assumption was not met. Hence we used a log-binomial regression to assess the factors associated with unsuccessful outcomes and calculated adjusted relative risks and 95% confidence intervals to measure associations. Since we used an exploratory approach, all the variables used in unadjusted analysis were included in multivariable model. A p value of <0.05 was considered statistically significant in all analyses.

2.6. Ethics Approval

Permission to conduct the study and access the data was obtained from the NTP. Ethics approval was obtained from the Scientific Committee at National Lung Hospital, Ha Noi, Vietnam (approval number 08/19) and the Ethics Advisory Group of International Union Against Tuberculosis and Lung Disease, Paris, France (approval number 16/19). As this study involved a review of existing records, the ethics committees waived the need for individual informed consent.

3. Results

3.1. Baseline Sociodemographic and Clinical Characteristics

A total of 302 MDR-TB patients received a levofloxacin-based STR during the study period. Sociodemographic and clinical characteristics are shown in Table 3. The mean (SD) age of the patients was 41.0 (14.3) years and 224 (74.2%) were men. Of the 302 patients, 117 (38.7%) were new TB cases. Sputum smear was positive among 210 (69.5%) and sputum culture was positive among 199 (65.9%) patients. About half of the patients belonged to the 33–50 kg weight band. The mean (SD) body mass index was 18.7 (2.7) kg/m2. A total of 256 (84.7%) patients were tested for HIV and of them, three (1%) were HIV-positive and only one received antiretroviral therapy (ART).

3.2. Adherence to Monthly Follow-Up Visits

Figure 1 depicts the extent of adherence to the follow-up visits among the study participants. The adherence rate among the study participants was more than 95% for all nine months.

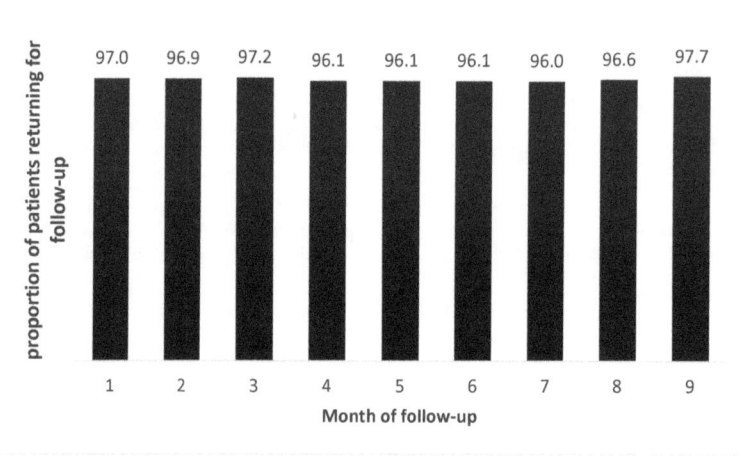

Figure 1. Monthly adherence to follow-up visit among MDR-TB patients who received STR from April 2016 to June 2018 in Vietnam. STR, Levofloxacin based shorter treatment regimen; MDR, Multi Drug resistance; NTP, National Tuberculosis Program.

3.3. Treatment Outcomes

Overall, 246 (81.5%) patients were cured and 13 (4.3%) completed the treatment (Table 4). Thus a total of 259 (85.8%) were successfully treated. Unsuccessful treatment outcomes such as treatment failure, loss to follow-up (LTFU) and death were observed in 16 (5.3%), 14 (4.6%) and 13 (4.3%) patients respectively. Among 275 patients with bacteriological outcome (excluding deaths and LTFU), 259 (94.2%) had a successful outcome. Patients who were culture positive at baseline had a worse outcome (due to higher failure rate) compared to those who were culture negative (Table 4).

HIV-positive TB patients, those aged ≥65 years and patients with a positive baseline culture were more likely to have unsuccessful outcomes (Table 5). The median (IQR) time to death from start of treatment was 95 (51–155) days and that to LTFU was 126 (57–214) days.

Table 3. Baseline sociodemographic and clinical characteristics of MDR-TB patients who received STR from April 2016 to June 2018 in Vietnam.

Characteristics	Number	(%)
Total	302	(100.0)
Age categories in years		
15–24	35	(11.6)
25–34	76	(25.2)
35–44	77	(25.5)
45–54	57	(18.9)
55–64	38	(12.6)
≥65	19	(6.2)
Gender		
Male	224	(74.2)
Female	78	(25.8)
Weight categories		
<33 kg	3	(1.0)
33–50 kg	133	(44.0)
51–70 kg	114	(37.8)
71–80 kg	3	(1.0)
Missing	49	(18.2)
Body Mass Index (kg/m^2)		
Underweight (<18.5)	113	(37.4)
Normal (18.5–22.9)	99	(32.8)
Overweight/obese (≥23.0)	17	(5.6)
Missing	73	(24.2)
HIV		
Negative	253	(84.0)
Positive	3	(1.0)
Missing	46	(15.0)
TB categories		
New	117	(38.7)
Relapse	112	(37.1)
Treatment after LTFU	2	(0.7)
Treatment after failure	60	(19.9)
Others	5	(1.6)
Missing	6	(2.0)
Sputum smear microscopy		
Negative	82	(27.1)
Scanty positive	35	(11.6)
1+ positive	77	(25.5)
2+ positive	45	(14.9)
3+ positive	53	(17.6)
Unknown/missing	10	(3.3)
Culture positive		
Negative	61	(20.2)
Positive	199	(65.9)
Unknown	42	(13.9)
Year of enrolment		
2016	99	(32.8)
2017	72	(23.8)
2018	131	(43.4)

Table 4. Treatment outcomes (disaggregated by baseline culture positivity) among patients who received STR from April 2016 to June 2018 in Vietnam.

Treatment Outcomes	Culture Positive		Culture Negative		Culture Unknown		Total	
	N	(%)	N	(%)	N	(%)	N	(%)
Total	199	(100)	61	(100)	42	(100)	302	(100)
Successful Outcomes	166	(83.4)	55	(90.2)	38	(90.5)	259	(85.8)
Cured	158	(79.4)	52	(85.3)	36	(85.7)	246	(81.5)
Completed	8	(4.0)	3	(4.9)	2	(4.8)	13	(4.3)
Unsuccessful Outcomes	33	(16.6)	6	(9.8)	4	(9.5)	43	(14.2)
Failure	13	(6.6)	1	(1.6)	2	(4.8)	16	(5.3)
LTFU	10	(5.0)	2	(3.3)	2	(4.8)	14	(4.6)
Died	10	(5.0)	3	(4.9)	0	(0)	13	(4.3)

Table 5. Factors associated with unsuccessful treatment outcome among MDR-TB patients who received STR from April 2016 to June 2018 in Vietnam.

Factors	Total	Unsuccessful Outcome		RR	(95%CI)	aRR	(95%CI)
	N	n	(%)#				
Total	302	43	(14.2)				
Age in years							
15–44	188	22	(11.7)	ref		ref	
45–64	95	17	(17.9)	1.53	(0.85–2.74)	1.57	(0.84–2.93)
≥ 65	19	4	(21.0)	1.80	(0.69–4.68)	2.97	(1.22–7.22) *
Gender							
Male	224	35	(15.6)	1.52	(0.74–3.14)	1.31	(0.71–2.44)
Female	78	8	(10.3)	ref		ref	
BMI							
Under weight (<18.5)	113	15	(13.3)	1.10	(0.54–2.23)	0.98	(0.46–2.06)
Normal (18.5–22.9)	99	12	(12.1)	ref		Ref	
Overweight/Obese (≥23.0)	17	3	(17.6)	1.46	(0.46–4.62)	1.52	(0.48–4.81)
Missing	73	13	(17.8)	1.47	(0.71–3.03)	1.82	(0.93–3.57)
TB category							
New	113	13	(11.5)	ref		ref	
Previously treated	175	26	(14.9)	1.29	(0.69–2.41)	1.22	(0.65–2.28)
Missing	6	2	(33.3)	2.9	(0.84–10.03)	3.21	(1.04–9.92) *
HIV							
Positive	3	2	(66.6)	4.82	(2.04–11.34)	7.14	(3.51–15.65) *
Negative	253	35	(13.8)	ref		ref	
Unknown	46	6	(13.0)	0.94	(0.42–2.11)	1.14	(0.52–2.51)
Year of enrolment							
2016	99	20	(20.2)	1.76	(0.95–3.27)	1.79	(0.99–3.25)
2017	72	8	(11.1)	0.97	(0.43–2.18)	0.90	(0.40–1.99)
2018	131	15	(11.4)	ref			
Culture							
Negative	61	6	(9.8)	ref		ref	
Positive	199	33	(16.6)	1.69	(0.74–3.83)	2.39	(1.09–5.24) *
Unknown	42	4	(9.5)	0.97	(0.29–3.22)	1.44	(0.41–4.99)

#Row percentage.RR, risk ratio; aRR– adjusted risk ratio; CI, confident interval; BMI, body mass index; * statistically significant.

3.4. One-Year TB Relapse

Relapse data was available only for patients enrolled in year 2016. Among 99 patients enrolled in 2016, 79 patients had a successful treatment outcome and were contacted after 12 months of treatment completion. Everyone was screened for TB symptoms and only four patients had cough of ≥2 weeks. Everyone was advised to undergo chest X-ray, though only 51 (64.5%) patients underwent chest X-ray. A total of 43 (84.3%) patients had either abnormality on chest X-ray and/or cough ≥2 weeks. 26 out of

43 (60.5%) patients were able to produce sputum samples, which were tested using Xpert MTB/RIF assay and sputum culture. None of the patients tested had TB.

4. Discussion

This is the first study from Vietnam providing information on treatment outcomes of a levofloxacin-based STR among RR/MDR-TB patients managed under routine program settings. Most studies on STR have used either gatifloxacin or moxifloxacin (in normal or high doses). Levofloxacin-based STR has rarely been used and the only other patient cohort that used a levofloxacin-based STR was from Bangladesh. Thus, this study adds to the limited global evidence on the effectiveness of levofloxacin-based STR.

One of the major limitations is that we are unable to report the information on adverse drug events in this paper. This is being assessed independently by the Vietnam Pharmacovigilance Center and will be reported in a separate paper. The other limitations include lack of information on acquired SLD resistance and relapses for the full cohort of patients.

We found high rates of treatment success (86%) and bacteriological effectiveness (94%) in our study with no relapse reported in a sub-group. This is comparable to the results of the Bangladesh cohort, which reported a bacteriological effectiveness of 96%. We were able to obtain these results using a relatively lower dose of levofloxacin (maximum dose of 1000 mg/day), unlike the study from Bangladesh which used a high-dose levofloxacin (maximum dose of 1750 mg/day) [25]. The treatment success rates obtained using STR are also higher than the reported treatment success rates among MDR-TB patients treated with long regimen in Vietnam (68%) [1]. This comparison should though be made with caution due to possible selection bias. First, not all eligible patients received STR, because the number of patients enrolled was limited by the number of treatment courses available [27]. Second, the profile of the patients treated with STR (where SLD resistance has been ruled out) is different from those treated with the long regimen (where there may be people with unknown SLD resistance). Despite these limitations, we feel the use of STR in carefully selected RR/MDR-TB patients have the potential to improve the overall treatment success rates in Vietnam.

The LTFU rates were low at 4.6% and this may probably be due to direct observation of treatment and several other patient-friendly initiatives which included free hospitalization, provision of food allowance and reimbursement of transport costs and use of patient clubs for improving treatment adherence. The death rates were also low at 4.3% and most of deaths occurred during the intensive phase (75%) indicating severity of illness.

Several factors were found to be associated with unsuccessful outcomes. We found that HIV-positive patients had higher risk of unfavorable outcomes. About 15% of the patients were not HIV tested and only one out of three HIV-positive TB patients received ART. This needs to be strengthened. In this era of 'test and treat' strategy, it is rather unacceptable to see gaps in ART uptake among HIV-infected MDR-TB patients at high risk of mortality. Also, for reasons that are unclear, people aged ≥65 years had a higher risk of unsuccessful outcome. The outcomes seem to be improving over the years with patients enrolled in 2017 and 2018 having better outcomes compared to 2016 cohort. This may be due to a higher proportion of heavily treatment-experienced chronic patients in the earlier cohort compared to the recent ones. A limitation of this analysis is that we did not have information on drug susceptibility status of other first line (like isoniazid, pyrazinamide, streptomycin) drugs at baseline, socio-economic status and education level of the patients and other confounders that may have accounted for unsuccessful outcomes. Also, the exact reasons for LTFU and death were not explored in this study. This needs to be studied in future research using qualitative research methods.

The evidence from this study adds to the debate on the choice of FLUOROQUINOLONE in the STR. A multi-country analysis published recently by Van Deun et al shows that patients treated with a Gatifloxacin-based STR (97%) had the best bacteriologic outcomes followed by Levofloxacin (96%) and Moxifloxacin (95%) [25]. The same ranking was also demonstrated in a pharmacodynamics study assessing the microbial killing capacity of fluoroquinolones [24]. Unfortunately, Gatifloxacin was withdrawn from the market in most countries in April 2006, following a study among elderly patients (mean age was 78 years and most of them had diabetes) from Canada which reported higher risk of dysglycaemia with use of Gatifloxacin [17]. These results have not been replicated since then [20]. We also feel that the results of this study cannot be applied directly to the MDR-TB patient cohorts in most settings, who are much younger and often undernourished with much less likelihood of dysglycaemia. Experience from Bangladesh and Niger shows that dysglycaemia is relatively rare (4–6%), and even when it occurs, is reversible, and can easily be diagnosed and managed under program settings [13]. In contrast, Moxifloxacin-based STRs have reported relatively lower bacteriological effectiveness (with higher rates of acquired FLUOROQUINOLONE resistance and relapses) and high incidence of QT prolongation (ranging from 11% to 15%) [15,28] and cardiac arrhythmias, which are more challenging to detect (requires an electrocardiogram) and manage in routine program conditions. This has led to calls for bringing back Gatifloxacin into the market and adding it in the WHO essential drugs list, which has generic versions available and is less expensive [18,19]. Levofloxacin is intermediate in effectiveness and seems to have a better safety profile: it is not associated with clinically significant QT prolongation (like Moxifloxacin) [23] and causes milder forms of dysglycemia when compared to Gatifloxacin. Thus, it seems levofloxacin is the next best alternative to be used in STRs, in the absence of Gatifloxacin.

In conclusion, we found high rates of treatment success among RR/MDR-TB patients treated with a levofloxacin-based regimen in Vietnam. These results add to the global body of knowledge about effectiveness of STRs in general and specifically on the effectiveness of levofloxacin-based STRs. These findings also vindicate the decision of Vietnam NTP to use Levofloxacin as the core drug in STRs. This regimen may be considered for nationwide scale-up after a detailed assessment of adverse drug events.

Author Contributions: Study design and protocol: L.T.N.A., A.M.V.K., G.R., T.H., T.T.H.T., G.H.N., H.B.N., N.V.N., M.Q., A.G.; Data collection: L.T.N.A.; Data analysis: L.T.N.A., A.M.V.K., G.R., T.H.; Drafting the paper: L.T.N.A., A.M.V.K., G.R.; Critical review and approval for submission: L.T.N.A., A.M.V.K., G.R., T.H., T.T.H.T., G.H.N., H.B.N., N.V.N. All authors have read and agreed to the published version of the manuscript.

Funding: The training programme, within which this paper was developed, was funded by the Department for International Development (DFID), London, UK. The data collection was funded by World Health Organization Representative Office in Vietnam. The funders had no role in study design, data collection and analysis, decision to publish or preparation of the manuscript. The open access publication costs were funded by the Department for International Development (DFID), UK and La Fondation Veuve Emile Metz-Tesch (Luxembourg).

Acknowledgments: This research was conducted through the Structured Operational Research and Training Initiative (SORT IT), a global partnership led by the Special Program for Research and Training in Tropical Diseases at the World Health Organization (WHO/TDR). The model is based on a course developed jointly by the International Union Against Tuberculosis and Lung Disease (The Union) and Medécins sans Frontières (MSF/Doctors Without Borders). The specific SORT IT program which resulted in this publication was jointly developed and implemented by: The Union South-East Asia Office, New Delhi, India; the Centre for Operational Research, The Union, Paris, France; The Union, Mandalay, Myanmar; The Union, Harare, Zimbabwe; MSF Luxembourg Operational Research (LuxOR); MSF Operational Center Brussels (MSF OCB); Jawaharlal Institute of Postgraduate Medical Education and Research (JIPMER), Puducherry, India; Post Graduate Institute of Medical Education and Research (PGIMER), Chandigarh, India; All India Institute of Medical Sciences (AIIMS), New Delhi, India; ICMR- National institute of Epidemiology, Chennai, India; Society for Education Welfare and Action (SEWA)—Rural, Jhagadia, India; Common Management Unit (AIDS, TB & Malaria), Ministry of National Health Services, Regulations and Coordination, Islamabad, Pakistan; and Kidu Mobile Medical Unit, His Majesty's People's Project and Jigme Dorji Wangchuck National Referral Hospital, Thimphu, Bhutan. We also thank the KNCV for the technical assistance offered during the conception and implementation of the pilot, and WHO for financial support for the conduct of this research.

Conflicts of Interest: The authors declare no conflict of interest.

References

1. World Health Organization (WHO). *Global Tuberculosis Report 2019*; World Health Organization: Geneva, Switzerland, 2019; Volume 66.

2. World Health Organization (WHO). *WHO Meeting Report of a Technical Expert Consultation: Non-Inferiority Analysis of Xpert MTB/RIF Ultra Compared to Xpert MTB/RIF*; WHO: Geneva, Switzerland, 2017.
3. Cepheid GeneXpert Omni. Available online: http://www.cepheid.com/en/genexpert-omni/47?view=products (accessed on 7 February 2019).
4. Xie, Y.L.; Chakravorty, S.; Armstrong, D.T.; Hall, S.L.; Via, L.E.; Song, T.; Yuan, X.; Mo, X.; Zhu, H.; Xu, P.; et al. Evaluation of a Rapid Molecular Drug-Susceptibility Test for Tuberculosis. *N. Engl. J. Med.* **2017**, *377*, 1043–1054.
5. World Health Organization (WHO). *The Use of Molecular Line Probe Assays for the Detection of Resistance to Second-Line Anti-Tuberculosis Drugs*; WHO: Geneva, Switzerland, 2016.
6. World Health Organization (WHO). *The Use of Bedaquiline in the Treatment of Multidrug-Resistant Tuberculosis Interim Policy Guidance*; WHO: Geneva, Switzerland, 2013.
7. World Health Organization (WHO). *The Use of Delamanid in the Treatment of Multidrug-Resistant Tuberculosis Interim Policy Guidance*; WHO: Geneva, Switzerland, 2014.
8. World Health Organization (WHO). *Rapid Communication: Key Changes to Treatment of Multidrug- and Rifampicin-Resistant Tuberculosis (MDR/RR-TB)*; WHO: Geneva, Switzerland, 2018.
9. World Health Organization (WHO). *WHO Treatment Guidelines for Drug-Resistant Tuberculosis. 2016 Updated*; WHO: Geneva, Switzerland, 2016.
10. Kuaban, C.; Noeske, J.; Rieder, H.L.; Aït-Khaled, N.; Abena Foe, J.L.; Trébucq, A. High effectiveness of a 12-month regimen for MDR-TB patients in Cameroon. *Int. J. Tuberc. Lung Dis.* **2015**, *19*, 517–524. [PubMed]
11. Piubello, A.; Harouna, S.H.; Souleymane, M.B.; Boukary, I.; Morou, S.; Daouda, M.; Hanki, Y.; Van Deun, A. High cure rate with standardised short-course multidrugresistant tuberculosis treatment in Niger: No relapses. *Int. J. Tuberc. Lung Dis.* **2014**, *18*, 1188–1194. [PubMed]
12. Aung, K.J.M.; Van Deun, A.; Declercq, E.; Sarker, M.R.; Das, P.K.; Hossain, M.A.; Rieder, H.L. Successful '9-month Bangladesh regimen' for multidrugresistant tuberculosis among over 500 consecutive patients. *Int. J. Tuberc. Lung Dis.* **2014**, *18*, 1180–1187.
13. Ahmad Khan, F.; Salim, M.A.H.; du Cros, P.; Casas, E.C.; Khamraev, A.; Sikhondze, W.; Benedetti, A.; Bastos, M.; Lan, Z.; Jaramillo, E.; et al. Effectiveness and safety of standardised shorter regimens for multidrug-resistant tuberculosis: Individual patient data and aggregate data meta-analyses. *Eur. Respir. J.* **2017**, *50*, 1–13.
14. Trébucq, A.; Schwoebel, V.; Kashongwe, Z.; Bakayoko, A.; Kuaban, C.; Noeske, J.; Hassane, S.; Souleymane, B.; Piubello, A.; Ciza, F.; et al. Treatment outcome with a short multidrug-resistant tuberculosis regimen in nine African countries. *Int. J. Tuberc. Lung Dis.* **2018**, *22*, 17–25. [PubMed]
15. Nunn, A.J.; Phillips, P.P.J.; Meredith, S.K.; Chiang, C.Y.; Conradie, F.; Dalai, D.; Van Deun, A.; Dat, P.T.O.; Lan, N.; Master, I.; et al. A trial of a shorter regimen for rifampin-resistant tuberculosis. *N. Engl. J. Med.* **2019**, *380*, 1201–1213. [PubMed]
16. Nunn, A.J.; Rusen, I.D.; Van Deun, A.; Torrea, G.; Phillips, P.P.J.; Chiang, C.Y.; Squire, S.B.; Madan, J.; Meredith, S.K. Evaluation of a standardized treatment regimen of anti-tuberculosis drugs for patients with multi-drug resistant tuberculosis (STREAM): Study protocol for a randomized controlled trial. *Trials* **2014**, *15*, 1–10.
17. Park-Wyllie, L.Y.; Juurlink, D.N.; Kopp, A.; Shah, B.R.; Stukel, T.A.; Stumpo, C.; Dresser, L.; Low, D.E.; Mamdani, M.M. Outpatient Gatifloxacin Therapy and Dysglycemia in Older Adults. *N. Engl. J. Med.* **2006**, *354*, 1352–1361. [PubMed]
18. Chiang, C.Y.; Van Deun, A.; Rieder, H.L. Gatifloxacin for short, effective treatment of multidrug-resistant tuberculosis. *Int. J. Tuberc. Lung Dis.* **2016**, *20*, 1143–1147. [PubMed]
19. Chiang, C.Y.; Trébucq, A.; Piubello, A.; Rieder, H.L.; Van Deun, A. Should gatifloxacin be included in the model list of essential medicines? *Eur. Respir. J.* **2018**, *51*, 1702329. [PubMed]
20. Chou, H.W.; Wang, J.L.; Chang, C.H.; Lee, J.J.; Shau, W.Y.; Lai, M.S. Risk of severe dysglycemia among diabetic patients receiving levofloxacin, ciprofloxacin, or moxifloxacin in Taiwan. *Clin. Infect. Dis.* **2013**, *57*, 971–980. [PubMed]
21. Cox, V.; Tommasi, M.; Sa, A.; Furin, J.; Quelapio, M.; Koura, K.G.; Padanilam, X.; Dravniece, G.; Piubello, A. QTc and anti-tuberculosis drugs: A perfect storm or a tempest in a teacup? Review of evidence and a risk assessment. *Int. J. Tuberc. Lung Dis.* **2018**, *18*, 0423.

22. Van Deun, A.; Decroo, T.; Piubello, A.; de Jong, B.C.; Lynen, L.; Rieder, H.L. Principles for constructing a tuberculosis treatment regimen: The role and definition of core and companion drugs. *Int. J. Tuberc. Lung Dis.* **2018**, *22*, 239–245. [PubMed]
23. Makaryus, A.N.; Byrns, K.; Makaryus, M.N.; Natarajan, U.; Singer, C.; Goldner, B. Effect of ciprofloxacin and levofloxacin on the QT interval: Is this a significant "clinical" event? *South. Med. J.* **2006**, *99*, 52–56. [PubMed]
24. Deshpande, D.; Pasipanodya, J.G.; Mpagama, S.G.; Bendet, P.; Srivastava, S.; Koeuth, T.; Lee, P.S.; Bhavnani, S.M.; Ambrose, P.G.; Thwaites, G.; et al. Levofloxacin Pharmacokinetics/Pharmacodynamics, Dosing, Susceptibility Breakpoints, and Artificial Intelligence in the Treatment of Multidrug-resistant Tuberculosis. *Clin. Infect. Dis.* **2018**, *67*, S293–S302. [PubMed]
25. Van Deun, A.; Decroo, T.; Kuaban, C.; Noeske, J.; Piubello, A.; Aung, K.J.M.; Rieder, H.L. Gatifloxacin is superior to levofloxacin and moxifloxacin in shorter treatment regimens for multidrug-resistant TB. *Int. J. Tuberc. Lung Dis.* **2019**, *23*, 965–971. [PubMed]
26. Piubello, A.; Aït-khaled, N.; Caminero, J.A.; Chiang, C.Y.; Dlodlo, R.A.; Fujiwara, P.I.; Heldal, E.; Koura, K.; Monedero, I.; Roggi, A.; et al. *Field Guide for the Management of Drug-Resistant Tuberculosis*, 1st ed.; International Union Against Tuberculosis and Lung Disease: Paris, France, 2018.
27. Id, G.B.; Nhung, N.V.; Skrahina, A.; Ndjeka, N.; Id, D.F.; Zignol, M. Advances in clinical trial design for development of new TB treatments—Translating international tuberculosis treatment guidelines into national strategic plans: Experiences from Belarus, South Africa, and Vietnam. *PLoS Med.* **2019**, *16*, e1002896.
28. Khan, F.; Ismail, M.; Khan, Q.; Ali, Z. Moxifloxacin-induced QT interval prolongation and torsades de pointes: A narrative review. *Expert Opin. Drug Saf.* **2018**, *17*, 1029–1039. [PubMed]

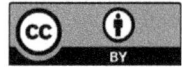

© 2020 by the authors. Licensee MDPI, Basel, Switzerland. This article is an open access article distributed under the terms and conditions of the Creative Commons Attribution (CC BY) license (http://creativecommons.org/licenses/by/4.0/).

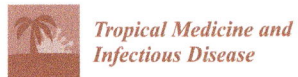 *Tropical Medicine and Infectious Disease*

Article

Can the High Sensitivity of Xpert MTB/RIF Ultra Be Harnessed to Save Cartridge Costs? Results from a Pooled Sputum Evaluation in Cambodia

Monyrath Chry [1], Marina Smelyanskaya [2], Mom Ky [1], Andrew J Codlin [2], Danielle Cazabon [3], Mao Tan Eang [4] and Jacob Creswell [2,*]

1. Cambodia Anti-Tuberculosis Association, Phnom Penh and Cambodia, Phnom Penh 12250, Cambodia; rath@thecata.org.kh (M.C.); momky@thecata.org.kh (M.K.)
2. Stop TB Partnership, TB REACH, 1218 Geneva, Switzerland; marinas@stoptb.org (M.S.); andrew.codlin@gmail.com (A.J.C.)
3. McGill International TB Centre, McGill University, Montreal, QC H4A 3J1, Canada; danielle.cazabon@gmail.com
4. National Center for Tuberculosis and Leprosy Control (CENAT), Phnom Penh 12250, Cambodia; mao@online.com.kh
* Correspondence: jacobc@stoptb.org

Received: 17 December 2019; Accepted: 11 February 2020; Published: 15 February 2020

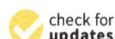

Abstract: Despite the World Health Organization recommending the use of rapid molecular tests for diagnosing tuberculosis (TB), uptake has been limited, partially due to high cartridge costs. Other infectious disease programs pool specimens to save on diagnostic test costs. We tested a sputum pooling strategy as part of a TB case finding program using Xpert MTB/RIF Ultra (Ultra). All persons were tested with Ultra individually, and their remaining specimens were also grouped with 3–4 samples for testing in a pooled sample. Individual and pooled testing results were compared to see if people with TB would have been missed when using pooling. We assessed the potential cost and time savings which different pooling strategies could achieve. We tested 584 individual samples and also grouped them in 153 pools for testing separately. Individual testing identified 91 (15.6%) people with positive Ultra results. One hundred percent of individual positive results were also found to be positive by the pooling strategy. Pooling would have saved 27% of cartridge and processing time. Our results are the first to use Ultra in a pooled approach for TB, and demonstrate feasibility in field conditions. Pooling did not miss any TB cases and can save time and money. The impact of pooling is only realized when yield is low.

Keywords: TB diagnostics; laboratory methods; case detection; Xpert Ultra

1. Introduction

Early and increased diagnosis of tuberculosis (TB) remains a key part of the World Health Organization's (WHO) End TB Strategy [1]. Almost a decade ago, the introduction of the Xpert MTB/RIF (Xpert) assay presented an opportunity to transform the ways in which TB is diagnosed and care is delivered. The Xpert assay can rapidly detect resistance to rifampicin and has demonstrated superior sensitivity in diagnosing pulmonary [2], extrapulmonary [3], and pediatric [4] TB when compared to its century-old predecessor—acid fast bacilli (AFB) smear microscopy. Xpert testing has led to an increase in multidrug-resistant (MDR) TB detection [5] and an increase in bacteriological confirmation of drug-sensitive TB where it has been scaled up [6,7]. Xpert was initially only recommended as the initial test for TB in people living with HIV and those at increased risk of MDR-TB [8]. However, the WHO now recommends that Xpert be used as a first-line test for everyone with presumptive TB [9].

Yet, in many settings, especially in countries with a high burden of TB, AFB smear microscopy remains the mainstay of TB testing despite missing 40%–50% of people with TB [10,11].

The high cost of installing and operationalizing a GeneXpert testing network is one of the reasons for the continued low levels of Xpert coverage in many countries. Despite an over 40% reduction in Xpert cartridge costs [12], the current USD 9.98 price per cartridge is still high when compared to AFB smear microscopy [13]. The impact of Xpert's higher cost is particularly acute in high TB burden countries, most of which are still highly dependent on international donor resources to fund their TB response [14]. The Global Fund to Fight AIDS, TB, and Malaria (Global Fund) is currently the largest donor for TB internationally, and has invested significantly in the procurement of GeneXpert systems and Xpert cartridges [14]. However, even with the Global Fund's substantial support for Xpert cartridges and machine procurement, the resources needed to test all people with presumptive TB using a rapid molecular test at current prices are well beyond available funding levels.

To reduce spending on diagnostic testing, other infectious disease programs have utilized a pooled testing strategy. Pooling involves combining several specimens of blood, urine, sputum etc. into a common pool which is then tested. If the pooled test result is negative, all of the individual specimens are declared as negative without being individually retested. If the pooled test result is positive, at least one of the pool's component specimens is positive, and all of the component specimens should be individually retested to identify which ones are positive and negative. This testing strategy has been used for screening in blood banks [15] and sexually transmitted infections including HIV [16–18]. While a pooled sputum specimen strategy has the potential to bring about significant cost savings, the technique has not been readily adopted as a TB testing strategy. However, the few studies which have been published on this approach show its promise. A study evaluating the pooled Xpert testing strategy in Nigeria showed that it would have identified 96% of individual specimens containing TB bacteria and could have reduced Xpert costs and usage by 30% [19]. Another evaluation in South Africa showed that Xpert identified 100% of pools containing AFB smear-positive specimens, but just 76% of pools with AFB smear-negative, culture-positive specimens [20].

One major concern with the testing of pooled sputum specimens from multiple people with presumptive TB is that TB bacteria may be diluted to a concentration which is below the detection limits of the Xpert assay, thus producing false negative results. Sputum pooling should be more feasible if the sensitivity of the test is very high, i.e., can identify disease even in diluted samples. In 2018, Cepheid released its next-generation Xpert test—the Xpert MTB/RIF Ultra (Ultra) assay. Initial reports indicate that the Ultra assay can improve sensitivity compared with Xpert. The Ultra assay improved sensitivity by 5% among all people enrolled. However, among groups with lower bacterial burdens such as individuals with smear-negative, culture-positive results and people with HIV infection, the gains in sensitivity were much higher (17% and 12% respectively) [21].

Cambodia is a high TB burden country, and only an estimated 58% of people with TB in the country are diagnosed and have access to treatment [14]. The 2011 Cambodia TB prevalence survey identified that the largest gaps are in diagnosing patients over 55 years of age, and highlighted that many people with TB presented no symptoms [22]. In addition, in rural areas access to TB testing and specifically molecular testing is limited. Our intervention took this into consideration, focusing on people aged 55 years and older, providing chest X-ray (CXR) screening in addition to a symptom screen, and bringing a mobile lab to rural areas to test with Ultra. Results presented in this paper evaluate the concordance of test results and potential cost implications of a pooling strategy embedded within an active case finding intervention in rural Cambodia using Ultra.

2. Methods

2.1. Active Case Finding Setting

This evaluation of a pooled testing strategy was embedded within an active TB case finding (ACF) initiative in Cambodia funded by the Stop TB Partnership's TB REACH initiative. The Cambodia

Anti-Tuberculosis Association (CATA) organized a series of mobile CXR screening days in rural operational districts (ODs) from 12 June 2017 to 16 May 2018. The TB screening activities were aimed at individuals aged 55 years and older, similar to what has been described elsewhere [23]. In addition to engaging older individuals, screenings also targeted other villagers who reported cough and/or other TB symptoms. Village Health Support Groups (VHSG) conducted door to door outreach and sensitization activities prior to testing days and referred older individuals and people presenting with TB symptoms and aged under 55 to local health centers. On testing days, the mobile unit equipped with an X-ray machine and a 4-module GeneXpert, was parked at the local health center to facilitate testing. As part of the larger ACF initiative, we pooled samples using Ultra on a subset of individuals as the Ultra assay was in limited supply and we wanted to evaluate the feasibility of using a pooled method in future ACF events. On certain days, the team would agree to use Ultra cartridges and pool the samples. During the other screening days, the ACF initiative proceeded as described.

All older individuals (55 years and over) attending the screening day received a CXR and those under 55 years of age were verbally screened and eligible for CXR if they reported a current cough of any duration. CXR results were read by a trained radiologist and classified into four categories: (1) active TB; (2) presumptive TB/suspected TB abnormality; (3) healed TB/other lung abnormality; (4) CXR normal. Any individual with an abnormal CXR and people with a reported cough were eligible for sputum collection, so CXR was not used to screen people out of the testing algorithm but rather for classification.

2.2. Pooling of Specimens and Ultra Testing

Sputum specimens were individually tested using the Ultra assay according to the manufacturer's instructions with a 1:2 sputum to reagent ratio. Individuals with an error, invalid, or no result in the Ultra test outcome were retested to obtain a valid positive or negative result for the detection of *Mycobacterium tuberculosis* (MTB). The individual result was used as the definitive result for this analysis and for treatment decisions. Anyone with an MTB-positive result including trace call results on the individual Ultra test were eligible for appropriate TB treatment according to the National Center for Tuberculosis and Leprosy Control (CENAT) guidelines.

Remnant specimens, a mixture of sputum, and Ultra Sample Reagent which was left over after individual Ultra testing were grouped into batches of three or four containers. We attempted to group remnant specimens from individuals by their CXR classification so that a pooled specimen would contain remnant specimens from all CXR abnormal or all CXR normal individuals. However, this was not always possible due to delays with CXR reading and variance in the types of participants who were mobilized and tested each day. Thus, a small subset of remnant specimen groupings contained a mix of individuals with CXR abnormal and CXR normal results. At the testing site, we took 0.75mL of each individual specimen (to ensure that 2.25–3mL of total specimen was available for testing) which was deposited into a new sputum container and swirled inside the container for 5–10 seconds to mix the sample thoroughly. The pooled specimen was then tested using the Ultra assay according to the manufacturer's instructions.

2.3. Data Management and Analysis

Individual and pooled Ultra test results were entered into a database using the coding scheme recommended by the Global Laboratory Initiative [24]. The data were cleaned, checked for inconsistencies, and analyzed using R version 3.5.1 (R Foundation for Statistical Computing, Vienna, Austria). We calculated the agreement between the individual Ultra results and the pooled Ultra results for detecting MTB, as well as rifampicin (RIF) resistance. We calculated the theoretical cost and time savings that could be achieved by using a pooling strategy with different approaches. For the analysis, the cost of an Ultra cartridge was estimated to be USD 10.36 (including shipping and import fees) based on shipping information from the Global Drug Facility at Stop TB Partnership, and we used a 90 minute runtime for the Ultra assay [25].

2.4. Ethical Approval

Approval to conduct this programmatic intervention was obtained from the National Center for Tuberculosis and Leprosy Control CENAT. Verbal consent was obtained; individuals were able to refuse participation at any point during the screening, diagnosis, or treatment process without compromising their access to the routine care provided by CENAT. De-identified data were used for this analysis.

3. Results

3.1. Individual Test Results

A total of 584 individual Ultra results were analyzed. These individuals were 50.5% (n = 295) female and 49.5% (n = 289) male; 89% (n = 522) were aged 55 and above. Basic demographic, screening, and TB risk characteristics are presented in Table 1. In total, 91 individual samples (15.6%) had positive results on Ultra. These included 3 (3.3%) with rifampicin resistance, 1 (1.1%) whose rifampicin result was indeterminate, and 13 (14.3%) individuals who had trace calls (see Table 2). Of the 13 people with individual trace call results, two had previous treatment history and 10 had CXRs that were read as 'active TB' or 'presumptive TB'.

Table 1. Demographic information for individuals tested with Xpert MTB/RIF Ultra (Ultra).

Individuals Tested with Ultra	n = 584	%	Individuals with Positive Ultra Results	n = 91	%
Sex			*Sex*		
Female	295	50.5%	Female	31	34%
Male	289	49.5%	Male	60	66%
Age			*Age*		
<35	9	1.5%	<35	2	2.2%
35<55	53	9.1%	35<55	16	17.6%
>55	522	89%	>55	71	78.0%
Employment Status			*Employment Status*		
Elderly/retired	78	13.4%	Elderly/retired	13	14.3%
Factory worker	2	0.3%	Farmer	55	60.4%
Farmer	413	70.7%	Government officer	2	2.2%
Government officer	9	1.5%	Unemployed	12	13.2%
Unemployed	59	10.1%	Own business	4	4.4%
Own Business	10	1.7%	Private company staff	1	1.1%
Private company staff	1	0.2%	Seller	4	4.4%
Seller	12	2.1%			
Symptom screen			*Symptom Screen*		
Any symptom	556	95.2%	Any symptom	86	94%
No symptoms	28	4.8%	No symptoms	5	5.5%
Cough alone	43	7.7%	Cough alone	5	5.5%
Chest X-ray (CXR) Results			*CXR Results*		
CXR active	115	19.7%	CXR active	47	51.6%
CXR presumptive Tuberculosis (TB)	112	19.2%	CXR presumptive TB	29	31.9%
CXR healed	45	7.7%	CXR healed TB	13	14.3%
CXR normal	301	51.5%	CXR normal	2	2.2%
CXR other	11	1.9%			
Other TB risk factors			*Other TB risk factors*		
TB contact	84	14.4%	TB contact	17	18.7%
PLHIV	5	0.86%	PLHIV	2	2.2%
Diabetes	34	5.8%	Diabetes	10	11.0%

A total of 227 individuals had a CXR reading of "active TB" or "presumptive TB" and 73 (32%) out of this subgroup were identified as being MTB-positive. By contrast, among 301 samples from individuals with normal CXR readings, only 2 were identified as being MTB-positive. Overall, samples from pools with CXR abnormalities (active, presumptive, or healed TB) contributed 78 out of 91 (85.7%) of all the MTB-positive cases (Table 3).

Table 2. Test results of individual and pooled Ultra testing in Cambodia.

Xpert MTB/RIF Ultra Result	Individual Results n = 584		Pooled Results n = 153	
Negative (N)	493	84.4%	80	52.3%
MTB with rifampicin resistance detected (RR)	3	0.5%	0	0%
MTB with no rifampicin resistance detected (T)	74	12.7%	59	38.6%
MTB with low rifampicin resistance detected (Ti)	1	0.2%	3	1.9%
MTB trace detected (TT)	13	2.2%	11	7.2%

MTB = *Mycobacterium tuberculosis*.

Table 3. Pooled and individual results *.

Results from Pooled Testing		Results from Individual Testing		
		Total	MTB-Negative	MTB-Positive
All pooled specimens	153	584	493 (84.4%)	91 (15.6%)
MTB-Negative	80 (52.3%)	304	304 (100.0%)	0 (0.0%)
MTB-Positive	73 (47.7%)	280	189 (67.5%)	91 (32.5%)
RIF-Resistant MTB	0 (0.0%)	-	-	3 (3.3%)
Pooled specimens with all CXR abnormal individuals	66	253	175 (69.2%)	78 (30.8%)
MTB-Negative	6 (9.1%)	22	22 (4.5%)	0 (0.0%)
MTB-Positive	60 (90.9%)	231	153 (31.0%)	78 (85.7%)
RIF-Resistant MTB	0 (0.0%)	-	-	3 (3.3%)
Pooled specimens with mixed CXR results	17	64	55 (85.9%)	9 (14.1%)
MTB-Negative	6 (35.3%)	23	23 (4.7%)	0 (0.0%)
MTB-Positive	11 (64.7%)	41	30 (6.1%)	11 (12.1%)
RIF-Resistant MTB	0 (0.0%)	-	-	0 (0.0%)
Pooled specimens with all CXR normal individuals	70	267	265 (99.3%)	2 (0.7%)
MTB-Negative	68 (97.1%)	259	259 (52.5%)	0 (0.0%)
MTB-Positive	2 (2.9%)	8	6 (1.2%)	2 (2.2%)
RIF-Resistant MTB	0 (0.0%)	-	-	0 (0.0%)

MTB = *Mycobacterium tuberculosis*, CXR = chest X-ray, RIF = Rifampicin. * For individual results based on CXR group and MTB-negative or MTB-positive pooled sample percentages refer to the proportion of the total positive or negative results.

3.2. Pooled Results

There were in total 153 pooled samples that were tested. There were 28 pools with three individual samples and 125 pools containing four individual samples. Of the 153 pools, 66 were made from samples from individuals with abnormal CXR readings ("active TB", "healed TB", "presumptive TB", "other CXR abnormality"), 70 were made from samples from individuals with normal CXR readings, and 17 were mixed (any CXR abnormality and CXR normal reading). Among the 153 pooled samples, 73 (47.7%) had an MTB-positive result and 80 were negative on Ultra. Of the 80 negative pools, 68 (85%) came from CXR normal sample pools and the other 12 came from CXR abnormal or mixed pools. All the 304 individual test results from the 80 negative pools tested negative, indicating 100% agreement, and no extra testing would have resulted in more MTB-positive individuals being detected. Table 2 summarizes the pooled and individual testing results.

All 73 pools with an MTB-positive result had at least one MTB-positive individual test result, indicating that no false positive results were found in the pooled samples. Seventeen (23%) of the 73 positive pools contained multiple individual samples that tested for MTB-positive; 16 pools had two positive individual samples, one pool had three individual positive samples, and the remaining 56 had one individual positive sample. Out of the 73 positive pools, 60 (82.2%) came from pools composed of CXR abnormal samples, 11(15.1%) came from pools composed of mixed abnormal and normal samples, and 2 (2.7%) came from pools containing only CXR normal samples.

Of these 73 pooled samples with MTB-positive results, 0 had rifampicin-resistant results, 3 (5.4%) had rifampicin indeterminate results, and 11 (15%) were trace calls (Table 2). The three pools with MTB-positive results with no rifampicin resistance detected, revealed rifampicin resistance in the individual sample during individual testing. These rifampicin-resistant samples would not have been missed, since all the positive pools were retested. The 11 pooled samples with trace call results contained 44 individual results of which 12 were positive. Among the 12 positive individuals, seven samples were MTB-positive, four had trace calls (two of these came from the same pool), and one was MTB-positive with indeterminate rifampicin resistance.

3.3. Cartridge Savings and Impact of CXR Screening on Costs

If this ACF initiative had only conducted direct, individual Ultra testing, it would have used 584 Ultra cartridges, requiring 876 h of testing run times and costing a total of USD 6050 for cartridge procurement (Table 4). Our pooled testing approach used 153 Ultra cartridges to test pooled specimens (229 h of testing run times and a cost of USD 1585). An additional 280 cartridges would have been required for all of the individual specimens from the 73 pooled specimens with positive results (420 h of testing run times and a cost of USD 2900). In total, 433 Ultra cartridges would have been used representing a 26.8% reduction in Ultra cartridge costs and testing workloads with no loss of yield.

Table 4. Cost and time estimates utilizing different testing approaches.

	Total Cartridges Used	Cartridges Saved (%)	Total Time Required (Hours)	Time Saved (Hours)	Total Cost	Costs Saved (%)
Individual approach	584	-	876		USD 6050	
Pooled approach	433	151 (27)	650	226	USD 4485	1565 (27)
Hybrid approach *	382	202 (35)	573	300	USD 3958	2092 (35)

* Hybrid approach includes pooling only those with normal CXR readings and individually testing those with CXR abnormalities.

Since the pooled specimens containing only individual samples from people with abnormal CXR results had such a high positivity rate (90.9%), the testing strategy which results in the largest reductions in costs and testing workloads is actually a hybrid strategy, where individuals with an abnormal CXR have their individual sputum specimens directly tested and where the sputum specimens from people with normal CXR results are pooled before testing. If this hybrid strategy had been used, we would have directly tested 304 specimens from people with abnormal results, 70 pooled specimens from people with normal CXR results, and just 8 individual specimens after a positive pooled test result. This testing strategy would have required a total of 382 Ultra cartridges (573 h of testing run time and USD 3958 in cartridge costs representing a 34.6% reduction in Ultra cartridge costs and testing workloads compared to direct, individual Ultra testing).

4. Discussion

Our study adds to a very small but intriguing body of literature on the possible benefits of pooling sputum specimens for testing with molecular assays. This is the first published account of pooling with the Ultra assay. Two previous studies from Nigeria [19] and South Africa [20] used the Xpert MTB/RIF assay, and while both of these studies document efficiency gains in terms of workloads and cost, they both also reported missing a small number of people with TB in the pooled specimens (only 4% in Nigeria, but pooling missed 24% of smear-negative, culture-positive samples in the South African study). By contrast, our pooled testing evaluation with the Ultra assay showed that no pooled specimens with a negative result contained individual MTB-positive samples.

The detection limit of the Ultra assay is much lower than Xpert MTB/RIF, which should reduce the risk that pooling dilutes TB DNA below the detection limits of the molecular assay [21]. A controlled laboratory study using spiked sputum demonstrated the Xpert MTB/RIF cycle threshold increased with the dilution of TB DNA, but still managed to detect the majority of MTB-positive specimens [26].

It would logically follow that the use of Ultra would improve these results and that pooling with Ultra may advance the access of more individuals to rapid TB testing.

Pooling has been successfully used in other infectious diseases, but the premise of pooling is only useful when testing yields are low. Our study demonstrates that if the pre-test probability of a positive result is high then pooling multiple specimens together only increases the likelihood that the pooled result will be positive, resulting in more instead of less testing. For example, at an MTB-positive prevalence of 16%, the probability of having a pooled test result combining four individuals which contains at least one positive individual specimen is roughly 50%, and at 10% prevalence, this probability drops to 34%. When MTB-positive prevalence is 5%, more than 80% of pooled specimens will contain all negative individual specimens, offering high rates of expected savings. A laboratory-controlled study on pooling samples found good results of Xpert when pooling up to 11 negative samples with one spiked positive sample, but the authors noted the logistical challenges of using more than four or five samples for each pool [26].

The relationship between the pre-test probability and potential cartridge and time savings is then modified by the use of other screening tools, such as CXR. Because the interpretation of CXR findings can greatly increase the pre-test probability of having MTB-positive results [27], programs may want to stratify the results of the CXR to maximize cost savings. In our study, the potential cost and cartridge savings of a universal pooling strategy was 26%, but even greater efficiencies could have been achieved by pooling only CXR normal samples, which would have saved 35% of costs and cartridges. Implementing a pooled testing approach would have been more costly if used among those with a CXR reading of active TB because so many pools would have required retesting. While traditional CXR equipment is expensive and challenging to take on the road, the advent of digital CXR with computer-aided reading (CAR) has the potential to reach wider population groups and be less costly over time. The ability of CAR to provide continuous probability scores gives TB screening and testing programs an opportunity to develop cutoff scores to maximize the cost savings for pooling based on the artificial intelligence scoring [28].

The main concern regarding the use of Ultra has been its loss of specificity when testing samples from individuals with previous history of TB treatment [21]. In our sample of 584 individuals, 11 samples demonstrated the lowest bacillary burden also identified as "trace call". Of these 11, only two individuals had been previously treated. These two had symptoms and CXR readings that suggested TB, so the decision was made to treat both individuals for TB. The other nine individuals had symptoms and suggestive CXR readings and were also treated for TB. More research and presentation of results on trace calls need to be published and considered to help programs understand the implications of trace call results. We were not able to conduct culture as part of the study nor do we have data on the cycle thresholds, which could potentially provide more insight into the trace call results as well as support the individual testing results, which is a limitation.

Our study accompanied an active TB screening and testing campaign, and we thus had access to a large quantity of samples and could test them almost immediately after obtaining them. We also had experienced lab technicians working on labeling and testing the samples who received specific training on the pooling protocols, and had access to an adequate number of GeneXpert systems. While the study was done in field conditions, certain preparations were made to ensure rapid testing of the samples and adequate recording of pooled and individual test results, including additional oversight from the research team, special templates for grouping samples and documenting results, and end of the day reports. Our time savings analysis does not take into account the extra time it takes to prepare a pooled sample, but this time was not considered substantial. Attempts at pooling specimens to increase laboratory throughput may consider such challenges as long-term storage of samples, inconsistencies in recording, contamination, and staff shortages. Thus, if the practice is to be adopted, further training and refining of procedures have to be developed. Our results are promising regarding the feasibility of pooling samples with Ultra in field conditions. Programs can decide to attempt to use pooling based on the expected or observed yield in the tested population.

5. Conclusions

Our results demonstrate that pooling specimens from multiple individuals with presumptive TB for testing with the Ultra assay is feasible in field conditions. Individual test results showed that no one with TB nor rifampicin resistance would have been missed by employing a pooled testing approach. TB screening and testing campaigns testing a large number of individuals with an expected low yield can pool sputum samples to save both cartridge costs and time. Additional research is needed to document results across different settings to ensure that similar results are obtainable, and that pooling use can be used at a larger scale.

Author Contributions: Conceptualization M.C., M.K., A.J.C. and J.C.; Methodology, M.C., M.K., A.J.C. and J.C.; Formal Analysis, M.C., M.S., D.C. and J.C.; Investigation, M.C., M.K. and M.T.E.; Resources, M.C., M.K. and M.T.E.; Data Curation, M.C., M.K., D.C., M.S. and J.C.; Writing—Original Draft Preparation, J.C., M.S., D.C. and A.J.C.; Writing—Review & Editing, M.C., M.S., M.K., A.J.C., D.C., M.T.E. and J.C.; Supervision, M.C., M.K. and M.T.E.; Funding Acquisition, M.C. and M.K. All authors have read and agreed to the published version of the manuscript.

Funding: The work was implemented under a TB REACH Wave 5 grant provided by Stop TB Partnership. TB REACH is generously supported by Global Affairs Canada—Grant 7062544.

Acknowledgments: The work was implemented under a TB REACH Wave 5 grant provided by Stop TB Partnership. TB REACH is generously supported by Global Affairs Canada. The authors would like to recognize the work of the Village Health Support Groups for their work in mobilizing the communities for the tuberculosis screening. MS, AJC & JC are members of Stop TB Partnership. The interpretations articulated in this work are their personal views and not necessarily represent the Stop TB Partnership's official position.

Conflicts of Interest: The authors declare that there is no conflict of interest.

References

1. World Health Organization. The End TB Strategy. 2015. Available online: https://www.who.int/tb/End_TB_brochure.pdf?ua=1 (accessed on 7 March 2018).
2. Steingart, K.R.; Schiller, I.; Horne, D.J.; Pai, M.; Boehme, C.C.; Dendukuri, N. Xpert® MTB/RIF assay for pulmonary tuberculosis and rifampicin resistance in adults. *Cochrane Database Syst. Rev.* **2014**, CD009593. [CrossRef]
3. Tortoli, E.; Russo, C.; Piersimoni, C.; Mazzola, E.; Dal Monte, P.; Pascarella, M.; Borroni, E.; Mondo, A.; Piana, F.; Scarparo, C.; et al. Clinical validation of Xpert MTB/RIF for the diagnosis of extrapulmonary tuberculosis. *Eur. Respir. J.* **2012**, *40*, 442–447. [CrossRef] [PubMed]
4. Nicol, M.P.; Workman, L.; Isaacs, W.; Munro, J.; Black, F.; Eley, B.; Boehme, C.C.; Zemanay, W.; Zar, P.H.J. Accuracy of the Xpert MTB/RIF test for the diagnosis of pulmonary tuberculosis in children admitted to hospital in Cape Town, South Africa: A descriptive study. *Lancet Infect. Dis.* **2011**, *11*, 819–824. [CrossRef]
5. World Health Organization. Global Tuberculosis Report 2013. 2013. Available online: https://apps.who.int/iris/bitstream/handle/10665/91355/9789241564656_eng.pdf?sequence=1&isAllowed=y (accessed on 22 November 2019).
6. Creswell, J.; Rai, B.; Wali, R.; Sudrungrot, S.; Adhikari, L.M.; Pant, R.; Pyakurel, S.; Uranw, D.; Codlin, A.J. Introducing new tuberculosis diagnostics: The impact of Xpert(®) MTB/RIF testing on case notifications in Nepal. *Int. J. Tuberc. Lung Dis.* **2015**, *19*, 545–551. [CrossRef] [PubMed]
7. Correction: Impact of Replacing Smear Microscopy with Xpert MTB/RIF for Diagnosing Tuberculosis in Brazil: A Stepped-Wedge Cluster-Randomized Trial. Available online: https://journals.plos.org/plosmedicine/article?id=10.1371/journal.pmed.1001928 (accessed on 25 November 2019).
8. World Health Organization. Automated Real-Time Nucleic Acid Amplification Technology for Rapid and Simultaneous Detection of Tuberculosis and Rifampicin Resistance: Xpert Mtb/Rif System: Policy Statement. 2011. Available online: https://apps.who.int/iris/handle/10665/44586 (accessed on 22 November 2019).
9. World Health Organization. Automated Real-Time Nucleic Acid Amplification Technology for Rapid and Simultaneous Detection of Tuberculosis and Rifampicin Resistance: Xpert Mtb/Rif Assay for the Diagnosis of Pulmonary and Extrapulmonary TB in Adults and Children: Policy Update. 2013. Available online: https://apps.who.int/iris/handle/10665/112472 (accessed on 22 November 2019).

10. Pinyopornpanish, K.; Chaiwarith, R.; Pantip, C.; Keawvichit, R.; Wongworapat, K.; Khamnoi, P.; Supparatpinyo, K.; Sirisanthana, T. Comparison of Xpert Mtb/Rif Assay and the Conventional Sputum Microscopy in Detecting Mycobacterium Tuberculosis in Northern Thailand. Tuberculosis Research and Treatment. 2015. Available online: https://www.hindawi.com/journals/trt/2015/571782/ (accessed on 22 November 2019).
11. Cuevas, L.E.; Al-Sonboli, N.; Lawson, L.; Yassin, M.A.; Arbide, I.; Al-Aghbari, N.; Sherchand, J.B.; Al-Absi, A.; Emenyonu, E.N.; Merid, Y.; et al. LED fluorescence microscopy for the diagnosis of pulmonary tuberculosis: A multi-country cross-sectional evaluation. *PLoS Med.* **2011**, *8*, e1001057. [CrossRef] [PubMed]
12. Albert, H.; Nathavitharana, R.R.; Isaacs, C.; Pai, M.; Denkinger, C.M.; Boehme, C.C. Development, roll-out and impact of Xpert MTB/RIF for tuberculosis: What lessons have we learnt and how can we do better? *Eur. Respir. J.* **2016**, *48*, 516–525. [CrossRef] [PubMed]
13. Pantoja, A.; Kik, S.V.; Denkinger, C.M. Costs of novel tuberculosis diagnostics–will countries be able to afford it? *J. Infect. Dis.* **2015**, *211*, S67–S77. [CrossRef] [PubMed]
14. World Health Organization. Global Tuberculosis Report 2019. 2019. Available online: https://apps.who.int/iris/bitstream/handle/10665/329368/9789241565714-eng.pdf?ua=1 (accessed on 22 November 2019).
15. Mine, H.; Emura, H.; Miyamoto, M.; Tomono, T.; Minegishi, K.; Murokawa, H.; Yamanaka, R.; Yoshikawa, A.; Nishioka, K. High throughput screening of 16 million serologically negative blood donors for hepatitis B virus, hepatitis C virus and human immunodeficiency virus type-1 by nucleic acid amplification testing with specific and sensitive multiplex reagent in Japan. *J. Virol. Methods* **2003**, *112*, 145–151. [CrossRef]
16. Emmanuel, J.C.; Bassett, M.T.; Smith, H.J.; Jacobs, J.A. Pooling of sera for human immunodeficiency virus (HIV) testing: An economical method for use in developing countries. *J. Clin. Pathol.* **1988**, *41*, 582–585. [CrossRef] [PubMed]
17. Morandi, P.A.; Schockmel, G.A.; Yerly, S.; Burgisser, P.; Erb, P.; Matter, L.; Sitavanc, R.; Perrin, L. Detection of human immunodeficiency virus type 1 (HIV-1) RNA in pools of sera negative for antibodies to HIV-1 and HIV-2. *J. Clin. Microbiol.* **1998**, *36*, 1534–1538. [CrossRef] [PubMed]
18. Lindan, C.; Mathur, M.; Kumta, S.; Jerajani, H.; Gogate, A.; Schachter, J.; Moncada, J. Utility of pooled urine specimens for detection of Chlamydia trachomatis and Neisseria gonorrhoeae in men attending public sexually transmitted infection clinics in Mumbai, India, by PCR. *J. Clin. Microbiol.* **2005**, *43*, 1674–1677. [CrossRef] [PubMed]
19. Abdurrahman, S.T.; Mbanaso, O.; Lawson, L.; Oladimeji, O.; Blakiston, M.; Obasanya, J.; Dacombe, R.; Adams, E.R.; Emenyonu, N.; Sahu, S.; et al. Testing Pooled Sputum with Xpert MTB/RIF for Diagnosis of Pulmonary Tuberculosis To Increase Affordability in Low-Income Countries. *J. Clin. Microbiol.* **2015**, *53*, 2502–2508. [CrossRef] [PubMed]
20. Zishiri, V.; Chihota, V.; McCarthy, K.; Charalambous, S.; Churchyard, G.J.; Hoffmann, C.J. Pooling sputum from multiple individuals for Xpert® MTB/RIF testing: A strategy for screening high-risk populations. *Int. J. Tuberc. Lung Dis.* **2015**, *19*, 87–90. [CrossRef] [PubMed]
21. World Health Organization. WHO Meeting Report of a Technical Expert Consultation: Non-Inferiority Analysis of Xpert Mtb/Rif Ultra Compared to Xpert Mtb/Rif. 2017. Available online: https://apps.who.int/iris/bitstream/handle/10665/254792/WHO-HTM-TB-2017.04-eng.pdf?sequence=1 (accessed on 1 November 2019).
22. National Tuberculosis Control Program, Kindgon of Cambodia. *Second National Tuberculosis Prevalence Survey, Cambodia 2011*; National Centre for TB and Leprosy Control: Phnom Penh, Cambodia, 2011.
23. Codlin, A.J.; Monyrath, C.; Ky, M.; Gerstel, L.; Creswell, J.; Eang, M.T. Results from a roving, active case finding initiative to improve tuberculosis detection among older people in rural cambodia using the Xpert MTB/RIF assay and chest X-ray. *J. Clin. Tuberc. Mycobact. Dis.* **2018**, *13*, 22–27. [CrossRef] [PubMed]
24. Global Laboratory Initiative. Module 4: Recording and Reporting. GLI Training Package: Diagnostic Network Strengthening and Xpert MTB/RIF (Ultra) Implementation. 2018. Available online: http://www.stoptb.org/wg/gli/assets/documents/M4%20Recording%20&%20reporting.zip (accessed on 22 November 2019).
25. Stop TB Partnership. Xpert®MTB/RIF and Ultra Techincal Information Note. 2019. Available online: http://www.stoptb.org/assets/documents/gdf/drugsupply/Xpert_info_note.pdf (accessed on 25 November 2019).
26. Ho, J.; Jelfs, P.; Nguyen, P.T.B.; Sintchenko, V.; Fox, G.J.; Marks, G.B. Pooling sputum samples to improve the feasibility of Xpert® MTB/RIF in systematic screening for tuberculosis. *Int. J. Tuberc. Lung Dis.* **2017**, *21*, 503–508. [CrossRef] [PubMed]

27. van't Hoog, A.H.; Onozaki, I.; Lonnroth, K. Choosing algorithms for TB screening: A modelling study to compare yield, predictive value and diagnostic burden. *BMC Infect. Dis.* **2014**, *14*, 532. [CrossRef] [PubMed]
28. Qin, Z.Z.; Sander, M.S.; Rai, B.; Titahong, C.N.; Sudrungrot, S.; Laah, S.N.; Adhikari, L.M.; Carter, E.J.; Puri, L.; Codlin, A.J.; et al. Using artificial intelligence to read chest radiographs for tuberculosis detection: A multi-site evaluation of the diagnostic accuracy of three deep learning systems. *Sci. Rep.* **2019**, *9*, 1–10. [CrossRef] [PubMed]

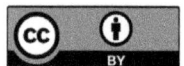

© 2020 by the authors. Licensee MDPI, Basel, Switzerland. This article is an open access article distributed under the terms and conditions of the Creative Commons Attribution (CC BY) license (http://creativecommons.org/licenses/by/4.0/).

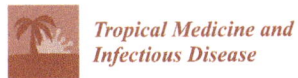

Article

An Innovative Public–Private Mix Model for Improving Tuberculosis Care in Vietnam: How Well Are We Doing?

Thuong Do Thu [1,*], Ajay M. V. Kumar [2,3,4], Gomathi Ramaswamy [5], Thurain Htun [6], Hoi Le Van [1], Luan Vo Nguyen Quang [7], Thuy Dong Thi Thu [7], Andrew Codlin [7], Rachel Forse [7], Jacob Crewsell [8], Hoi Nguyen Thanh [9], Hai Nguyen Viet [1], Huy Bui Van [1], Hoa Nguyen Binh [1,3,10] and Nhung Nguyen Viet [1,10]

1. Vietnam Integrated Center for Tuberculosis and Respirology Research, Vietnam National Lung Hospital, Vietnam Tuberculosis Control Programme, Hanoi 100000, Vietnam; hoilv@yahoo.com (H.L.V.); nguyenviethai.hmu@gmail.com (H.N.V.); vhcapri@gmail.com (H.B.V.); nguyenbinhhoatb@yahoo.com (H.N.B.); VietNhung@yahoo.com (N.N.V.)
2. International Union Against Tuberculosis and Lung Disease, South-East Asia Office, New Delhi 110016, India; akumar@theunion.org
3. International Union Against Tuberculosis and Lung Disease, Paris 75006, France
4. Yenepoya Medical College, Yenepoya (Deemed to be University), Mangaluru 575018, India
5. National Centre of Excellence and Advanced Research on Anemia Control, Centre for Community Medicine, All India Institute of Medical Sciences, New Delhi 110029, India; gmthramaswamy@gmail.com
6. International Union Against Tuberculosis and Lung Disease, Mandalay 05021, Myanmar; thurainhtun30111990@gmail.com
7. Friends for International Tuberculosis Relief, Ho Chi Minh City 700000, Vietnam; luan.vo@tbhelp.org (L.V.N.Q.); thuy.dong@tbhelp.org (T.D.T.T.); Andrew.codlin@tbhelp.org (A.C.); rachel.forse@tbhelp.org (R.F.)
8. Stop TB Partnership, Geneva 1218, Switzerland; jacobc@stoptb.org
9. Haiphong International General Hospital, Haiphong 180000, Vietnam; hoinguyenthanhbm@gmail.com
10. Hanoi Medical University, Hanoi 100000, Vietnam
* Correspondence: thuthuong0308@gmail.com; Tel.: +84-343007914 (ext. 235); Fax: +84-438326162

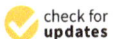

Received: 14 November 2019; Accepted: 10 February 2020; Published: 14 February 2020

Abstract: To improve tuberculosis (TB) care among individuals attending a private tertiary care hospital in Vietnam, an innovative private sector engagement model was implemented from June to December 2018. This included: (i) Active facility-based screening of all adults for TB symptoms (and chest x-ray (CXR) for those with symptoms) by trained and incentivized providers, with on-site diagnostic testing or transport of sputum samples, (ii) a mobile application to reduce dropout in the care cascade and (iii) enhanced follow-up care by community health workers. We conducted a cohort study using project and routine surveillance data for evaluation. Among 52,078 attendees, 368 (0.7%) had symptoms suggestive of TB and abnormalities on CXR. Among them, 299 (81%) were tested and 103 (34.4%) were diagnosed with TB. In addition, 195 individuals with normal CXR were indicated for TB testing by attending clinicians, of whom, seven were diagnosed with TB. Of the 110 TB patients diagnosed, 104 (95%) were initiated on treatment and 97 (93%) had a successful treatment outcome. Given the success of this model, the National TB Programme is considering to scale it up nationwide after undertaking a detailed cost-effectiveness analysis.

Keywords: public–private mix model; public–private partnership; missing cases; operational research; SORT IT

1. Introduction

Tuberculosis (TB) is the leading cause of mortality from a single infectious agent globally, accounting for 1.45 million deaths annually [1]. The global community has pledged to end the TB epidemic by 2030 [2]. While there has been progress, the rate of decline of TB incidence has been modest at ~2% each year [3]. At this rate, we will not be able to realize the goal of ending TB by 2030. To accelerate progress, the Stop TB Partnership recommends that countries should strive to achieve 90-(90)-90 targets (diagnosing 90% of all people with TB including 90% among key populations and treating 90% of them successfully) [4].

One of the major challenges in TB control is "missing cases". Globally, of the 10 million people estimated to have developed TB in 2018, only 7 million were notified [1]. The gap of 3 million includes people who are not diagnosed and treated, and those managed in the private health sector, but not notified to National Tuberculosis Programmes (NTP).

A multi-country study found that in more than 60% of TB patients, the private sector was the first point of contact, yet the proportion of cases notified to NTP was less than 10% [5]. Also, health care provision in the private sector is not standardized and poorly regulated in many countries. These may lead to delays in diagnosis and treatment, improper case management, increased risk of developing drug resistance, disease transmission, and catastrophic health expenditure [6]. Engagement and collaboration with private sector in those countries where a large proportion of care seeking is sought with private providers in critical [2].

Vietnam is one among the 30 high TB burden countries and has strong private health care sector. It is estimated that approximately 50% of TB patients seek initial care in the private sector before visiting the public health system [7,8]. In 2018, only 57% of estimated incident cases were notified to NTP, meaning there is no information about the rest of the patients and a majority of these may be receiving care in the private sector [1]. Mirroring the global picture, previous studies from Vietnam have also reported mismanagement in diagnosis and treatment of TB in the private health sector [9–11]. All these findings underline the need to engage the private health care providers in Vietnam's TB care and prevention efforts.

To engage the private sector, several public–private mix (PPM) models have been implemented by the Vietnam NTP since 2001. One such model involved training of private health care providers and strengthening referral mechanisms between the private sector and NTP. This yielded an increase in overall TB case detection rate of Ho Chi Minh City by 7% [12], but there were several gaps. About 30% of presumptive TB patients referred to NTP for sputum microscopy did not reach the diagnostic facility and nearly 60% of the patients diagnosed were lost to follow-up before starting treatment. Of those started on treatment, only 60% successfully completed it [13].

To address these gaps, a new model was implemented in Haiphong International General Hospital (HIGH) in 2018 as part of the TB REACH-funded Zero TB Vietnam initiative. This model included three unique components: (i) active facility-based screening of all adults for TB symptoms (and chest x-ray (CXR) for those with symptoms) by trained and incentivized providers, with on-site diagnostic testing or transport of sputum samples, (ii) an innovative mobile application to reduce dropout in the care cascade and iii) enhanced follow-up care through engagement of a local network of community health workers (CHWs). However, this model has not yet been systematically evaluated. In this study, we aimed to evaluate the performance of this private sector engagement model by tracking the cascade of tuberculosis care among the individuals attending the HIGH in Vietnam from June to December 2018.The specific objectives were to determine, (i) the number (proportion) with presumptive tuberculosis and among them, the number (proportion) who were investigated for tuberculosis (ii) the number (proportion) diagnosed with tuberculosis and initiated on treatment (iii) the treatment outcomes among those initiated on treatment and (iv) the delays involved at different steps of the care cascade.

2. Materials and Methods

2.1. Study Design

This was a cohort study involving analysis of routine surveillance data.

2.2. Setting

Vietnam is a South-East Asian country with a population of 93.7 million. The country is divided into 63 provinces, which are further divided into districts, communes, and sub-communes. About 34.4% of the population live in urban areas and about 10% people are below the poverty line [14]. Healthcare services are provided by both public and private sectors.

2.2.1. TB Control Program in Vietnam

The public health facilities for TB care and prevention are managed either directly by the NTP or indirectly through the Department of Health (DOH). Under the NTP, TB diagnosis, treatment, and control activities are carried out by the national level unit, 63 TB and lung disease hospitals or provincial TB units, and 707 TB management units (TBMUs) at the district level.

2.2.2. PPM Models

There has been significant progress in the implementation of PPM initiatives for TB care and prevention in Vietnam. There are four types of PPM models. PPM Model 1 entails the referral of presumptive TB patients identified by the private providers to NTP for further evaluation. PPM Model 2 encompasses the diagnosis of TB and referral to the NTP. PPM Model 3 entails the provision of directly-observed treatment. PPM model 4 provides both diagnostic and treatment services similar to a TBMU. Private providers participating in PPM initiatives are trained for TB screening, diagnosis with sputum smear microscopy, and recording and reporting as per NTP guidelines.

2.2.3. PPM Model at HIGH

PPM model at HIGH is similar to the model 4. HIGH was chosen for the intervention because it is the biggest tertiary care private hospital in Haiphong province (considered a poor-performing province by NTP) and there was political commitment from the director of the HIGH to collaborate with the NTP. Three departments from the HIGH (Endocrinology, Otolaryngology, and Respiratory medicine) were targeted for systematic screening. These three departments were chosen because they were expected to account for the majority of pulmonary presumptive TB patients visiting HIGH. The doctors and nurses of these departments were trained on the management of TB cases as per NTP guidelines and were given incentives for TB screening, diagnosis and treatment, and systematic recording and reporting.

A total of 110 USD of fixed allowance per month was provided to the hospital. About 70 USD was provided every month for conducting the monthly review meetings and printing of forms. In addition, performance-based incentives were provided: (i) 0.5 USD given to the nurse for each chest X-ray conducted (ii) 1 USD given to the nurse for each sample transported for Xpert MTB/RIF testing (iii) 2 USD given to the doctor for each patient diagnosed with TB (iv) 3 USD given to the doctor for each TB patient completing treatment. The project was supervised by a focal point (@45 USD per month), PPM coordinator (@130 USD per month) and a PPM supervisor (@130 USD per month). These incentives were on top of the salaries they received. Thus, the total cost incurred on the project for six months was 4100 USD. All costs were incurred in Viet Nam Dong and translated to USD based on the average exchange rate during the implementation period.

All out-patients attending the selected departments (Endocrinology, Otolaryngology, and Respiratory medicine) were screened for symptoms such as cough, hemoptysis, chest pain and dyspnea, fever, fatigue and unexpected weight loss. Individuals who had any of these symptoms or who had a history of contact with TB were requested to undergo chest radiography. Contacts were defined as people living in the same household with a TB patient for at least two nights per week during the last 6 months. Individuals with symptoms suggestive of TB or exposure to a person with TB and parenchymal abnormalities suggestive of TB on chest X-ray were considered 'presumptive TB' and evaluated further for bacteriologic confirmation. The chest radiographs of the presumptive TB patients were examined by the radiologists at HIGH. Patients with TB symptoms and no abnormalities on chest X-ray were also offered tests for bacteriological confirmation based on the discretion of the attending physician. Spot sputum samples (without induction) were collected from the patients. For those who were not able to produce sputum, bronchoscopy was suggested by the treating physician and the bronchial washings were used for further testing. Patients with lymphadenopathy were referred for histopathological examination for confirmation of TB.

Individuals with a positive symptom screen were counselled by the treating physician about the different diagnostic tests available and their costs and were offered one of more of the following tests in the hospital for bacteriological confirmation: (i) Transcription Concerted Reaction (TRC) Ready 80 test (ii) sputum microscopy (iii) liquid culture and drug susceptibility test for first-line drugs. The TRC Ready 80 test is an automated molecular assay designed to detect mycobacterium tuberculosis (MTB) complex 16S rRNA present in clinical specimens (pulmonary and extra-pulmonary) or culture isolates. This has been described in greater detail elsewhere [15]. Though this test not endorsed by the WHO yet, it has been approved for use in Vietnam by the MOH for diagnosing TB. Chest X-ray screening and diagnostic tests at HIGH were paid by the patient at the following rates: 3 USD for chest X-ray, 3 USD for microscopy, 12 USD for culture, and 36 USD for TRC Ready 80. For patients unable to afford these tests, sputum samples were collected and transported to a nearby NTP facility for TB diagnosis using Xpert MTB/RIF assay, which was offered free of charge. The nurses in HIGH were trained on the procedures of sputum collection in falcon tubes, packaging and transportation in cold chain to the nearby NTP facility (which is located at a distance of 1.5 kms from HIGH). Nurses transported the sputum specimens in-person at the end of the day to the NTP facility.

Patients diagnosed with TB disease either through bacteriologic confirmation or clinical diagnosis were initiated on anti-TB treatment at an NTP facility or a private health facility of the patient's choice. Patients diagnosed with drug-susceptible TB were treated with first-line drugs and those with rifampicin resistance were referred to the NTP's provincial TB hospital for further evaluation. While drugs were provided free of charge to the patients at NTP facilities, patients paid out of pocket at private health facilities.

The CHWs were notified immediately after the diagnosis of each TB patient for linkage to care and follow-up from treatment start until completion. CHWs were motivated volunteers identified from each commune and recruited to support TB care and prevention activities in the Zero TB project (under funding support of TB REACH grant). They were mostly women and received formal training (for two days by NTP staff) on screening, counselling, follow-up care and support of TB patients. In the community, CHWs performed household contact tracing and counseling on treatment adherence and infection control. They received performance-based incentives as part of another project and did not receive any specific incentives for the project described in this study. The study's case definitions and treatment outcomes were in accordance with NTP and WHO guidelines.

2.2.4. Recording and Reporting

All patient details were entered in the ACIS (Access to Care Information System, Clinton Health Access Initiative/TechUp, Vietnam) application, a data collection and case management tool for persons with presumptive TB in the community. Dedicated tablets with preinstalled software were procured and provided to the nurses and were trained on its use. Nurses captured data about presumptive TB patients using this tool. This application is bi-directionally connected with the NTP's electronic recording and reporting system, the Vietnam TB Information Management Electronic System (VITIMES), which enabled the electronic referral of case files of persons with suspected or diagnosed TB to NTP facilities.

2.3. Study Population

All patients aged ≥15 years attending the three outpatient departments of HIGH between 24 June, 2018 and 31 December, 2018 were included.

2.4. Data Variables and Sources

Case-level covariates were extracted from the ACIS and VITIMES systems. These included TB symptoms, chest X-ray findings, diagnostic test results, diagnoses, treatment initiation dates, and treatment outcomes. We used name, age, and sex to merge the two databases, but removed names and other personal identifiers before analysis to ensure confidentiality of data.

2.5. Analysis and Statistics

Data was analyzed using Stata software (version 14.0, Statacorp, Texas, TX, USA). We have depicted the cascade of care in the form of a flowchart with dropouts at every stage summarized as frequencies and percentages. To calculate the proportion with presumptive TB, we chose all people attending the three out patient departments (OPD) as the denominator, because information on who among them were screened was not available in the records. TB treatment outcomes were categorized into successful (cured and treatment completed) and unsuccessful (failure, lost to follow-up, died, not evaluated) outcomes. The time delays between screening, undergoing diagnostic test and initiation of treatment were summarized using median and interquartile range (IQR). Factors associated with 'not getting investigated for TB' among presumptive TB patients were assessed using adjusted risk ratios and 95% confidence intervals (CI) calculated using log-binomial regression. We also assessed factors associated with TB diagnosis among patients investigated for TB using the same effect measures.

2.6. Ethics Approval

Ethics approval was obtained from the Scientific Ethics Committee of the National Lung Hospital, Hanoi, Vietnam (approval number 954/QD-BVPTU) and the Ethics Advisory Group of the International Union Against Tuberculosis and Lung Disease, Paris, France (approval number 22/19). Since this was a review of existing records with no direct interaction with human participants, the need for individual informed consent was waived by the ethics committees. Confidentiality of the patient data was ensured by (i) providing restricted access to patient data only to the research team (ii) using password protection to access the electronic files and (iii) removing all the personal identifiers (such as name, address, phone number) before analysis.

3. Results

A total of 52,078 adults attended the three OPDs at HIGH during the study period. Of them, 2739 (5.3%) had either symptoms suggestive of TB or were exposed to someone with TB. Of these, 1372 (50%) were male and mean (SD) age was 49 (17) years. The profile of these patients is depicted in Table 1. Cough was the predominant symptom present in 2240 (82%) individuals, followed by chest pain and dyspnea in 1926 (70%), fatigue in 1521 (56%) and fever in 418 (15%). Contact with a person with TB was reported by 34 (1%) patients.

Table 1. Socio-demographic and clinical profile of people with tuberculosis (TB) symptoms or contact history attending the Haiphong International General Hospital in Vietnam, from June to December 2018.

Characteristic	Number	(%)
Total	2739	(100.0)
Age group (years)		
15-44	1170	(42.7)
45-64	1084	(39.6)
≥ 65	485	(17.7)
Gender		
Male	1372	(50.1)
Female	1367	(49.9)
Self-reported HIV status		
Negative	596	(21.8)
Positive	4	(0.1)
Unknown	2139	(78.1)
Self-reported diabetes		
No	1699	(62.0)
Yes	161	(5.9)
Unknown	879	(32.1)
Presenting symptoms		
Cough (any duration) *	2240	(81.8)
Chest pain and dyspnea	1926	(70.3)
Fever	418	(15.3)
Fatigue	1521	(55.5)
Sweating at night	51	(1.9)
Unexplained weight loss	133	(4.9)
History of contact of TB	34	(1.2)

HIV = Human immunodeficiency virus infection, TB = Tuberculosis; * 125 of these patients had hemoptysis.

3.1. Cascade of Care

The cascade of care among study participants is depicted in Figure 1. Of the 2739 symptomatic individuals or those with contact history, 368 (13.4%) had chest X-ray suggestive of TB and were identified as having presumptive TB (i.e., 368/52,078 [0.7%]). Of these, 299 (81%) underwent at least one of the diagnostic tests for TB and 103 (34.4%) were diagnosed with TB. In addition, 195/2371 (8%) patients with normal chest X-ray also underwent tests for TB, of whom 7 (4%) cases were diagnosed. In total, 110 people were diagnosed with TB. Of the 110 TB patients, 92 (84%) had bacteriologically confirmed TB and the rest were either clinically diagnosed or based on the results of other histopathological investigations. Of them, 104 (95%) were initiated on anti-TB treatment. All, except one, received treatment at an NTP health facility. Two individuals had rifampicin-resistant TB and were referred to the Provincial Lung Hospital and subsequently treated with second-line drugs. The majority of patients had pulmonary TB (n = 98, 88%), while the remaining 12 patients had extra-pulmonary TB (09 pleural TB and 3 lymph node TB).

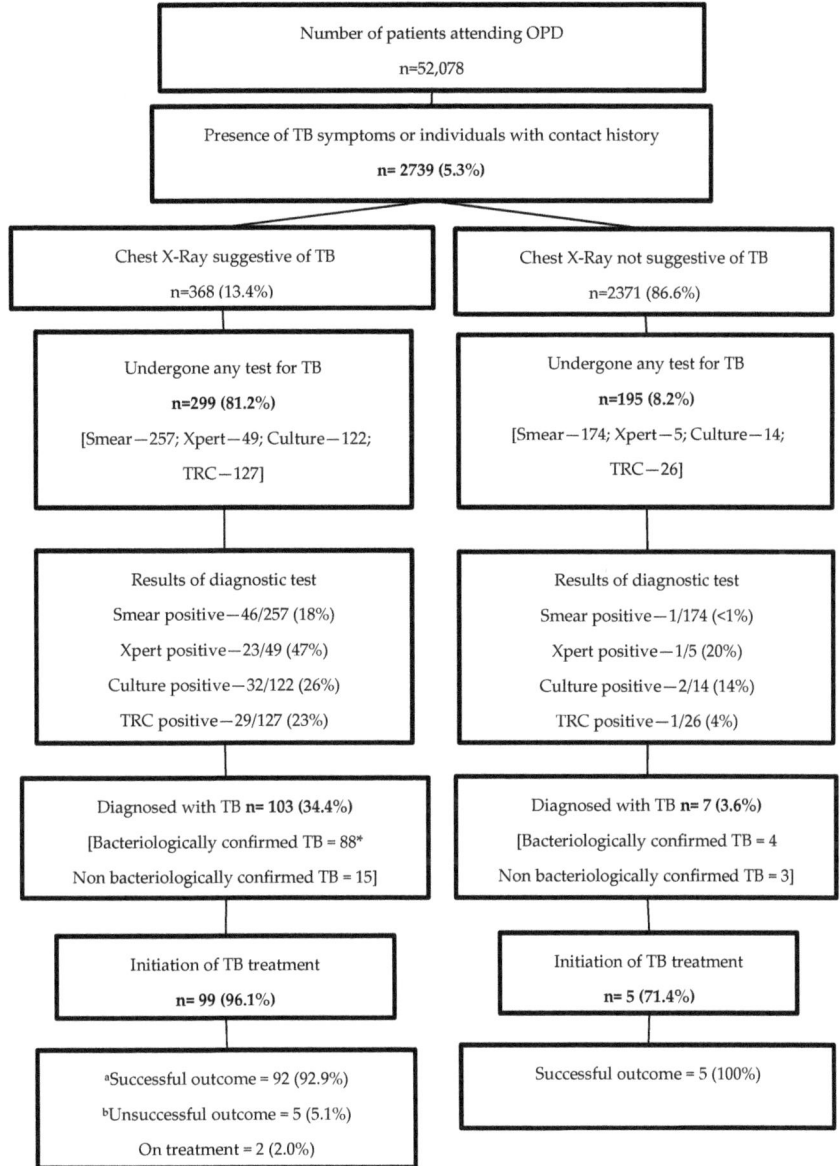

Figure 1. Cascade of tuberculosis care (from screening to treatment outcome) among the patients attending the Haiphong International General Hospital in Vietnam, from June to December 2018. OPD = Outpatient Department; TB = tuberculosis; TRC = transcription concerted reaction. a: successful outcome: cured and treatment completed. B: unsuccessful outcome: death, loss to follow-up, failure, and not evaluated. *Two individuals had rifampicin resistance and were started on second-line drugs.

3.2. Factors Associated with 'Not Getting Tested for TB'

Of the 368 individuals with presumptive TB, 69 (19%) did not undergo any diagnostic testing. Patients without cough, without fever, without night sweats, without weight loss, and without TB contact history were less likely to be tested for TB (Table 2).

Table 2. Factors associated with 'not getting tested for TB' among presumptive TB patients attending the Haiphong International General Hospital in Vietnam, from June to December 2018.

Characteristic	Total	Not Tested for TB# n	(%)	RR	(95%CI)	aRR	(95%CI)
Total	368	69	(18.7)	-		-	
Age (years)							
15–44	138	27	(19.6)	0.89	(0.52–1.51)	1.06	(0.97–1.08)
45–64	148	24	(16.2)	0.74	(0.43–1.28)	1.01	(0.96–1.07)
65 and above	82	18	(21.9)	1		1	
Gender							
Male	203	30	(14.8)	1		1	
Female	165	39	(23.6)	1.60	(1.04–2.46)	1.02	(0.99–1.06)
Self-reported HIV status							
Negative	195	24	(12.3)	-		-	
Positive	1	0	(0.0)	-		-	
Unknown	172	45	(25.2)	-		-	
Self-reported diabetes							
No	280	49	(17.5)	0.72	(0.39–1.34)	1.03	(0.94–1.13)
Yes	37	9	(24.3)	1		1	
Unknown	51	11	(21.6)	0.89	(0.41–1.92)	1.17	(1.06–1.28)
Cough							
No	68	20	(29.4)	1.80	(1.15–2.82)	1.07	(1.02–1.28)
Present	300	49	(16.3)	1		1	
Fever							
No	267	59	(22.1)	2.23	(1.19–4.19)	1.20	(1.12–1.29)
Present	101	10	(9.9)	1		1	
Chest pain and dyspnea							
No	128	23	(18.0)	0.94	(0.60–1.47)	0.99	(0.96–1.04)
Present	240	46	(19.2)	1		1	
Fatigue							
No	159	38	(23.9)	1.61	(1.05–2.47)	0.95	(0.91–0.98)
Present	209	31	(14.8)	1		1	
Night sweat							
No	343	68	(19.8)	4.96	(0.72–34.21)	1.37	(1.08–1.77)
Present	25	1	(4.0)	1		1	
Weight loss *							
No	311	65	(20.9)	2.93	(1.11–7.71)	1.38	(1.20–1.62)
Present	56	4	(7.1)	1		1	
Contact history of TB							
No	355	67	(18.8)	1.23	(0.34–4.47)	1.31	(1.01–1.71)
Present	13	2	(15.4)	1		1	

* Data missing for one; HIV = human immunodeficiency virus; TB = tuberculosis; CI = confidence interval; aRR = adjusted relative risk.

3.3. Factors Associated with TB Diagnosis

Of the 494 patients who underwent diagnostic tests, 110 (22%) were diagnosed with TB. Patients with self-reported diabetes and those with weight loss had a significantly higher chance of getting diagnosed with TB (Table 3).

Table 3. Factors associated with diagnosis of TB among the patients who were investigated in the Haiphong International General Hospital in Vietnam, from June to December 2018.

Characteristic	Number Tested	Confirmed TB[#] n	(%)	RR	(95%CI)	aRR	(95%CI)
Total	494	110	(22.3)	-		-	
Age (years)							
15–44	191	45	(23.6)	1.32	(0.81–2.16)	1.59	(0.93–2.72)
45–64	202	47	(23.3)	1.31	(0.80–2.13)	1.33	(0.80–2.21)
65 and above	101	18	(17.8)	1		1	
Gender							
Male	267	63	(23.6)	1.14	(0.82–1.59)	1.01	(0.73–1.39)
Female	227	47	(20.7)	1		1	
Self-reported HIV status							
Negative	218	70	(32.1)	-		-	
Positive	2	0	(0.0)	-		-	
Unknown	274	40	(14.6)	-		-	
Self-reported diabetes							
No	375	83	(22.1)	1		1	
Yes	40	16	(40.0)	1.81	(1.18–2.76)	2.13	(1.31–3.48)
Unknown	79	11	(13.9)	0.63	(0.35–1.12)	0.78	(0.44–1.39)
Cough							
No	66	10	(15.1)	1		1	
Present	428	100	(23.4)	1.54	(0.85–2.80)	1.42	(0.82–2.46)
Fever							
No	355	69	(19.4)	1		1	
Present	139	41	(29.5)	1.52	(1.08–2.13)	1.32	(0.95–1.83)
Chest pain and dyspnea							
No	162	44	(27.2)	1		1	
Present	332	66	(19.9)	0.73	(0.53–1.02)	0.78	(0.56–1.08)
Fatigue							
No	224	40	(17.9)	1		1	
Present	270	70	(25.9)	1.45	(1.03–2.05)	1.18	(0.82–1.69)
Night sweat							
No	469	100	(21.3)	1		1	
Present	25	10	(40.0)	1.88	(1.12–3.13)	1.31	(0.76–2.25)
Weight loss *							
No	433	83	(19.2)	1		1	
Present	60	27	(45.0)	2.35	(1.67–3.30)	2.06	(1.44–2.96)
Contact history of TB							
No	480	105	(21.9)	1		1	
Present	14	5	(35.7)	1.63	(0.79–3.36)	1.51	(0.75–3.04)

* Data missing for one; HIV = human immunodeficiency virus; TB = tuberculosis; CI = confidence interval; aRR = adjusted relative risk.

3.4. Treatment Outcomes

The TB treatment outcomes are shown in Table 4. Among 104 patients initiated on treatment, 97 (93%) had successful treatment outcome, while 5 (5%) had unsuccessful outcome and 2 (2%) were still on treatment.

Table 4. Treatment outcomes among tuberculosis patients started on treatment in Haiphong International General Hospital in Vietnam, from June to December 2018.

Treatment Outcomes	N	(%)
Total	104	(100)
Cured	58	(55.8)
Treatment completed	39	(37.5)
Died	2	(1.9)
Lost to follow-up	3	(2.9)
On treatment *	2	(1.9)

* Two patients are on second-line treatment and are likely to complete by April 2020.

3.5. Median Delays

The delays at different steps of the cascade are shown in Table 5. The median (IQR) duration from visiting the HIGH to undergoing TB diagnostic test was 0 (0–1) day and from diagnosis to initiation of treatment was 6 (1–17) days.

Table 5. Delays in the TB care cascade among the patients attending the Haiphong International General Hospital in Vietnam, from June to December 2018.

Duration	Number Eligible	Number (%) with Valid Dates	Median Days	(IQR)
From visiting the HIGH to receiving the TB diagnosis test	494	487 (99)	0	(0–1)
From TB diagnosis to initiation of treatment	103	99 (93)	6	(1–17)

TB = Tuberculosis; IQR = Interquartile Range; HIGH = Haiphong International General Hospital.

4. Discussion

This is the first report from Vietnam evaluating an innovative PPM model using an information technology based tool for improving tuberculosis care in private health sector. While there are many studies evaluating the specific components of the TB care cascade in the private sector, very few have comprehensively examined all the steps of the cascade in a single study [16]. This is one such effort. Overall, the performance of the model was excellent in plugging the gaps in TB care cascade in the private sector and substantially better than previous PPM models implemented in Vietnam [13]. About 80% of the presumptive TB patients were investigated for TB. Nearly 95% of the cases diagnosed were initiated on treatment, which is significantly better than previous studies from Vietnam and Pakistan, where nearly 60% were lost to follow-up before treatment [13,17]. All the cases were notified to NTP. More than 90% of all TB patients completed the treatment successfully, in line with the global 90-(90)-90 targets. These results were better than those reported from India [18], Pakistan [17], Thailand [19], and Vietnam [9,13] and were on par with outcomes reported from Myanmar [20].

In our view, the success of the model may be attributed to the following aspects. First, unlike earlier PPM initiatives which predominantly used a 'referral model' for investigation of tuberculosis (wherein presumptive TB patients were referred to an NTP facility), the new model offered TB tests on-site or arranged for transportation of sputum samples. This might have reduced the gaps and delays in testing. Second, the use of a mobile application enabled notification of every TB case diagnosed. This alerted the health care system and the last-mile service providers like CHWs to proactively track and provide follow-up care to the patients, thus reducing gaps in treatment initiation and completion. Third, all the providers were trained and performance-based incentives were offered for every successful event in the care cascade. The total costs incurred were modest at 4100 USD for the six-month pilot period (equivalent to ~37 USD per TB case diagnosed). However, we have not undertaken a detailed cost-effectiveness analysis. This should be a topic of future research.

There were some other notable findings. First, only 0.7% of patients attending the OPD were identified as 'presumptive TB' patients. This is substantially lower than that reported from other settings like Pakistan (which varied from 2.9% to 7.5%) [21,22]. This difference is likely due to many differences between the settings which include (i) a stricter definition used for 'presumptive TB' (both symptom positive and chest X-ray abnormality) and (ii) the denominator being all patients attending OPD rather than the number screened in our study. It is possible that some of the patients attending the OPD might not have been screened and there was no documentation to find out the exact numbers screened.

Second, about one in five presumptive TB patients did not undergo investigations and people without symptoms were less likely to undergo investigation. This is concordant with the observations by Creswell et al. in Karachi, Pakistan [22]. Patients without symptoms may have low risk perception or may have been accorded lower priority for testing by attending clinicians. Some patients may not have been able to produce a sputum sample. The high costs of the diagnostic tests for which patients had to pay out of pocket may have been another deterrent for uptake of tests. Also, people with symptoms but normal chest X-ray were less likely to be tested. This may be again related to the definition of presumptive TB used in this project, which required an abnormal X-ray in addition to symptoms. This may also be the reason for the high yield of TB (33%) among people with presumptive TB.

Had we tested everyone with symptoms, we might have had lower yield in terms of percentage, but more cases in terms of absolute numbers. Of course, this would have had additional cost implications. One possible way to increase the number of cases detected without too much additional effort will be to use the duration of symptoms to prioritize investigation for TB—like investigating only those with cough of more than or equal to 2 weeks rather than testing everyone with cough of any duration [23]. Unfortunately, we did not have information on duration of symptoms and hence we cannot comment on this issue any further. All these call for revisiting the definition of presumptive TB used in the project.

Third, a standard diagnostic algorithm was not followed in the project. The nature and the number of tests offered to each patient seemed to vary. While we do not know the exact reasons for this variation, we speculate that this was dependent on the ability of individual patients to afford the high costs of the tests and based on the physician's choice of diagnostic test. This aspect needs to be studied further using qualitative research methods. We recommend that all patients undergo a standard diagnostic algorithm, preferably using tests approved globally for use and, if possible, at subsidized costs.

The study had some limitations. First, we relied on routinely collected data and hence errors in documentation cannot be ruled out. However, we estimate that such errors are limited in number and impact given real-time and post hoc data validation mechanisms in the ACIS software and by data management team. Second, there was no documentation about the number of people screened. As a result, we were unable to calculate the 'number needed to screen' to detect an additional TB case. Also, the patients attending only three OPDs were screened. Hence the number of TB cases diagnosed may not reflect the true burden of TB among patients attending HIGH. We may have missed many patients, especially those with extrapulmonary TB because departments such as surgery, gynecology and urology were not involved in the project. We may also have missed many patients because of the strict definition of presumptive TB used in our study. In a national TB prevalence survey from Vietnam, only 10% of all presumptive TB patients fulfilled such strict criteria and accounted for only 27% of all TB patients [24]. Third, the study was conducted in a single hospital thereby limiting its generalizability. For this reason, we have refrained from the assessing the impact of this intervention on case notification at the community level. This kind of impact has been demonstrated by previous studies elsewhere [18,21,25]. Fourth, we did not have data for the pre-intervention period to enable before–after comparisons. There was no systematic recording and reporting of TB-related indicators before the study. The data obtained in this study may act as a baseline for any future evaluations. Finally, the exact reasons for the gaps at each step of the cascade were not investigated in this study. Future research should look into this aspect using qualitative research methods.

In conclusion, the new PPM model in Vietnam performed well with high levels of testing, diagnosis, treatment start and completion among TB patients. Given the success of this model in plugging the gaps in TB care cascade, the NTP in Vietnam is considering to scale-up this model nationwide after undertaking a detailed cost-effectiveness analysis. The lessons learned from this study may be useful to make amendments in the PPM model and optimize project implementation going forward.

Author Contributions: Conceptualization and protocol development: T.D.T., A.M.V.K., G.R., T.H., H.L.V., L.V.N.Q., H.N.T., A.C., R.F., T.D.T.T., T.H., H.N.V., H.B.V., H.N.B., and N.N.V. Data Collection: T.D.T., T.D.T.T., and A.C. Data Analysis or interpretation: T.D.T., A.M.V.K., G.R., T.H., and J.C. Writing the first draft: T.D.T., A.M.V.K., and G.R. Critical review of the paper and final approval: T.D.T., A.M.V.K., G.R., H.L.V., L.V.N.Q., H.N.T., A.C., R.F., T.D.T.T., H.N.V., H.B.V., H.N.B., N.N.V., and J.C. All authors have read and agreed to the published version of the manuscript.

Funding: This research study was generously supported by a grant from the Stop TB Partnership's TB REACH initiative, with funding from Global Affairs Canada. The training program, within which this paper was developed, and the open access publication costs were funded by Department for International Development (DFID), UK and La Fondation Veuve Emile Metz-Tesch (Luxembourg). The funders had no role in study design, data collection and analysis, decision to publish, or preparation of the manuscript.

Acknowledgments: This research was conducted through the Structured Operational Research and Training Initiative (SORT IT), a global partnership led by the Special Program for Research and Training in Tropical Diseases at the World Health Organization (WHO/TDR). The model is based on a course developed jointly by the International Union Against Tuberculosis and Lung Disease (The Union) and Medécins sans Frontières (MSF/Doctors Without Borders). The specific SORT IT program which resulted in this publication was jointly developed and implemented by: The Union South-East Asia Office, New Delhi, India; the Centre for Operational Research, The Union, Paris, France; The Union, Mandalay, Myanmar; The Union, Harare, Zimbabwe; MSF Luxembourg Operational Research (LuxOR); MSF Operational Center Brussels (MSF OCB); Jawaharlal Institute of Postgraduate Medical Education and Research (JIPMER), Puducherry, India; Post Graduate Institute of Medical Education and Research (PGIMER), Chandigarh, India; All India Institute of Medical Sciences (AIIMS), New Delhi, India; Velammal Medical College Hospital and Research Institute, Madurai, India; Society for Education Welfare and Action (SEWA)—Rural, Jhagadia, India; Common Management Unit (AIDS, TB & Malaria), Ministry of National Health Services, Regulations and Coordination, Islamabad, Pakistan; and Kidu Mobile Medical Unit, His Majesty's People's Project and Jigme Dorji Wangchuck National Referral Hospital, Thimphu, Bhutan. The authors would also like to thank the Vietnam National Tuberculosis Control Programme, Friends for International Tuberculosis Relief, Ho Chi Minh City, Vietnam, Haiphong International General Hospital for their support, the Stop TB Partnership's TB REACH for providing grant, and the community health workers for their help with data collection and follow-up of TB patients.

Conflicts of Interest: The authors declare no conflict of interest.

References

1. World Health Organization (WHO). Global Tuberculosis Report. 2019. Available online: https://www.who.int/tb/publications/global_report/en/ (accessed on 18 October 2019).
2. World Health Organization. The End TB Strategy. Available online: https://www.who.int/tb/strategy/end-tb/en/ (accessed on 14 October 2019).
3. Ortblad, K.F.; Lozano, R.; Murray, C.J. An alternative estimation of tuberculosis incidence from 1980 to 2010: Methods from the Global Burden of Disease 2010. *Lancet* **2013**, *381*, S104. [CrossRef]
4. World Health Organization (WHO). Stop TB Partnership. In *The Paradigm Shift 2016–2020: Global Plan to End TB*; World Health Organization: Geneva, Switzerland, 2015.
5. Chin, D.P.; Hanson, C.L. Finding the Missing Tuberculosis Patients. *J. Infect. Dis.* **2017**, *216*, S675–S678. [CrossRef]
6. Sulis, G.; Pai, M. Missing tuberculosis patients in the private sector: Business as usual will not deliver results. *Public Health Action* **2017**, *7*, 80–81. [CrossRef] [PubMed]
7. Lönnroth, K.; Uplekar, M.; Arora, V.K.; Juvekar, S.; Lan, N.T.N.; Mwaniki, D.; Pathania, V. Public-private mix for DOTS implementation: What makes it work? *Bull World Health Organ* **2004**, *82*, 580–586.
8. Oanh, T.T.M.; Phượng, H.T.; Phương, N.K.; Tuấn, K.A.; Thủy, N.T.; Mai, V.L.; My, Đ.T. *Current Situation Assessment and Recommended Solutions to Strengthen Public Private Partnership in Health Sector*; Health Strategy and Policy Institute: Ha Noi, Vietnam, 2011.
9. Lönnroth, K.; Thuong, L.M.; Lambregts, K.; Quy, H.T.; Diwan, V.K. Private tuberculosis care provision associated with poor treatment outcome: Comparative study of a semi-private lung clinic and the NTP in two urban districts in Ho Chi Minh City, Vietnam. National Tuberculosis Programme. *Int. J. Tuberc. Lung. Dis.* **2003**, *7*, 165–171. [PubMed]
10. Lönnroth, K.; Lambregts, K.; Nhien, D.T.; Quy, H.T.; Diwan, V.K. Private pharmacies and tuberculosis control: A survey of case detection skills and reported anti-tuberculosis drug dispensing in private pharmacies in Ho Chi Minh City, Vietnam. *Int. J. Tuberc. Lung. Dis.* **2000**, *4*, 1052–1059. [CrossRef] [PubMed]
11. Lönnroth, K.; Thuong, L.M.; Linh, P.D.; Diwan, V.K. Delay and discontinuity—A survey of TB patients' search of a diagnosis in a diversified health care system. *Int. J. Tuberc. Lung. Dis.* **1999**, *3*, 992–1000. [PubMed]
12. Quy, H.T.; Lan, N.T.N.; Lönnroth, K.; Buu, T.N.; Dieu, T.T.N.; Hai, L.T. Public-private mix for improved TB control in Ho Chi Minh City, Vietnam: An assessment of its impact on case detection. *Int. J. Tuberc. Lung. Dis.* **2003**, *7*, 464–471. [PubMed]

13. Quy, H.T.; Lönnroth, K.; Lan, N.T.N.; Buu, T.N. Treatment results among tuberculosis patients treated by private lung specialists involved in a public-private mix project in Vietnam. *Int. J. Tuberc. Lung. Dis.* **2003**, *7*, 1139–1146. [PubMed]
14. The World Bank Vietnam Continues to Reduce Poverty, According to WB Report. Available online: https://www.worldbank.org/en/news/press-release/2018/04/05/vietnam-continues-to-reduce-poverty-according-to-world-bank-report (accessed on 14 October 2019).
15. UNITAID. Tuberculosis Diagnostics Technology Lanscape. 2017, pp. 1–90. Available online: https://unitaid.org/assets/2017-Unitaid-TB-Diagnostics-Technology-Landscape.pdf (accessed on 6 November 2019).
16. Lei, X.; Liu, Q.; Escobar, E.; Philogene, J.; Zhu, H.; Wang, Y.; Tang, S. Public–private mix for tuberculosis care and control: A systematic review. *Int. J. Infect. Dis.* **2015**, *34*, 20–32. [CrossRef] [PubMed]
17. Khan, B.J.; Kumar, A.M.V.; Stewart, A.; Khan, N.M.; Selvaraj, K.; Fatima, R.; Samad, Z. Alarming rates of attrition among tuberculosis patients in public-private facilities in Lahore, Pakistan. *Public Health Action* **2017**, *7*, 127–133. [CrossRef] [PubMed]
18. Lal, S.S.; Sahu, S.; Wares, F.; Lönnroth, K.; Chauhan, L.S.; Uplekar, M. Intensified scale-up of public-private mix: A systems approach to tuberculosis care and control in India. *Int. J. Tuberc. Lung. Dis.* **2011**, *15*, 97–104. [PubMed]
19. Chengsorn, N.; Bloss, E.; Anekvorapong, R.; Anuwatnonthakate, A.; Wattanaamornkiat, W.; Komsakorn, S.; Moolphate, S.; Limsomboon, P.; Kaewsa-ard, S.; Nateniyom, S.; et al. Tuberculosis services and treatment outcomes in private and public health care facilities in Thailand, 2004–2006. *Int. J. Tuberc. Lung. Dis.* **2009**, *13*, 888–894. [PubMed]
20. Thet Lwin, Z.M.; Sahu, S.K.; Owiti, P.; Chinnakali, P.; Majumdar, S.S. Public-private mix for tuberculosis care and control in Myanmar: A strategy to scale up? *Public Health Action* **2017**, *7*, 15–20. [CrossRef] [PubMed]
21. Khan, A.J.; Khowaja, S.; Khan, F.S.; Qazi, F.; Lotia, I.; Habib, A.; Mohammed, S.; Khan, U.; Amanullah, F.; Hussain, H.; et al. Engaging the private sector to increase tuberculosis case detection: An impact evaluation study. *Lancet Infect. Dis.* **2012**, *12*, 608–616. [CrossRef]
22. Creswell, J.; Khowaja, S.; Codlin, A.; Hashmi, R.; Rasheed, E.; Khan, M.; Durab, I.; Mergenthaler, C.; Hussain, O.; Khan, F.; et al. An evaluation of systematic tuberculosis screening at private facilities in Karachi, Pakistan. *PLoS ONE* **2014**, *9*, e93858. [CrossRef] [PubMed]
23. Van't Hoog, A.H.; Onozaki, I.; Lonnroth, K. Choosing algorithms for TB screening: A modelling study to compare yield, predictive value and diagnostic burden. *BMC Infect. Dis.* **2014**, *14*, 532. [CrossRef] [PubMed]
24. Hoa, N.B.; Sy, D.N.; Nhung, N.V.; Tiemersma, E.W.; Borgdorff, M.W.; Cobelens, F.G.J. National survey of tuberculosis prevalence in Viet Nam. *Bull World Health Organ* **2010**, *88*, 273–280. [CrossRef] [PubMed]
25. Kumar, M.K.A.; Dewan, P.K.; Nair, P.K.J.; Frieden, T.R.; Sahu, S.; Wares, F.; Laserson, K.; Wells, C.; Granich, R.; Chauhan, L.S. Improved tuberculosis case detection through public-private partnership and laboratory-based surveillance, Kannur District, Kerala, India, 2001–2002. *Int. J. Tuberc. Lung. Dis.* **2005**, *9*, 870–876. [PubMed]

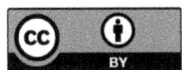

© 2020 by the authors. Licensee MDPI, Basel, Switzerland. This article is an open access article distributed under the terms and conditions of the Creative Commons Attribution (CC BY) license (http://creativecommons.org/licenses/by/4.0/).

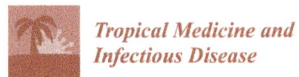

Article

Contact Investigation of Multidrug-Resistant Tuberculosis Patients: A Mixed-Methods Study from Myanmar

Aye Mon Phyo [1,*], Ajay M. V. Kumar [2,3,4], Kyaw Thu Soe [5], Khine Wut Yee Kyaw [2,6], Aung Si Thu [1], Pyae Phyo Wai [1], Sandar Aye [1], Saw Saw [7], Htet Myet Win Maung [8] and Si Thu Aung [8]

1. TB Department, International Union Against Tuberculosis and Lung Disease (The Union), Mandalay 15021, Myanmar; aungsithu1984@gmail.com (A.S.T.); dr.p.p.wai2012@gmail.com (P.P.W.); sandaraye213@gmail.com (S.A.)
2. Centre for Operational Research, International Union Against Tuberculosis and Lung Disease (The Union), 75006 Paris, France; AKumar@theunion.org (A.M.V.K.); dr.khinewutyeekyaw2015@gmail.com (K.W.Y.K.)
3. Centre for Operational Research, International Union Against Tuberculosis and Lung Disease (The Union), South-East Asia Office, New Delhi 110016, India
4. Department of Community Medicine, Yenepoya Medical College, Yenepoya (Deemed to be University), Mangaluru 575022, India
5. Department of Medical Research (Pyin Oo Lwin Branch), Ministry of Health and Sports, Pyin Oo Lwin 05081, Myanmar; kyawthusoe.dmr@gmail.com
6. Department of Operational Research, International Union against Tuberculosis and Lung Disease (The Union), Mandalay 15021, Myanmar
7. Department of Medical Research, Ministry of Health and Sports, Yangon 11191, Myanmar; sawsawsu@gmail.com
8. National Tuberculosis Programme, Ministry of Health and Sports, Nay Pyi Taw 15011, Myanmar; htetmyetwinmaung@gmail.com (H.M.W.M.); sithuaung@mohs.gov.mm (S.T.A.)
* Correspondence: ayemonphyoe8@gmail.com or ayemonphyo@theunion.org; Tel.: +95-9969830209

Received: 20 October 2019; Accepted: 22 November 2019; Published: 26 December 2019

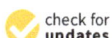

Abstract: There is no published evidence on contact investigation among multidrug-resistant tuberculosis (MDR-TB) patients from Myanmar. We describe the cascade of contact investigation conducted in 27 townships of Myanmar from January 2018 to June 2019 and its implementation challenges. This was a mixed-methods study involving quantitative (cohort analysis of programme data) and qualitative components (thematic analysis of interviews of 8 contacts and 13 health care providers). There were 556 MDR-TB patients and 1908 contacts, of whom 1134 (59%) reached the health centres for screening (chest radiography and symptoms). Of the latter, 344 (30%) had presumptive TB and of them, 186 (54%) were investigated (sputum microscopy or Xpert MTB/RIF®). A total of 27 TB patients were diagnosed (six bacteriologically-confirmed including five with rifampicin resistance). The key reasons for not reaching township TB centres included lack of knowledge and lack of risk perception owing to wrong beliefs among contacts, financial constraints related to loss of wages and transportation charges, and inconvenient clinic hours. The reasons for not being investigated included inability to produce sputum, health care providers being unaware of or not agreeing to the investigation protocol, fixed clinic days and times, and charges for investigation. The National Tuberculosis Programme needs to note these findings and take necessary action.

Keywords: contacts; contact tracing; contact investigation; MDR-TB

1. Introduction

Tuberculosis (TB) is one of the top ten leading causes of deaths in the world. In 2017, there were an estimated 10 million TB patients including 558,000 with resistance to rifampicin (RR-TB), of which 82% had multidrug-resistant TB (MDR-TB, defined as resistance to at least rifampicin and isoniazid) [1]. Myanmar is one of the 30 countries classified as having a 'high MDR-TB burden' by the World Health Organization (WHO). There were an estimated 14,000 patients with MDR/RR-TB in 2017 in Myanmar, of whom only 3281 (23%) were reported to be diagnosed by the national TB programme (NTP) [1]. This means that a vast majority of MDR-TB patients remain undiagnosed or not reported to the NTP in Myanmar.

The "End TB strategy" of the WHO emphasizes early diagnosis and prompt treatment of all TB patients, including drug-resistant TB, to break the chain of transmission and prevent further spread of disease in the community [2]. In line with this, the STOP TB partnership proposes 90-(90)-90 targets (diagnosing and treating 90% of all people with TB, including 90% of the key populations at risk of TB, and achieving 90% treatment success for all people diagnosed with TB) [3]. One such key population group at high risk of TB is 'household contacts', living in close contact with source TB patients. Systematic reviews report that the pooled yield of active TB among the contacts is 4.5% [4,5]. A study from New York city reported a yield of active TB of 1% among household contacts investigated [6]. A systematic review among contacts of drug resistant TB patients showed a higher yield of 7.8%, with the majority of secondary cases having the same drug resistance or genotyping pattern as the source case, indicating primary transmission of drug-resistant strains of tuberculosis bacilli [7].

Hence, the WHO recommends 'contact investigation'—systematic investigation of all household contacts of source TB patients for active and latent tuberculosis and institution of appropriate curative and preventive treatment, respectively [8]. This strategy is endorsed by the NTP in Myanmar and it has been recommended that household contacts of MDR-TB patients with TB symptoms are investigated using Xpert MTB/RIF® assay since 2016 [9].

However, the implementation of this policy is poor and aggregate programme data indicate that contact investigation was done in only 30% of all bacteriologically-confirmed TB patients notified [10]. There is no published evidence about contact investigation among MDR-TB patients from Myanmar, as there is no structured, case-based, recording, reporting, and monitoring of this activity.

The International Union Against Tuberculosis and Lung Disease (The Union), an international non-governmental organization, started implementing a community-based MDR-TB care project in selected townships of Myanmar [11]. As part of this project, community volunteers have been trained and incentivized to conduct many activities including 'contact investigation' among MDR-TB patients. This provides an opportunity to assess the extent of implementation of contact investigation, as well as its barriers and possible solutions to address them.

Therefore, we undertook a mixed-methods operational research study with the following objectives: (1) Among the household contacts of MDR-TB patients registered from January 2018 to June 2019, to assess (i) the number and proportion of presumptive TB patients identified, investigated, diagnosed, and treated for TB; (ii) demographic and clinical factors associated with getting or not getting investigated; and (iii) the median duration between the various steps in the cascade. (2) To explore the barriers in implementing contact investigation from the perspective of household contacts and health care providers.

2. Methods

2.1. Study Design

This was an explanatory mixed-methods study design involving a quantitative component (a cohort analysis of routinely collected programme data) followed by a qualitative component (descriptive study) involving interviews of providers and contacts [12].

2.2. Study Setting

2.2.1. General Setting

Myanmar is the second largest country in Southeast Asia, with a population of 52 million people (2014 Census) [13]. About two-thirds of the population lives in rural areas, while the urban populations are concentrated in Yangon and Mandalay regions. Administratively, Myanmar is divided into seven states, seven regions, and one union territory (Nay Pyi Taw), and subdivided into 74 districts with 330 townships [13].

2.2.2. Specific Setting

The study was conducted in 27 selected townships of Mandalay Region, Magway Region, Sagaing Region, and Shan State of Myanmar, implementing the MDR-TB care project with funding support from the Global Fund for AIDS, Tuberculosis, and Malaria. Under this project, the key activities include evening direct observation of treatment for MDR-TB patients, provision of financial incentives to patients, counselling and monitoring of patients for adverse drug effects, health education to family members, and contact investigation. These activities are undertaken by the community volunteers or the project nurses hired and trained for this purpose. Community volunteers are people living in the same ward/village as the patients, but not family members; have reasonable education background (being able to read and write in Myanmar language); have time and interest to learn; and are committed to the care of patients. Peers who have had TB in the past are preferred as volunteers. Community volunteers are supervised by a project focal nurse (one per township) who coordinates with the staff at township level. Every volunteer is assigned a maximum of three MDR-TB patients for providing care. For MDR-TB patients who are not assigned a community volunteer, the project nurse of the respective township conducts the contact investigation, wherever possible.

Both community volunteers and focal nurses receive periodic training on contact investigation and its recording and reporting. The training includes steps to identify household contacts; conduct symptom screening; and refer for investigations, follow-up, and linkage to treatment if required.

2.2.3. Household Contact Investigation

The process of contact investigation is described in Figure 1. First, the volunteer or the project nurse visits the home of MDR-TB patients and educates them about the importance of contact investigation. Then, the contacts are screened for TB symptoms (cough, fever, weight loss, night sweats, or enlarged lymph nodes) and, regardless of symptoms, they are referred to the township TB centre for chest radiography. If the patient is unable to visit, sputum samples are collected and transported. Irrespective of symptoms or chest radiography findings, people who are able to produce a sputum specimen are investigated further using sputum microscopy for acid-fast bacilli (AFB) and Xpert MTB/RIF® assay. People who are positive for AFB and/or positive for TB bacilli on Xpert MTB/RIF® assay are diagnosed as having TB and are started on first-line or second-line TB treatment, depending on the results of rifampicin resistance. Contacts who are unable to produce sputum or those with 'negative sputum results, but shadows suggestive of TB on chest radiography', are referred for further management to the physician, who makes a decision on clinical diagnosis of TB and treatment. In some township TB centres, the facilities for Xpert MTB/RIF® assay and chest radiography are not available. In such situations, contacts are referred to the nearest TB centre or hospital for investigation.

Household contacts are provided a maximum incentive of 7000 MMK (~5 US$) if they undergo investigation. This is intended to cover the costs of transportation and some investigations like chest radiography, which may not be available free of charge in some townships.

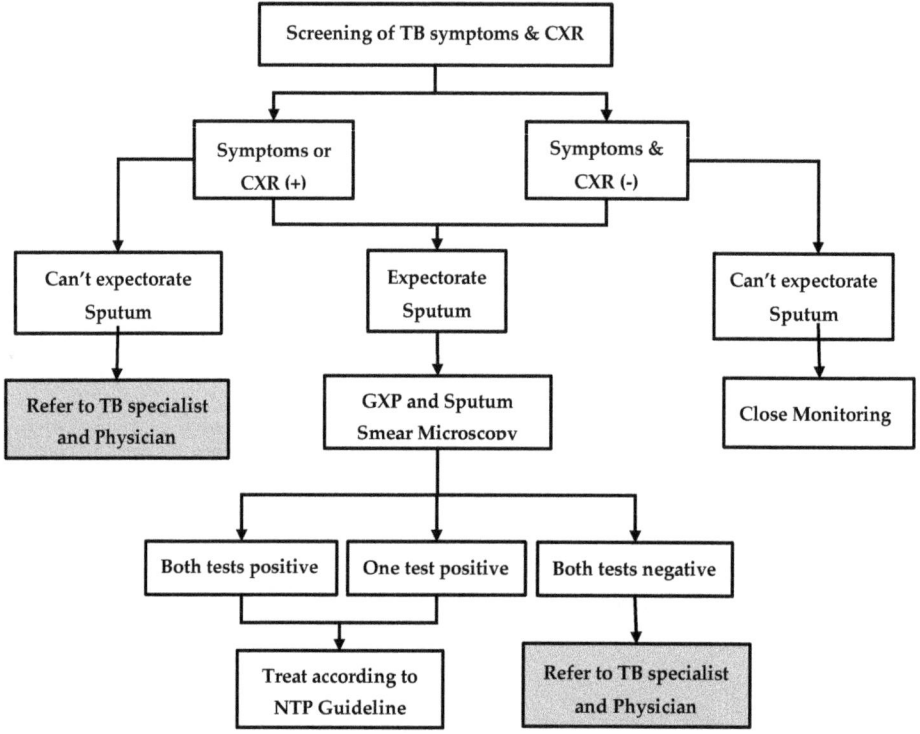

Figure 1. Systematic screening and investigation algorithm for household contacts of index MDR-TB patients in the community-based MDR-TB care project in Myanmar, 2018–19. MDR-TB = multidrug resistant tuberculosis; TB = tuberculosis; CXR = chest X-ray; GXP = Xpert MTB/RIF®; TB symptoms = cough, fever, loss of weight, night sweat, and lymph node enlargement.

2.3. Recording

The information of index MDR-TB patients including the number of household contacts for each patient is captured in an MS Excel database. There is a "contact register" maintained at the township TB centres, which captures all the details of investigation, TB diagnosis, and treatment of contacts. This information is captured electronically in a quality-assured EpiData database by trained data entry operators and validated periodically by the project supervisors.

2.4. Study Population

2.4.1. Quantitative

All household contacts of index MDR-TB patients newly registered in 27 project townships from January 2018 to June 2019 were included. In line with WHO guidelines, a household contact was defined as "a person who shares the same enclosed living space for one or more nights or for frequent or extended periods during the day with the source patient during the treatment or during the three months before commencement of the current treatment".

2.4.2. Qualitative

The study population includes a purposive sample (maximum variation) of household contacts of MDR-TB patients, community volunteers, and project nurses from selected townships from each region/state. First, we calculated the township-wise Xpert MTB/RIF® testing rates among contacts with presumptive TB. We selected the township with the highest testing coverage and three townships with the lowest testing coverage in such a way that one township was selected from each region/state. In each selected township, two household contacts of MDR-TB patients (one who was investigated and one who was not), two community volunteers, and one project nurse were selected for interviews. In addition, we also interviewed the project supervisor. Thus, a total of 21 interviews were conducted. Participants who were knowledgeable, vocal, and willing to express were purposively selected. The sample size was guided by the saturation of the findings.

2.5. Data Variables, Sources of Data, and Data Collection

2.5.1. Quantitative

The data were extracted from electronic databases of the project. The variables included symptoms, chest radiography findings, and results of sputum microscopy and Xpert MTB/RIF® assay. In addition, dates of start of treatment among index patients, contact registration, TB investigation, diagnosis, and treatment start among contacts were collected.

2.5.2. Qualitative

Data collection was done between February and March 2019. Interviews were conducted at a time and place convenient to participants using an interview guide by K.T.S. (a medical doctor from the Department of Medical Research), and K.W.Y.K. (an operational research fellow from The Union), who are trained and experienced in qualitative research (Supplementary File S1) [14]. The guide was pilot tested before implementing in the field. Audio recording was done after receiving consent from participants. Verbatim notes were taken during interview. The average duration of interviews was approximately 45 min. After the interview was over, the summary of the interviews was read back to the participants to ensure participant validation.

2.6. Data Analysis

2.6.1. Quantitative

We analysed using STATA software (version 14.2 STATA Corp., College Station, TX, USA). The demographic and clinical characteristics of the household contacts were summarized using median (inter-quartile range) for continuous variables and frequencies and proportions for categorical variables. The median time between the different stages of the process was calculated.

2.6.2. Operational Definitions

People with either symptoms of TB and/or abnormal shadows on chest radiograph were considered as presumptive TB for this analysis. People who had undergone any of the diagnostic tests (sputum microscopy, Xpert MTB/RIF® assay, or fine needle aspiration cytology) were considered as having been investigated for TB. The date when these investigations were carried out was considered as 'date of investigation'. If a person underwent more than one investigation, the earlier date was considered. For bacteriologically-confirmed TB patients, the date of the positive test was considered as the date of diagnosis, whereas for clinically diagnosed patients, the date of chest radiography was considered as the date of diagnosis.

Factors associated with not being investigated for TB and getting tested with Xpert MTB/RIF® assay were measured using adjusted relative risks (RR) and 95% confidence intervals (CI). We initially tried to perform a log-binomial regression. As we did not obtain convergence, a modified Poisson regression with robust error variance was used. Variables that were significant (p value < 0.05) in unadjusted analysis or that were known to be associated with the outcome from published literature were included in the multivariable model.

2.6.3. Qualitative

Transcripts were prepared in Myanmar language on the same day of interview based on the audio recordings and verbatim notes. Manual descriptive thematic analysis was performed by the principal investigator [15]. It was reviewed by a second investigator to reduce bias and subjectivity in interpretation. The decision of coding rules and theme generation was done in consensus among investigators. The analysis was done in Burmese language and only the final result was translated into English. The themes are presented for barriers and solutions with the corresponding quotes. Any difference between the investigators was resolved by discussion. We have adhered to the Strengthening the Reporting of Observational Studies in Epidemiology (STROBE) guidelines and 'Consolidated Criteria for Reporting Qualitative Research (COREQ) in conducting and reporting the study [16,17].

2.7. Ethics Issues

Ethics approval was obtained from the Ethics Review Committee, Department of Medical Research, Ministry of Health and Sports, Myanmar (Ethics/DMR/2018/159) and the Ethics Advisory Group of The Union, Paris, France (EAG number 48/18). Permission to conduct the study was obtained from the National Tuberculosis Programme, Ministry of Health and Sports, Myanmar. We obtained written informed consent for conducting the interviews and audio recording. A waiver of informed consent was obtained from the ethics committees for quantitative component as this included secondary data analysis.

3. Results

3.1. Quantitative

There were 556 MDR-TB patients who had 1908 contacts living with them. Of the latter, 1134 (59%) reached the township TB centre for screening (Figure 2). The median (inter quartile range, IQR) age of contacts was 30 (14–50) years and 664 (59%) were female.

3.1.1. Cascade of Contact Investigation

Of the 1134 contacts, 344 (30%) had presumptive TB and of them, 186 (54%) were investigated. However, 213 individuals were found to be investigated even though they did not have any symptoms or abnormal chest radiography. Thus, a total of 399 people were investigated for TB and among them, 27 TB patients were diagnosed. Most of the clinically diagnosed cases belonged to the group with 'no symptoms, but positive findings on chest radiography' and nearly half of them were children. There was no TB patient diagnosed in the group without TB symptoms that had normal chest radiography. Barring one patient who died, all the remaining 26 (96%) patients started on the treatment (Figure 2).

The characteristics of TB patients are shown in Table 1. Of the 27 patients, six had bacteriologically-confirmed TB, while the rest were clinically diagnosed. Of the six bacteriologically-confirmed, five had pulmonary TB (all with rifampicin resistance) and one had extrapulmonary TB who was AFB-positive on Fine Needle Aspiration Cytology aspirate. All were new cases, barring one who reported a previous history of TB. A total of 362 contacts underwent sputum microscopy and only one was AFB-positive. Xpert MTB/RIF® assay was conducted among 176 contacts and 5 were diagnosed as TB (this included the one case diagnosed by sputum microscopy).

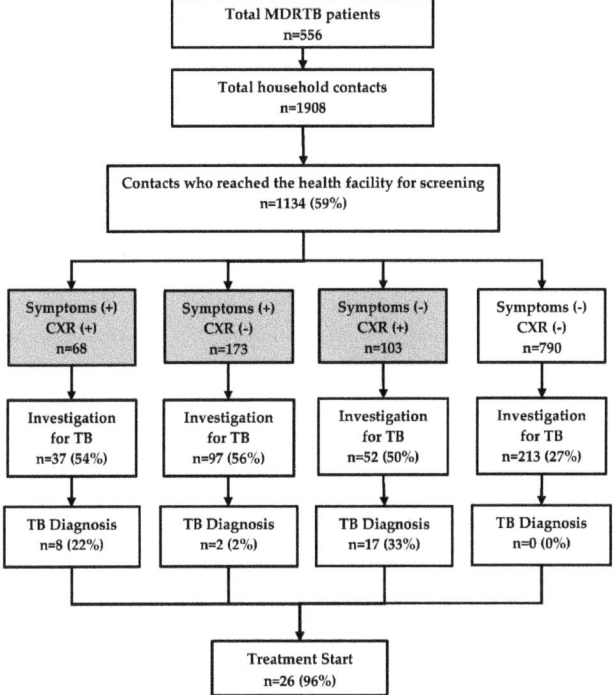

Figure 2. TB investigation, diagnosis, and treatment of household contacts of MDR-TB patients registered in a community based MDR-TB care project in Myanmar, between January 2018 and June 2019. TB = tuberculosis; MDR-TB = multidrug resistant tuberculosis; CXR = chest X-ray. The numbers in the shaded boxes indicate people with presumptive TB defined as those with symptoms (cough, fever, weight loss, and night sweats) and/or abnormal shadows on the chest radiograph.

Table 1. Characteristics of TB patients diagnosed among household contacts of MDR-TB patients registered in a community based MDR-TB care project in Myanmar, between January 2018 and June 2019.

Characteristics	TB Patients	
	N	(%)
Total	27	(100)
Age group (years)		
≤14	10	(37.0)
15–44	12	(44.4)
45–64	4	(14.8)
≥65	1	(3.70)
Sex		
Male	12	(44.4)
Female	15	(55.6)
Rifampicin resistance		
Not tested	7	(25.9)
No	15	(55.6)
Yes	5	(18.5)
Type of TB		
Bacteriologically-confirmed	6	(22.2)
Clinically diagnosed	21	(77.8)
Site of TB		
Pulmonary TB	26	(96.3)
Extrapulmonary TB	1	(3.7)

TB = tuberculosis; MDR-TB = multidrug resistant tuberculosis.

3.1.2. Factors Associated with Not Being Investigated for TB

Of 344 presumptive TB patients, 158 (46%) were not investigated for TB. In adjusted analysis, failure to do TB investigation was significantly higher among the contacts who were less than 15 years old, those who were registered in health facilities without an Xpert MTB/RIF® machine, and those who were referred when compared with those whose sputum was collected and transported to health facilities by project staff (Table 2).

Table 2. Factors associated with not being investigated for TB among household contacts with presumptive TB registered in a community-based MDR-TB care project in Myanmar, between January 2018 and June 2019.

Characteristics	Total	Not Investigated		RR	(95%CI)	aRR	(95%CI)
	N	N	(%)				
Total	344	158	(45.9)				
Age (years)							
≤14	93	62	(66.7)	1.77	(1.37–2.28) *	1.47	(1.15–1.89) *
15–44	143	54	(37.8)	Ref		Ref	
45–64	82	34	(41.5)	1.10	(0.79–1.53)	1.13	(0.83–1.53)
≥65	26	8	(30.8)	0.81	(0.44–1.51)	0.90	(0.52–1.58)
Gender							
Male	145	64	(44.1)	Ref		Ref	
Female	199	94	(47.2)	1.07	(0.85–1.35)	1.14	(0.92–1.42)
Cough							
Yes	185	71	(38.4)	Ref		Ref	
No	159	87	(54.7)	1.43	(1.13–1.80) *	1.08	(0.87–1.34)
Fever							
Yes	27	17	(63)	1.42	(1.03–1.94) *	NE	
No	317	141	(44.5)	Ref			
Loss of weight							
Yes	65	35	(53.8)	1.22	(0.94–1.59)	NE	
No	279	123	(44.1)	Ref			
Health Facility							
Without GXP	40	28	(70)	1.64	(1.29–2.08) *	1.60	(1.24–2.07) *
With GXP	304	130	(42.8)	Ref		Ref	
Refer type							
Patient	299	157	(52.5)	23.63	(3.39–164.6) *	20.46	(2.88–145.53) *
Sputum Sample	45	1	(2.2)	Ref		Ref	
State/Region							
Mandalay	196	83	(42.3)	Ref		Ref	
Sagaing	76	37	(48.7)	1.15	(0.87–1.53)	1.20	(0.89–1.62)
Shan	38	19	(50)	1.18	(0.83–1.69)	1.18	(0.85–1.65)
Magway	34	19	(55.9)	1.32	(0.94–1.85)	1.06	(0.74–1.51)

TB = tuberculosis; MDR-TB = multidrug resistant tuberculosis; GXP = Xpert MTB/RIF® machine; CI = confidence interval; RR = relative risk; aRR = adjusted relative risk; n = number; NE = not estimated.* = statistically significant. The variables that were significant in the unadjusted analysis and that were found to be associated in previous studies were included in the adjusted analysis. Fever was not included in the adjusted model owing to collinearity with cough.

3.1.3. Factors Associated with Getting Tested for Xpert MTB/RIF®

Of 344 presumptive TB patients, 121 (35%) were tested using Xpert MTB/RIF®. In the adjusted analysis, the Xpert MTB/RIF® testing was significantly lower among contacts aged less than 15 years and significantly higher in health facilities with an Xpert MTB/RIF® machine on-site (Table 3).

Table 3. Factors associated with GXP testing among household contacts with presumptive TB registered in a community-based MDR-TB care project in Myanmar, between January 2018 and June 2019.

Characteristics	Total	GXP Tested		RR	(95%CI)	aRR	(95%CI)
	N	N	(%)				
Total	344	121	(35.2)				
Age (Years)							
≤14	93	22	(23.7)	0.53	(0.35–0.79) *	0.54	(0.35–0.82) *
15–44	143	64	(44.8)	Ref		Ref	
45–64	82	28	(34.1)	0.76	(0.54–1.08)	0.75	(0.53–1.05)
≥65	26	7	(26.9)	0.60	(0.31–1.16)	0.59	(0.31–1.12)
Gender							
Male	145	53	(36.6)	Ref		Ref	
Female	199	68	(34.2)	0.93	(0.70–1.25)	0.95	(0.72–1.25)
Cough							
Yes	185	75	(40.5)	1.40	(1.04–1.89) *	1.06	(0.78–1.45)
No	159	46	(28.9)	Ref		Ref	
Health Facility							
Without GXP	40	7	(17.5)	Ref		Ref	
With GXP	304	114	(37.5)	2.14	(1.08–4.27) *	2.14	(1.1–4.17)
Refer type							
Patient	299	101	(33.8)	Ref		Ref	
Sputum Sample	45	20	(44.4)	1.32	(0.92–1.89)	1.16	(0.8–1.69)
State/Region							
Mandalay	196	76	(38.8)	Ref		Ref	
Sagaing	76	21	(27.6)	0.71	(0.48–1.07)	0.67	(0.44–1.03)
Shan	38	18	(47.4)	1.22	(0.84–1.78)	1.21	(0.85–1.73)
Magway	34	6	(17.6)	0.46	(0.22–0.96) *	0.51	(0.24–1.08)
Symptoms							
No Symptom	103	31	(30.1)	Ref		NE	
Any Symptom	241	90	(37.3)	1.24	(0.89–1.74)		

TB = tuberculosis; MDR-TB = multidrug resistant tuberculosis; GXP = Xpert MTB/RIF® machine; CI = confidence interval; RR = relative risk; aRR = adjusted relative risk, n = number; NE = not estimated. * = statistically significant. The variables that were significant in the unadjusted analysis and that were found to be associated in previous studies were included in the adjusted analysis.

3.1.4. Delays

The median (IQR) duration between treatment start of index case to contact screening at the township TB centre was 81 (28–208) days. Among those investigated, 75% underwent the investigation within a day. The median time to treatment from diagnosis was 8 days—this was 14 days among bacteriologically-confirmed patients, but 4 days among clinically diagnosed patients (Table 4).

Table 4. Median duration (days) between different steps in the cascade of contact investigation among household contacts registered in community-based MDR-TB care project in Myanmar, between January 2018 and June 2019.

Duration (Days)	Total Eligible	Number (%) with Valid Dates	Median Days	(IQR)
Treatment start of index MDR-TB case and contact screening	1134	1005 (89)	81	(28–208)
Contact screening and investigation	399	380 (95)	0	(0–1)
TB diagnosis and treatment initiation	26	26 (100)	8	(2–14)
Bacteriologically-confirmed TB	5	5 (100)	14	(14–15)
Clinically diagnosed TB	21	21 (100)	4	(2–10)

TB = tuberculosis; MDR-TB = multidrug resistant tuberculosis; IQR = inter quartile range.

3.2. Qualitative

Implementation barriers in contact investigation were multi-factorial and inter-related with each other. We organized the barriers under two broad themes—household contacts-related barriers and health system-related barriers. The barriers summarized here reflect the perspectives of both the household contacts and health care providers. Overall, the participants from the townships with low testing coverage reported a greater number of barriers and, more predominantly, health system barriers. The verbatim quotes (translated in English) are italicized and placed within double quotes.

3.2.1. Household Contact-Related Barriers

Unable to Visit the Clinic

Working people and school-going children were unable to visit the township TB centre for investigation because the clinic times conflicted with the work/school timings.

"Some contacts were students. So they have to attend school from Monday to Friday. They can't come on these days for taking CXR (Chest X ray)."

(Community volunteer-5)

"Contacts did not want to go to OPD (Outpatient Department) because they didn't want to absent their jobs."

(Project Nurse-3)

The other barrier was related to distance requiring a long time to travel, which was compounded by personal problems.

"Some contacts couldn't come because they were very old and they lived far away"

(Project Nurse-1)

"I feel motion sickness when I travel ... Therefore, I rarely travel"

(tested household contact-1)

Inability to Produce Sputum

Some contacts could not produce sputum at all or only an inadequate amount of sputum for investigation.

"Sayarma (The Nurse) gave the sputum cup to me and told to produce sputum. But I can't produce the sputum."

(Non-tested Household contacts-4)

Financial Constraints

Some contacts, especially daily wage labourers, were reported to have financial constraints associated with visiting the township TB centre, as it meant absence from work and loss of daily wages, in addition to transportation charges. Although the project supported their travel allowance, it was a fixed amount and did not cover all the expenses.

"They could not spend time for investigation. They are daily-wages workers. Therefore, they need to work for their daily income."

(Project Nurse-4)

"For the contacts who lived far away from township TB centre, there are higher transportation costs. Although project supports this cost, it is not enough for them."

(Project Nurse-3)

Beliefs and Attitude

Some contacts refused to do contact investigation because they did not have any signs and symptoms and strongly believed that they do not have the disease. Others did not want to undergo investigation because they were afraid of possible side-effects of the TB drugs in the eventuality that they were diagnosed to have TB. One person mentioned that *God will take care of her illness*, even if it existed.

"*Contacts said that they believed that they have no disease (TB). So they don't want to test.*"

(Community volunteer-8)

"*I heard TB patients are afraid of the injections and they can't withstand the side-effects, so do I.*"

(Not-tested household contacts-3)

3.2.2. Health System-Related Barriers

Lack of or Inadequate Counselling

Not all MDR-TB patients were assigned a volunteer in the project. So, the contact investigation may not have been done in such patients. The project nurse reported that some volunteers were not able to communicate and counsel effectively and convince the contacts to undergo TB screening.

"*Volunteers could not explain well about the importance of TB screening to contacts*"

(Project Nurse-2)

"*No one told me how to produce sputum*"

(non-tested contact-4)

The project supervisor reported that some of the contacts had already been investigated by the time volunteer visited the home, and hence were not referred. Such contacts were not recorded in the project database.

Do Not Know

Some of the health care providers at the township TB centre were not aware of the contact investigation protocol. So, chest radiography was not provided for asymptomatic contacts.

"*Even if the contacts reached the health facility, health care providers at TB centre did not offer chest X ray, because they had no signs and symptom of TB*"

(Project Nurse-3)

Do Not Agree

Some of the health care providers were aware of the protocol followed in the project, but did not agree, because it did not align with the NTP guidelines. While the project protocol advocated for screening using chest radiography in addition to symptom screening, NTP recommends only symptom screening and further investigation is limited to those with symptoms.

"*The TB focal person informed us that if there are no symptoms, we cannot do any investigation*"

(Project nurse-3)

They Do Not Do: High Workload

It was reported that investigations were not offered to contacts by the staff of the TB centre for various reasons. One was related to the high workload and shortage of human resources in laboratory unit in the township TB centre. Some of the staff at the township TB centre were unable to pay attention to the contact investigation as they were engaged with multiple responsibilities.

> "The laboratory technician position is vacant in TB centre"
>
> *(Project Nurse-2)*

> "The focal person does not involve fully in TB related activity as he also worked for other public health programmes. He is always busy"
>
> *(Project Nurse-4)*

They Do, But on Fixed Days and Times

Some laboratories had a fixed time to receive sputum specimens from the patients. If the patients arrived outside the times, they were asked to return the next day. Sputum specimens received outside the fixed times were discarded and this meant requesting contacts for additional specimens. In some health facilities, the chest X-ray unit imposed restrictions on the number of chest radiographs that could be taken on a given day (such as a maximum of 10 persons per day). All of the others were asked to come on the next day. This was very inconvenient for the contacts who had travelled from far off places. Similarly, there was a fixed day in a week for doctors to examine presumptive TB patients and make a decision about clinical diagnosis.

> "The laboratory accepts sputum sample between 9 am and 10 am only. Specimens received outside this time are discarded and then it is difficult to request for additional specimens from contacts."
>
> *(Project Nurse-4)*

> "Chest X ray unit opens at 9 am and they allow only 10 persons per day to take chest X ray from TB department. Therefore, when the contact came and if it is beyond their maximum number, this person is asked to return the next day. And, the contact may not return."
>
> *(Project Nurse-1)*

They Do, But They Charge

It was reported that the contacts had to pay to undergo chest radiography in some places.

> "Chest X-ray fee is high. Here, it is 1500 MMK and this charge is higher in other township hospitals."
>
> *(Project Nurse-3)*

4. Discussion

This is the first study from Myanmar providing information on contact investigation among MDR-TB patients and its implementation challenges. We discuss the magnitude of gaps at each step of the cascade and their reasons below.

One of the main gaps was that nearly four in ten contacts did not reach the health facility for screening. This is higher than that reported from South Africa and similar to Ethiopia [18,19]. The possible reasons included lack of knowledge about the need for contact investigation, lack of risk perception owing to wrong beliefs, financial problems related to loss of wages and high transportation charges not entirely reimbursed by the project, and conflicts of clinic times with work/school times. It is possible that home visits and educating about contact investigation may not have happened in some MDR-TB patients. An interesting observation revealed during key informant interviews was that several contacts had already been investigated for TB by the time the project staff made home visits. Such people were not included in the numerator, but were counted in the denominator, when calculating this indicator, thus marginally overestimating the proportion not reached.

The next gap was at the level of screening and investigating the contacts who had reached the health facility. Only half of the presumptive TB patients received any investigation for bacteriological confirmation. The children were less likely to be tested, mostly because they were unable to produce sputum, and the gastric lavage was not routinely done in our setting, which requires hospitalization.

Access to health facilities was another factor. The contacts who lived in townships that had Xpert MTB/RIF® facility were more likely to be tested as it reduced the travel cost and time.

Contacts whose sputum samples were collected at home and transported by project staffs were more likely to be investigated than contacts who had reached the health facility. Because investigation required two sputum samples, as per NTP guidelines, contacts referred to health facilities had to make multiple visits. Sometimes, the nearest health facility (to where the contacts were referred) did not have Xpert MTB/RIF assay services. In such instances, contacts had to be referred to another health facility with Xpert services. All these were reported as inconvenient and may have led to the losses in the cascade. While some TB focal persons at the township TB centre were unaware about the contact investigation protocol, some disagreed with the requirement of screening all contacts with chest radiography. There was also confusion among the providers about the eligibility criteria for prescribing the Xpert MTB/RIF® assay. The other barriers included fixed times and days for receiving sample or patients and demanding charges for investigations.

This study had several strengths and some limitations. First, we included a large sample of contacts covering 27 project townships of four states and regions. Thus, the findings are likely to be representative of the situation in these areas. Second, we used a mixed-methods study design, which helped in understanding the underlying reasons for the gaps in care cascade. Third, we used quality-assured data collected by project staff, which is routinely monitored and validated. Fourth, we achieved saturation in our qualitative interviews. Fifth, we followed the STROBE and COREQ guidelines for reporting the quantitative and qualitative components, respectively [16,17]. One limitation was that we had no information on 40% of household contacts who did not reach the health facility for screening; hence, we do not know if they were similar to those who reached the health facility. The impact of this on overall findings is unclear. Another limitation was that we did not interview the health care providers responsible for providing TB services and include their perspectives. This should be considered in future research.

Despite this limitation, our findings have many implications for programme policy and practice. First, we recommend that chest radiography be used for screening all household contacts regardless of TB symptoms, wherever possible, because the yield of TB was highest in the group with 'no symptoms, but abnormal chest radiograph'. Although most of the cases in this group were clinically diagnosed, there was one case of rifampicin resistance too. We may have diagnosed more cases of TB, had we tested everyone with Xpert MTB/RIF® assay. However, the feasibility of this recommendation needs to be tested before wider scale-up.

Second, we recommend that contacts 'without TB symptoms and normal chest radiograph' should not be investigated any further because there was zero TB in this group. This is also supported by evidence from systematic reviews [19]. A substantial number of patients were unnecessarily investigated and the resources could have been used elsewhere to increase the testing rates among presumptive TB patients.

Third, as shown in our study, the prevalence of drug resistant TB among contacts of MDR-TB patients is high in studies conducted elsewhere [7,20–22]. Hence, Xpert MTB/RIF® test should be the first diagnostic test of choice, as recommended by WHO [23]. There was no additional yield of TB owing to sputum microscopy in our study. Hence, we recommend discontinuing sputum microscopy for contacts of MDR-TB patients and focusing on the Xpert MTB/RIF® assay, as it can reduce the workload at township laboratories. This strategy can also be more convenient for the contacts, because sputum microscopy requires two specimens requiring multiple visits, whereas Xpert MTB/RIF® testing requires only one specimen.

Fourth, refresher training should be conducted periodically for community volunteers to improve their knowledge about contact investigation and counselling skills. The training content can be tailored to resolve the specific myths and beliefs among the contacts.

Fifth, efforts should be made to bring the contact investigation services closer to the community. This includes strengthening of sputum collection and transportation to township TB centres. However, this alone will not obviate the need for visiting health facility, as contacts also have to undergo chest radiography. To address this, we recommend exploring the possibility of using new technologies such as digital chest radiography with automated computer-aided detection of tuberculosis, which can be mounted in a mobile van for greater outreach [24].

In conclusion, we identified the magnitude of gaps in the cascade of contact investigation among MDR-TB patients in Myanmar, as well as reasons for the same. We hope these findings can be shaped into practical recommendations that will inform the NTP in Myanmar.

Supplementary Materials: The following are available online at http://www.mdpi.com/2414-6366/5/1/3/s1, S1: Interview Guide for Key Informant Interview.

Author Contributions: Conceptualization and protocol development: A.M.P., A.M.V.K., K.T.S., K.W.Y.K., A.S.T., P.P.W., S.A., S.S., H.M.W.M., and S.T.A.; Data Collection: A.M.P., K.T.S., and K.W.Y.K.; Data Analysis: A.M.P., A.M.V.K., K.T.S., and K.W.Y.K.; Writing the first draft: A.M.P., A.M.V., and K.T.S.; Critical review of the paper and final approval: A.M.P., A.M.V.K., K.T.S., K.W.Y.K., A.S.T., P.P.W., S.T.A., S.S., H.M.W.M., and S.T.A. All authors have read and agreed to the published version of the manuscript.

Funding: This research received no external funding. The training programme, within which this paper was developed, was funded by the Department for International Development (DFID), London, UK. The funders had no role in study design, data collection and analysis, decision to publish, or preparation of the manuscript.

Acknowledgments: This research was conducted through the Structured Operational Research and Training Initiative (SORT IT), a global partnership led by the Special Programme for Research and Training in Tropical Diseases at the World Health Organization (WHO/TDR). The model is based on a course developed jointly by the International Union Against Tuberculosis and Lung Disease (The Union) and Medecins Sans Frontieres (MSF/Doctors Without Borders). The specific SORT IT programme that resulted in this publication was jointly organised and implemented by The Centre for Operational Research, The Union, Paris, France; Department of Medical Research, Ministry of Health and Sports, Yangon; Department of Public Health, Ministry of Health and Sports, Nay Pyi Taw; The Union Country Office, Mandalay, Myanmar; The Union South-East Asia Office, New Delhi, India and London School of Hygiene and Tropical Medicine, London, UK.

Conflicts of Interest: The authors declare no conflict of interest.

References

1. World Health Organization. *Global Tuberculosis Report 2018*; World Health Organization: Geneva, Switzerland, 2018.
2. Uplekar, M.; Weil, D.; Lonnroth, K.; Jaramillo, E.; Lienhardt, C.; Dias, H.M.; Falzon, D.; Floyd, K. The End TB Strategy. *Lancet* **2015**, *6736*, 1–3.
3. Stop TB Partnership; UNOPS. *The Paradigm Shift (2016–2020), Global Plan To End TB*; Stop TB Partnership: Geneva, Switzerland; UNOPS: Geneva, Switzerland, 2015.
4. Morrison, J.; Pai, M.; Hopewell, P.C. Tuberculosis and latent tuberculosis infection in close contacts of people with pulmonary tuberculosis in low-income and middle-income countries: A systematic review and meta-analysis. *Lancet Infect. Dis.* **2008**, *8*, 359–368. [CrossRef]
5. Fox, G.J.; Barry, S.E.; Britton, W.J.; Marks, G.B. Contact investigation for tuberculosis: A systematic review and meta-analysis. *Eur. Respir. J.* **2013**, *41*, 140–156. [CrossRef] [PubMed]
6. Anger, H.A.; Proops, D.; Harris, T.G.; Li, J.; Kreiswirth, B.N.; Shashkina, E.; Ahuja, S.D. Active case finding and prevention of tuberculosis among a cohort of contacts exposed to infectious tuberculosis cases in New York City. *Clin. Infect. Dis.* **2012**, *54*, 1287–1295. [CrossRef] [PubMed]
7. Shah, N.S.; Yuen, C.M.; Heo, M.; Tolman, A.W.; Becerra, M.C. Yield of contact investigations in households of patients with drug-resistant tuberculosis: Systematic review and meta-analysis. *Clin. Infect. Dis.* **2014**, *58*, 381–391. [CrossRef] [PubMed]
8. World Health Organization. *Recommendations for Investigating Contacts of Persons with Infectious Tuberculosis in Low-and Middle-Income Countries*; World Health Organization: Geneva, Switzerland, 2012.
9. National Tuberculosis Programme; Ministry of Health and Sports; Government of Myanmar. *Guidelines for the Manangement of Drug Resistant Tuberculosis (DR-TB) in Myanmar*; National Tuberculosis Programme; Ministry of Health and Sports, Government of Myanmar: Nay Pyi Taw, Myanmar, 2017.

10. National Tuberculosis Program; Ministry of Health and Sports; Government of Myanmar. *National Strategic Plan for Tuberculosis (2016–2020)*; National Tuberculosis Programme; Ministry of Health and Sports, Government of Myanmar: Nay Pyi Taw, Myanmar, 2015.
11. Wai, P.P.; Shewade, H.D.; Kyaw, N.T.T.; Thein, S.; Si Thu, A.; Kyaw, K.W.Y.; Aye, N.N.; Phyo, A.M.; Maung, H.M.W.; Soe, K.T.; et al. Community-based MDR-TB care project improves treatment initiation in patients diagnosed with MDR-TB in Myanmar. *PLoS ONE* **2018**, *13*, e0194087. [CrossRef] [PubMed]
12. Creswell, J.; Plano Clark, V. *Designing and Conducting Mixed Methods Research*; Sage Publications Ltd.: London, UK, 2007.
13. Department of Population; Ministry of Immigration and Population; Government of Myanmar. *The 2015 Myanmar Population and Housing Census, The Union Report*; Department of Population, Ministry of Immigration and Population, Government of Myanmar: Nay Pyi Taw, Myanmar, 2014.
14. Kvale, S. Dominance through interviews and dialogues. *Qual. Inq.* **2006**, *12*, 480–500. [CrossRef]
15. Attride-Stirling, J. Thematic networks: An analytic tool for qualitative research. *Qual. Res.* **2001**, *1*, 385–405. [CrossRef]
16. Tong, A.; Sainsbury, P.; Craig, J. Consolidated criteria for reporting qualitative research (COREQ): A 32-item checklist for interviews and focus groups. *Int. J. Qual. Health Care* **2007**, *19*, 349–357. [CrossRef] [PubMed]
17. Von Elm, E.; Altman, D.G.; Egger, M.; Pocock, S.J.; Gøtzsche, P.C.; Vandenbroucke, J.P. The strengthening the reporting of observational studies in epidemiology (STROBE) statement: Guidelines for reporting observational studies. *Int. J. Surg.* **2014**, *12*, 1495–1499. [CrossRef] [PubMed]
18. Kigozi, G.; Engelbrecht, M.; Heunis, C.; Janse van Rensburg, A. Household contact non-attendance of clinical evaluation for tuberculosis: A pilot study in a high burden district in South Africa. *BMC Infect. Dis.* **2018**, *18*, 1–8. [CrossRef] [PubMed]
19. Ramos, J.M.; Biru, D.; Tesfamariam, A.; Reyes, F.; Górgolas, M. Screening for tuberculosis in family and household contacts in a rural area in Ethiopia over a 20-month period. *Int. J. Mycobact.* **2013**, *2*, 240–243. [CrossRef] [PubMed]
20. Hiruy, N.; Melese, M.; Habte, D.; Jerene, D.; Gashu, Z.; Alem, G.; Jemal, I.; Tessema, B.; Belayneh, B.; Suarez, P.G. Comparison of the yield of tuberculosis among contacts of multidrug-resistant and drug-sensitive tuberculosis patients in Ethiopia using GeneXpert as a primary diagnostic test. *Int. J. Infect. Dis.* **2018**, *71*, 4–8. [CrossRef] [PubMed]
21. Javaid, A.; Khan, M.A.; Khan, M.A.; Mehreen, S.; Basit, A.; Khan, R.A.; Ihtesham, M.; Ullah, I.; Khan, A.; Ullah, U. Screening outcomes of household contacts of multidrug-resistant tuberculosis patients in Peshawar, Pakistan. *Asian Pac. J. Trop. Med.* **2016**, *9*, 269–273. [CrossRef] [PubMed]
22. Saw, S.; Win, K.S.; Aung, S.T.; Aung, P.P.; Soe, K.T.; Tun, Z.L.; Thu, M.K. *Assessment of Community-based MDR TB Care in Yangon Region: An Operational Research February 2018*; Department of Medical Research, Myanmar Medical Association, Natioanl Tuberculosis Programme, Department of Public Health: Yangon, Myanmar, 2018.
23. World Health Organization Tuberculosis Diagnostics. *Automated Real-Time DNA Amplification Test for Rapid and Simultaneous Detection of TB and Rifampicin Resistance*; Xpert® MTB/RIF Assay; Factsheet; World Health Organization: Geneva, Switzerland, 2016; pp. 1–2.
24. Zaidi, S.M.A.; Habib, S.S.; Van Ginneken, B.; Ferrand, R.A.; Creswell, J.; Khowaja, S.; Khan, A. Evaluation of the diagnostic accuracy of Computer-Aided Detection of tuberculosis on Chest radiography among private sector patients in Pakistan. *Sci. Rep.* **2018**, *8*, 1–9. [CrossRef] [PubMed]

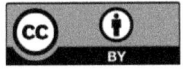

© 2019 by the authors. Licensee MDPI, Basel, Switzerland. This article is an open access article distributed under the terms and conditions of the Creative Commons Attribution (CC BY) license (http://creativecommons.org/licenses/by/4.0/).

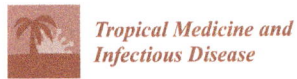

Article

Outcomes of Community-Based Systematic Screening of Household Contacts of Patients with Multidrug-Resistant Tuberculosis in Myanmar

Nang Thu Thu Kyaw [1,*], Aung Sithu [1], Srinath Satyanarayana [2,3], Ajay M. V. Kumar [2,3,4], Saw Thein [5], Aye Myat Thi [1], Pyae Phyo Wai [1], Yan Naing Lin [1], Khine Wut Yee Kyaw [1], Moe Myint Theingi Tun [1], Myo Minn Oo [1], Si Thu Aung [5] and Anthony D. Harries [3,6]

1. Center for Operational Research, International Union Against Tuberculosis and Lung Disease, Myanmar Office, Mandalay 05021, Myanmar; aungsithu@theunion.org (A.S.); drayemyatthi@gmail.com (A.M.T.); pyaephyowai@theunion.org (P.P.W.); nainglinn.zhaohong.yan@gmail.com (Y.N.L.); dr.khinewutyeekyaw2015@gmail.com (K.W.Y.K.); dr.moemyint86@gmail.com (M.M.T.T.); dr.myominnoo@gmail.com (M.M.O.)
2. Center for Operational Research, International Union Against Tuberculosis and Lung Disease, South-East Asia Office, New Delhi 110016, India; SSrinath@theunion.org (S.S.); AKumar@theunion.org (A.M.V.K.)
3. Center for Operational Research, International Union Against Tuberculosis and Lung Disease, 75006 Paris, France; adharries@theunion.org
4. Yenepoya Medical College, Yenepoya (Deemed to be University), Mangaluru 575018, India
5. National Tuberculosis Programme, Department of Public Health, Nay Pyi Taw 15011, Myanmar; dr.sawthein2010@gmail.com (S.T.); sta.ntp@gmail.com (S.T.A.)
6. Department of Infectious and Tropical Diseases, London School of Hygiene and Tropical Medicine, London WC1E 7HT, UK
* Correspondence: nangthu82@gmail.com; Tel.: +95-02-284-8046

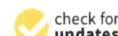

Received: 16 October 2019; Accepted: 13 November 2019; Published: 25 December 2019

Abstract: Screening of household contacts of patients with multidrug-resistant tuberculosis (MDR-TB) is a crucial active TB case-finding intervention. Before 2016, this intervention had not been implemented in Myanmar, a country with a high MDR-TB burden. In 2016, a community-based screening of household contacts of MDR-TB patients using a systematic TB-screening algorithm (symptom screening and chest radiography followed by sputum smear microscopy and Xpert-MTB/RIF assays) was implemented in 33 townships in Myanmar. We assessed the implementation of this intervention, how well the screening algorithm was followed, and the yield of active TB. Data collected between April 2016 and March 2017 were analyzed using logistic and log-binomial regression. Of 620 household contacts of 210 MDR-TB patients enrolled for screening, 620 (100%) underwent TB symptom screening and 505 (81%) underwent chest radiography. Of 240 (39%) symptomatic household contacts, 71 (30%) were not further screened according to the algorithm. Children aged <15 years were less likely to follow the algorithm. Twenty-four contacts were diagnosed with active TB, including two rifampicin- resistant cases (yield of active TB = 3.9%, 95% CI: 2.3%–6.5%). The highest yield was found among children aged <5 years (10.0%, 95% CI: 3.6%–24.7%). Household contact screening should be strengthened, continued, and scaled up for all MDR-TB patients in Myanmar.

Keywords: multidrug-resistant tuberculosis; household contact; screening; TB diagnosis; yield; operations research

1. Introduction

Myanmar is one of the 30 high tuberculosis (TB) and multidrug-resistant TB (MDR-TB) burden countries in the world. In 2017, of the estimated 14,000 MDR-TB cases in Myanmar, 3281 were diagnosed and 2666 were enrolled for treatment, indicating a significant gap in case detection and treatment [1]. Similarly, of the estimated 191,000 TB cases, only 132,025 were notified and treated. To reduce the TB and MDR-TB burden, it is essential to diagnose TB and MDR-TB early and provide quality assured treatment [2,3]. Early diagnosis and treatment reduce morbidity, mortality, and transmission of TB and MDR-TB in the community.

Close contacts of active TB and MDR-TB patients are at high risk of TB infection and disease. A systematic review reported a pooled yield of 3.4% active TB among close contacts of active TB, with the incidence being highest during the first year of exposure [4]. Another systematic review reported that the prevalence of active TB among household contacts of drug-resistant TB was as high as 7.8% [5]. Hence, there is a strong recommendation to screen all household contacts of MDR-TB patients for active TB, and if they are diagnosed with active TB, to initiate them on treatment as soon as possible [6].

The International Union against TB and Lung Disease (The Union) has been implementing a community-based MDR-TB care (CBMDR-TBC) project in Myanmar to support the National Tuberculosis Programme's (NTP) programmatic management of DR-TB since 2015. Due to the high presumed prevalence of TB among household contacts of MDR-TB patients, a systematic screening algorithm including a combination of screening methods (symptoms and chest radiography) and diagnostic tests (sputum smear microscopy and Xpert MTB/RIF assay) to screen for active TB and MDR-TB was incorporated as a key component of the CBMDR-TBC project. In early 2016, community volunteers and focal nurses were trained under the CBMDR-TBC project to implement this screening for all household contacts of index MDR-TB patients in project townships, and the project started systematic data collection (which included dedicated recording and reporting systems) of this activity in March 2016.

To date, there has been no published report from Myanmar describing the process of screening household contacts of MDR-TB patients, how well the screening algorithm was followed, and the yield of active TB among those screened. Therefore, in this study we assessed: (a) the proportion of household contacts who were screened for active TB using the systematic screening algorithm (the proportion who were screened using symptoms and chest radiography and those with TB symptoms who were investigated for active TB using sputum smear microscopy and/or Xpert MTB/RIF assay), (b) the socio-demographic characteristics associated with screening of TB according to the algorithm, (c) the yield of active TB, and (d) socio-demographic characteristics associated with the diagnosis of active TB during one year of the implementation of the project.

2. Materials and Methods

2.1. Study Design

This was an analysis of routinely collected program data.

2.2. Setting

2.2.1. Country Setting

Myanmar is a lower middle-income country with a population of 51 million. Geographically, the country is divided into 15 states/regions, which are further administratively divided into 412 townships. The country bears a high burden of MDR-TB along with its neighboring countries such as China, India, Bangladesh, and Thailand. The Programmatic Management of DR-TB was initiated in 2011 as part of the NTP's National Strategic Plan (2011–2015) to control TB in Myanmar [7]. Systematic contact tracing for all household contacts of MDR-TB patients is one of the key activities of the NTP's National Strategic Plan (2016–2020) [8]. The NTP recommends active screening of all household contacts of index MDR-TB patients and upfront use of Xpert MTB/RIF for investigating those with presumptive TB [9]. In order to facilitate Xpert MTB/RIF testing, the NTP has rolled out Xpert MTB/RIF machines in Myanmar since 2012, and by 2016 there were 65 Xpert MTB/RIF functional machines in the country.

2.2.2. Project Description and the Implementation of Systematic Screening

The CBMDR-TBC project was started in 2015 in collaboration with The Union and NTP to support the treatment initiation and adherence among MDR-TB patients in 33 townships across four states/regions in the upper part of Myanmar. Details of the CBMDR-TBC project have been described elsewhere [10]. Briefly, under the project, each township has a focal nurse who visits the index MDR-TB patients' house monthly to monitor treatment adherence and side effects and provide health education and psychosocial support. The project also assigns a community volunteer for each patient who visits the patient's house daily in the evening to provide directly observed treatment. Focal nurses supervise the volunteers, and the project managers of the CBMDR-TBC project in turn supervise the focal nurses.

In 2016, a systematic screening of the household contacts of MDR-TB patients was incorporated into the project. The focal nurses and community volunteers were trained to implement the TB screening for all household contacts of index MDR-TB patients and the systematic data collection. A household contact is defined as "a person who shares the same enclosed living space for one or more nights or for frequent or extended periods during the day with the index case during the treatment or during the three months before the commencement of the current treatment".

The trained focal nurse facilitates the screening of household contacts for TB once the MDR-TB patients are diagnosed and every six months thereafter using a screening and investigation algorithm as described in Figure 1. During the home visit to the MDR-TB patients, the focal nurse screens each household member using a symptom-based questionnaire and refers these members for a chest radiograph. Those with symptoms and/or abnormal chest radiograph submit one early morning sputum sample for Xpert MTB/RIF and two samples, one spot and one early morning sputum, for smear microscopy for acid-fast bacilli (AFB). The focal nurses are trained to instruct contacts on how to expectorate sputum according to the guidelines. The instruction includes: First, rinse the mouth with clean water; second, take a deep breath in and out for three times; third, take one deep breath and cough forcefully; and finally, spit the sputum into the sputum container provided. Those with no symptoms are closely monitored unless the chest radiograph is abnormal, at which point the patient is referred to a TB specialist for further assessment. The contacts who are positive on smear microscopy for AFB and/or Xpert MTB/RIF assay are diagnosed with active TB. Those with negative results on smear microscopy or the Xpert MTB/RIF assay but have an abnormal chest radiograph are referred to the TB specialist for clinical evaluation and a decision on whether there is a clinical diagnosis of active TB. Each household contact is line listed and given a unique contact registration number. The nurse records the results of this screening process in the MDR-TB household contact screening register (Annex S1).

The focal nurses are responsible for screening the household contacts of MDR-TB patients as soon as the index MDR-TB patients are diagnosed. However, not all household contacts of index MDR-TB patients are screened immediately for several reasons, and therefore there could be a considerable delay between the diagnosis of an index case and the initial screening of contacts. In addition to 6-monthly systematic screening, the volunteers and nurses also check whether any TB-related symptoms have developed in household contacts during their regular home visits. If a household contact reports any TB-related symptom before the scheduled screening appointment, the focal nurse facilitates the evaluation of such patients for active TB in line with the algorithm. In addition, the focal nurses and volunteers provide TB health education and support for household infection control measures. They receive periodic training on systematic screening and investigation of active TB in household contacts conducted by the project managers using a standardized training package. The training includes steps to identify household contacts, the conduct of symptom screening, the referral of persons for diagnostic investigations for active TB and drug-resistant TB, follow up, linkage to treatment if required, education, and support for infection control measures.

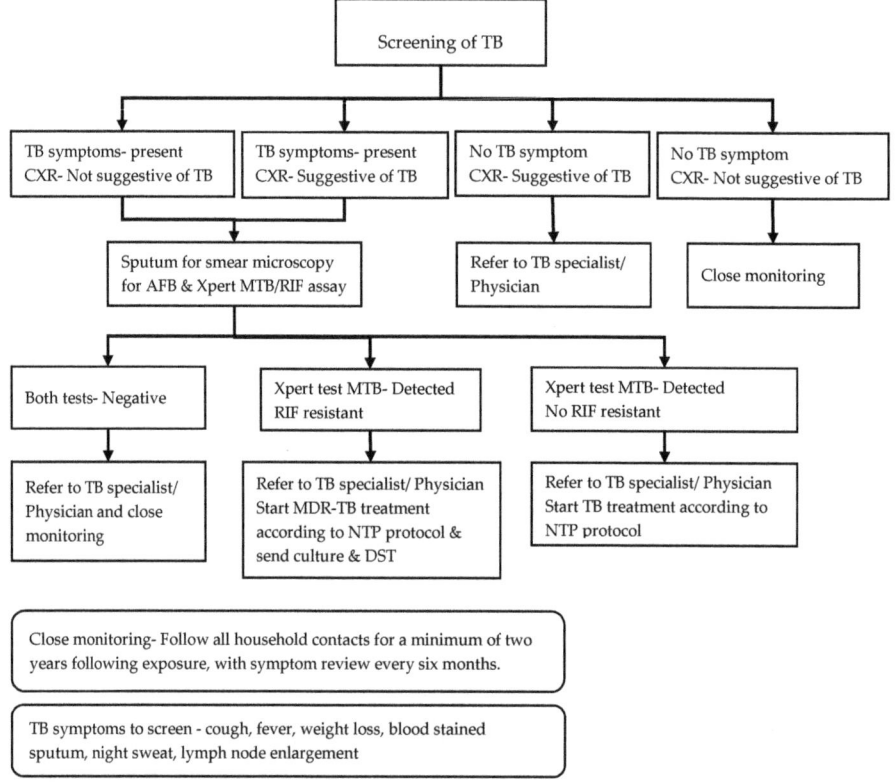

Figure 1. Systematic screening and investigation algorithm for household contacts of index multidrug-resistant tuberculosis (MDR-TB) patients in the community-based MDR-TB care project in Myanmar. TB = tuberculosis; CXR = chest radiography; AFB = acid-fast bacilli; NTP = National TB Programme; DST = drug sensitivity testing.

Every month, the information from the MDR-TB household contact screening register is entered into an electronic database (developed using EpiInfo version 7.2 software) by the project's data entry operators, and the data are checked and validated by the monitoring and evaluation officer of the project.

2.3. Study Sites and Population

The study population includes all household contacts of index MDR-TB patients enrolled for TB screening in 33 townships of the CBMDR-TBC project in Upper Myanmar between April 2016 and March 2017. The index MDR-TB patients of the contacts included in this study were MDR-TB patients who were newly initiated on treatment between April 2016 and March 2017 as well as those who were already on treatment before April 2016.

2.4. Sources of Data, Data Variables, and Data Collection

We used secondary data routinely collected in the electronic database. Data variables of household contacts of index MDR-TB patients included: Contact registration number; registration date for contact screening; age; sex; history of previous TB; HIV status; history of diabetes mellitus; clinical information on symptoms such as cough, fever, weight loss, hemoptysis, lymph node enlargement, and night sweats; and results of diagnostic investigations such as sputum smear microscopy, Xpert MTB/RIF assay, and chest radiography and the treatment registration number of their index case. These data were extracted from the electronic database.

2.5. Analysis and Statistics

The demographic and clinical characteristics of the household contacts were described using numbers (proportions) and medians (interquartile ranges). We assessed the proportion of the household contacts with TB symptoms and of those, the proportion who underwent further sputum evaluation (smear AFB and/or Xpert test MTB/RIF). We used binomial logit models to study the association between measured demographic and clinical characteristics and the odds of further sputum evaluation according to the screening algorithm.

The yield/proportion of TB was calculated by dividing the number of TB or MDR-TB cases diagnosed by the number of household contacts screened for TB. We also calculated the yield of active TB across various measured demographic and clinical characteristics. The prevalence ratios of active TB across various measured demographic and clinical characteristics were estimated using binomial log models. STATA software (version 12.1, copyright 1985–2011 StataCorp LP, College Station, TX, USA) was used for all analysis. The 95% confidence intervals (CIs) for proportions, odds ratios, and prevalence ratios were adjusted for clustering at the township and household level using cluster robust standard error estimates.

2.6. Ethics

Ethics approval was received from the Myanmar Ethics Review Committee, Department of Medical Research, Ministry of Health and Sports, Myanmar (Approval number: Ethics/DMR/2017/084) and the Ethics Advisory Group of International Union Against Tuberculosis and Lung Disease, Paris, France (EAG number: 120/16). Permission to conduct the study was granted from the National Tuberculosis Programme, Ministry of Health and Sports, Myanmar.

3. Results

There were 620 household contacts of 210 index MDR-TB patients who were enrolled for systematic screening for active TB. Of those enrolled, all were screened for symptoms and 505 (81%) also underwent chest radiography. There were 240 (39%) contacts who had one or more TB symptoms and were eligible for sputum smear microscopy and Xpert MTB/RIF testing. Of those eligible, 169 (70%) underwent sputum smear microscopy and/or an Xpert MTB/RIF assay. The remaining 71 (30%) contacts did not undergo either of these tests, though some were evaluated clinically by the TB specialist (Figure 2). As a result of all these investigations and clinical evaluations, 24 contacts (3.9%, 95% CI: 2.3%–6.5%) were diagnosed with active TB (seven were bacteriologically confirmed, including two with Rifampicin-resistant TB, and 17 were clinically diagnosed). The number of household contacts screened to diagnose one case of active TB was 26 (95% CI: 15–44).

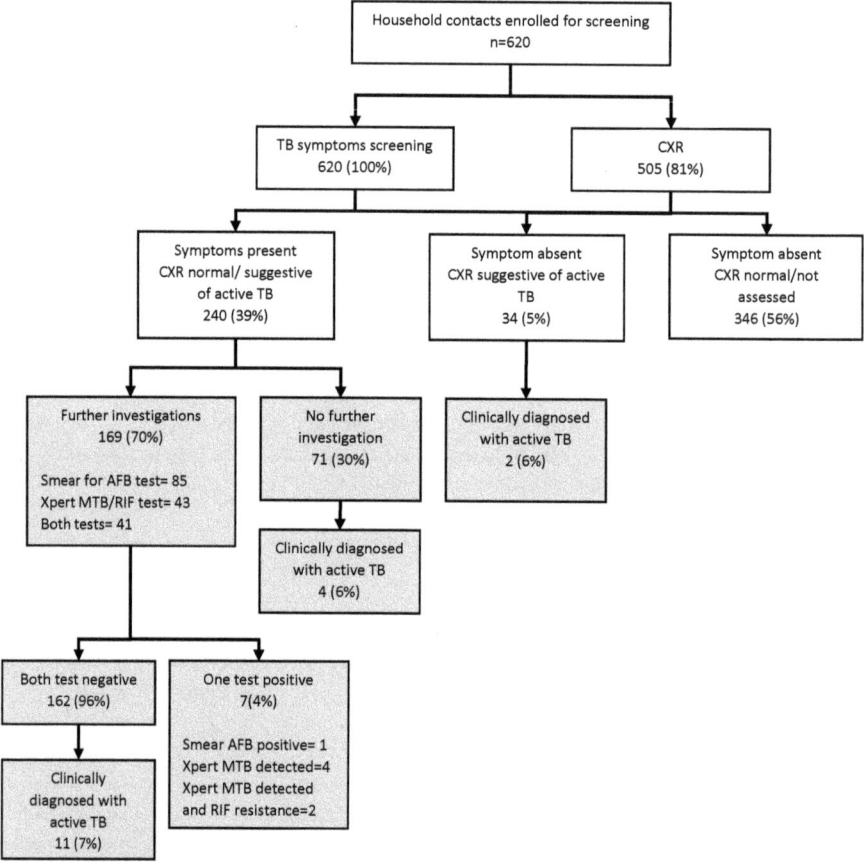

Figure 2. Number of household contacts of MDR-TB patients who underwent TB screening and investigations under the community-based MDR-TB Care Project in 33 townships in Myanmar, April 2016–March 2017. TB = tuberculosis; CXR = chest radiography; AFB = acid-fast bacilli.

3.1. Characteristics Associated with Following the Systematic Screening Algorithm among Symptomatic Contacts

The demographic and clinical characteristics of contacts with TB symptoms (n = 240) who underwent further evaluation by sputum tests (n = 169) versus those who did not undergo further evaluation by sputum tests (n = 71) are presented in Table 1. The age of the contact was the only characteristic that was statistically associated with whether contacts underwent further evaluation by sputum examination or not. Children aged less than 15 years were less likely to have had a sputum examination (either smear for AFB or Xpert test MTB/RIF), and contacts older than 49 years were more likely to have had a sputum examination when compared to contacts in the 15–49 year age group.

Table 1. Characteristics of symptomatic household contacts of MDR-TB patients, and their association with following the systematic screening algorithm under the community-based MDR-TB Care Project in 33 townships in Myanmar, April 2016–March 2017.

Characteristics	Total		Followed the Systematic Screening Algorithm			
	n	(%) †	n	(%) §	OR	(95% CI) *
Total	240	(100)	169	(70.4)		
Sex						
Male	105	(43.7)	70	(66.7)	Ref	
Female	135	(56.3)	99	(73.3)	0.7	(0.3–1.5)
Age						
<5 years	16	(6.7)	2	(12.5)	0.3	(0.0–0.2)
5–14 years	44	(18.3)	15	(34.1)	0.2	(0.0–0.4)
15–49 years	117	(48.8)	95	(81.2)	Ref	
>49 years	58	(24.2)	56	(96.5)	6.5	(2.2–18.9)
Missing	5	(2.1)	1	(20.0)	0.1	(0.0–0.8)
History of previous TB						
Yes	11	(4.6)	9	(81.8)	1.9	(0.5–6.6)
No	229	(95.4)	160	(69.9)	Ref	
HIV status						
Positive	3	(1.3)	3	(1.8)	NA	
Unknown	237	(98.7)	166	(98.2)		
History of diabetes mellitus						
Yes	2	(0.8)	1	(50.0)	0.4	(0.0–6.8)
Unknown	238	(99.2)	168	(70.6)	Ref	

OR = odds ratio; CI = confidence interval; Ref = reference group; * CIs are adjusted for clustering at household level as well as township level. † Column percentage; § Row percentage of total contact number. NA = not applicable.

3.2. Characteristics Associated with Diagnosed with Active TB among Registered Contacts

The demographic and clinical characteristics of 610 household contacts screened for active TB and the yield/prevalence of active TB in association with these characteristics are shown in Table 2. Overall 58% of the contacts were female, the median age of all contacts (IQR) was 31 (16–46) years and 40 (7%) contacts were children aged less than 5 years. Seventeen (3%) contacts had a previous history of TB, 6 (1%) had positive HIV status, and <1% of the contacts had a history of diabetes mellitus. Children aged less than 5 years had a significantly higher yield of TB when compared to contacts in the adult age groups. Since a small number of contacts were diagnosed with TB ($n = 24$), we did not perform a multivariable analysis to calculate the adjusted prevalence ratios.

Table 2. Demographic and clinical characteristics of household contacts of MDR-TB patients and the yield of TB among household contacts under the community-based MDR-TB Care Project in 33 townships in Myanmar, April 2016–March 2017.

Characteristics	Total		Diagnosed with Active TB				
	n	(%) †	n	%	(95% CI) §,*	PR	(95% CI) *
Total	610	100	24	3.9	(2.3–6.5)	-	
Sex							
Male	258	(41.6)	12	4.7	(1.9–10.8)	1.4	(0.6–3.4)
Female	362	(58.4)	12	3.3	(2.1–5.2)	ref	
Age							
<5 years	40	(6.5)	4	10.0	(3.6–24.7)	3.7	(1.2–11.4)
5–14 years	98	(15.8)	4	4.1	(1.2–13.4)	1.5	(0.4–5.5)
15–49 years	337	(54.4)	8	2.7	(1.4–5.1)	ref	
>49 years	137	(22.1)	5	4.4	(1.8–10.0)	1.6	(0.6–4.6)
Missing	8	(1.3)	1	12.5	(1.3–60.7)	4.7	(0.6–34.9)
History of previous TB							
Yes	17	(2.7)	0	-			

Table 2. Cont.

Characteristics	Total		Diagnosed with Active TB				
	n	(%) [†]	n	%	(95% CI) [§,*]	PR	(95% CI) *
No	603	(97.3)	24	4.0	(2.3–6.7)	NA	
HIV status							
Positive	6	(1.0)	1	16.7	(1.8–67.9)	4.4	(0.6–32.0)
Unknown	614	(99.0)	23	3.7	(2.2–6.4)	ref	
History of diabetes mellitus							
Yes	3	(0.5)	0	-			
Unknown	617	(99.5)	24	3.9	(2.3–6.6)	NA	

PR = prevalence ratio; CI = confidence interval; Ref = reference group; * CIs are adjusted for clustering at household level as well as township level. [†] Column percentage. [§] Row percentage of total contact number. NA = not applicable as PR cannot be calculated as there is zero prevalence in one of the two groups.

4. Discussion

This is the first study describing and evaluating the process of the systematic screening and investigation of household contacts of index MDR-TB patients in Myanmar. The study identified major gaps in the implementation of the screening as per the contact investigation algorithm. About 20% of all contacts enrolled were not screened by chest radiography. A third of the contacts with TB symptoms were not investigated by any sputum examination, and only one-fifth of contacts with TB symptoms were investigated by both sputum smear microscopy and the Xpert MTB/RIF assay. About 4% of contacts were diagnosed as having active TB disease. Children under 5 years of age who were contacts were more likely to be diagnosed with active TB. Since the study used routinely collected project data, we strongly believe that the findings can inform the national program in scaling up MDR-TB household contact screening in Myanmar.

There are a few limitations to the study. First, we did not have information on the total number of contacts of 210 index cases (the denominator) of which 620 were enrolled. This was due to a gap in our recording system that may have led to the focal nurses enrolling only those who they were able to meet and perform the symptom screening. Therefore, the gap between the number of contacts eligible and the number screened is likely to be higher than shown in our study. Second, as this study was cross-sectional in design, the results only provide an estimate of the prevalence of TB cases among contacts at a certain time period. Since the household contacts are more likely to develop TB anytime following exposure to the index case, a longitudinal study that provides information on both prevalent and incident cases would have provided much better estimates of the actual yield of TB among contacts. Third, due to the cross-sectional nature of the study and also since genotyping of contact's mycobacterial specimens was not done, we are unable to assess the temporal relationship between the exposure to the index patients and development of TB in the contacts, and therefore we cannot make any inferences about whether the TB disease diagnosed among contacts is due to TB transmission within the households. Fourth, about one-third of contacts did not undergo diagnostic evaluation according to the screening algorithm, and therefore the yield of MDR-TB cases among household contacts of MDR-TB patients in our study is an underestimate of the true yield. Finally, the study was based on routinely collected program data, and therefore there could be some errors in recording and reporting. We did not estimate the magnitude of these errors. However, we believe that due to the supervision and monitoring protocols in place, these errors are likely to be minimal and random, and therefore these errors are unlikely to have a major influence on the study results.

Despite these limitations, the study has some key findings to inform the program and future research. About 80% of contacts as per the screening algorithm underwent chest radiography. Anecdotally we were informed by the field-level health workers that this required substantial resources, time, and effort from them as well as the household contacts. Therefore, the large proportion of contacts who underwent chest radiography in our study may not be sustainable or replicable in routine practice.

Therefore, whether chest radiography is required for all household contacts irrespective of the presence of symptoms is a subject matter for further exploration and future study. In this future study, we suggest that different screening and investigation algorithms are compared and tested for their efficacy and cost-effectiveness in detecting active TB among household contacts of MDR-TB patients [11].

One-third of household contacts with TB symptoms did not undergo further sputum evaluation. A study from South Africa also showed that less than half of the symptomatic household contacts of MDR-TB underwent further TB diagnosis evaluation [12]. Similarly, many other studies have reported high drop-out rates during TB contact investigation [13]. There are possible patient-level and health system-level barriers that prevent the systematic contact investigation algorithm from being followed. A study conducted in Vietnam reported that contacts and patients' knowledge, attitude, and practices regarding TB influenced continued engagement in the TB investigation process [14]. Another study from Uganda reported that stigma about TB, the constraint on time and space in clinics for counselling, mistrust of health-center staff by patients and contacts, and high travel costs for health staff to conduct contact screening and for contacts to travel to health facilities were barriers to implement TB contact screening [15].

In addition, not all contacts who were tested by sputum smear examination were tested by Xpert MTB/RIF. Studies have shown that Xpert MTB/RIF can detect up to 59% additional TB cases when compared to sputum smear microscopy [16–18]. It can also detect RR-TB as well as reduce the turnaround time from sample collection to diagnosis and treatment [19]. Inadequate access or lack of access to Xpert MTB/RIF machines was one of the main barriers for Xpert MTB/RIF testing for all eligible patients. During the study period, there were only 65 Xpert MTB/RIF machines in the country while there were 330 townships with an MDR-TB center. Many townships did not have Xpert MTB/RIF machines, and some of the townships were far from those that had a functioning machine for referral. The national program has a plan to increase the number of machines in the country (85 machines by the end of 2018), and the NTP's drug-resistant TB guidelines (February 2017) also recommend screening of household contacts of MDR-TB using Xpert MTB/RIF [9]. This could substantially reduce the barriers for Xpert MTB/RIF testing and increase the number of TB cases detected among the household contacts. Other patient- and provider-level barriers for accessing Xpert MTB/RIF should be explored in this context.

The prevalence of TB among household contacts in our study is similar to other studies conducted in high TB and MDR-TB burden countries [4,20–22]. However, we believe that due to several gaps in implementation and the limitations mentioned above, the prevalence in our setting is likely to be higher than what we observed in this study. In order to obtain more accurate estimates of the burden of TB among household contacts, the gaps and limitations identified in our study must be addressed. This includes close and active surveillance for 24 months for early detection of active disease in those who may be infected [23]. In addition, there is a need to support index patients to improve infection control measures at the household level, such as simple measures to improve cross-ventilation so that further transmission can be minimized [20,23,24].

We found that child contacts younger than five years had the highest risk of being diagnosed with TB. Although some studies and systematic reviews have reported that the yield among children is comparable to that seen in adult contacts [5,25], some studies have shown that there is a high prevalence of TB in children among contacts, as seen in our study [26,27]. This can be explained by the fact that young children are more likely to stay at home, which can increase exposure time especially if the index cases are their first-degree relatives [28]. Hence, it would be worthwhile to consider chemoprophylaxis in children after active TB is excluded to prevent the development of TB or MDR-TB [29–31]. Currently, we do not have national guidelines on how to manage TB infection in child contacts of MDR-TB, and there is no consensus on the preventive regimen for contacts of MDR-TB. Therefore, there is a need to develop guidelines to manage childhood contacts of patients with MDR-TB and to provide preventive therapy in Myanmar. In the meantime, as per the existing strategy, the program should maintain active surveillance of all contacts so as to detect and treat cases early [32].

Policy and Practice Implications

The project needs to (1) strengthen the listing of all household contacts in the contact register and continue to record the results of the screening process in a systematic manner; (2) evaluate the efficacy and effectiveness of different contact screening algorithms and identify the most cost-effective and convenient algorithm that can be used in this setting; and (3) identify and address individual and system-level barriers for sputum smear examination and Xpert MTB/RIF testing.

5. Conclusions

The yield of TB (~4%) from screening household contacts of index MDR-TB patients was similar to what has been reported from other parts of the world. However, there were major gaps in screening according to the algorithm, and sputum smear microscopy and Xpert MTB/RIF testing were not done in all of the eligible contacts. The project should strengthen the systematic screening and investigation of TB in household contacts of MDR-TB patients, and the NTP should scale up the contact screening for all MDR-TB patients countrywide in order to achieve early detection and treatment of TB and MDR-TB.

Supplementary Materials: The following are available online at http://www.mdpi.com/2414-6366/5/1/2/s1, Annex S1: Household contact screening register used in the community-based MDR-TB Care Project in 33 townships.

Author Contributions: Conceptualization and protocol development: N.T.T.K., A.S., S.S., A.M.V.K., S.T., A.M.T., K.W.Y.K., S.T.A., A.D.H.; Data Collection: N.T.T.K., A.S.T., S.T., A.M.T., P.P.W., Y.N.L., K.W.Y.K., M.M.T.T., M.M.O.; Data Analysis: N.T.T.K., S.S., A.M.V.K., Y.N.L., K.W.Y.K., M.M.O., A.D.H.; Writing the first draft: N.T.T.K., S.S., A.D.H.; Critical review of the paper and final approval: N.T.T.K., A.S., S.S., A.M.V.K., S.T., A.M.T., P.P.W., Y.N.L., K.W.Y.K., M.M.T.T., M.M.O., S.T.A., A.D.H. All authors have read and agreed to the published version of the manuscript.

Funding: This research received no external funding.

Acknowledgments: We thank all the clinical, administrative and program staff from the National Tuberculosis Programme, Department of Public Health and The Union office in Myanmar for their dedication in caring for patients and community and their contribution in collecting and providing data. We thank the Department for International Development (DFD), UK, for funding the Global Operational Research Fellowship Programme in which first author and co-authors (N.T.T.K., K.W.Y.K. M.M.O.) work as operational research fellows.

Conflicts of Interest: The authors declare no conflict of interest.

References

1. World Health Organization. Global Tuberculosis Report 2018. Available online: http://www.who.int/tb/publications/global_report/en/ (accessed on 29 December 2018).
2. World Health Organization. Guidelines for Treatment of Drug-Susceptible Tuberculosis and Patient Care. Available online: http://www.who.int/tb/publications/2017/dstb_guidance_2017/en/ (accessed on 3 May 2017).
3. World Health Organization. Systematic Screening for Active Tuberculosis: Principles and Recommendations. Available online: https://www.who.int/tb/tbscreening/en/ (accessed on 11 October 2019).
4. Fox, G.J.; Barry, S.E.; Britton, W.J.; Marks, G.B. Contact investigation for tuberculosis: A systematic review and meta-analysis. *Eur. Respir. J.* **2013**, *41*, 140–156. [CrossRef] [PubMed]
5. Shah, N.S.; Yuen, C.M.; Heo, M.; Tolman, A.W.; Becerra, M.C. Yield of contact investigations in households of patients with drug-resistant tuberculosis: Systematic review and meta-analysis. *Clin. Infect. Dis.* **2014**, *58*, 381–391. [CrossRef] [PubMed]
6. World Health Organization. Companion Handbook to the WHO Guidelines for the Programmatic Management of Drug-Resistant Tuberculosis. 2014. Available online: http://www.who.int/tb/publications/pmdt_companionhandbook/en/ (accessed on 5 December 2016).
7. National Tuberculosis Programme Five Year National Strategic Plan for Tuberculosis Control 2011–2015. Available online: http://www.searo.who.int/myanmar/documents/en/ (accessed on 3 December 2018).
8. National Tuberculosis Programme National Strategic Plan for Tuberculosis 2016. Available online: http://mohs.gov.mm/Main/content/publication/list?pagenumber=1&pagesize=9 (accessed on 3 December 2018).

9. National Tuberculosis Programme Guidelines for the Management of Multi-Drug Resistant Tuberculosis (MDR-TB) in Myanmar. Available online: http://www.searo.who.int/myanmar/areas/tuberculosis/en/ (accessed on 27 May 2017).
10. Wai, P.P.; Shewade, H.D.; Kyaw, N.T.T.; Thein, S.; Thu, A.S.; Kyaw, K.W.Y.; Aye, N.N.; Phyo, A.M.; Maung, H.M.W.; Soe, K.T.; et al. Community-based MDR-TB care project improves treatment initiation in patients diagnosed with MDR-TB in Myanmar. *PLoS ONE* **2018**, *13*, e0194087. [CrossRef] [PubMed]
11. World Health Organization. Chest Radiography in Tuberculosis Detection. Available online: http://www.who.int/tb/publications/chest-radiography/en/ (accessed on 2 July 2017).
12. Kigozi, N.G.; Heunis, J.C.; Engelbrecht, M.C. Yield of systematic household contact investigation for tuberculosis in a high-burden metropolitan district of South Africa. *BMC Public Health* **2019**, *19*, 867. [CrossRef] [PubMed]
13. Armstrong-Hough, M.; Turimumahoro, P.; Meyer, A.J.; Ochom, E.; Babirye, D.; Ayakaka, I.; Mark, D.; Ggita, J.; Cattamanchi, A.; Dowdy, D.; et al. Drop-out from the tuberculosis contact investigation cascade in a routine public health setting in urban Uganda: A prospective, multi-center study. *PLoS ONE* **2017**, *12*, e0187145. [CrossRef]
14. Fox, G.J.; Loan, L.P.; Nhung, N.V.; Loi, N.T.; Sy, D.N.; Britton, W.J.; Marks, G.B. Barriers to adherence with tuberculosis contact investigation in six provinces of Vietnam: A nested case–control study. *BMC Infect. Dis.* **2015**, *15*, 103. [CrossRef]
15. Ayakaka, I.; Ackerman, S.; Ggita, J.M.; Kajubi, P.; Dowdy, D.; Haberer, J.E.; Fair, E.; Hopewell, P.; Handley, M.A.; Cattamanchi, A.; et al. Identifying barriers to and facilitators of tuberculosis contact investigation in Kampala, Uganda: A behavioral approach. *Implement. Sci.* **2017**, *12*, 33. [CrossRef]
16. Durovni, B.; Saraceni, V.; Hof, S.V.D.; Trajman, A.; Cordeiro-Santos, M.; Cavalcante, S.; Menezes, A.; Cobelens, F. Impact of Replacing Smear Microscopy with Xpert MTB/RIF for Diagnosing Tuberculosis in Brazil: A Stepped-Wedge Cluster-Randomized Trial. *PLoS Med.* **2014**, *11*, e1001766. [CrossRef]
17. Churchyard, G.J.; Stevens, W.S.; Mametja, L.D.; McCarthy, K.M.; Chihota, V.; Nicol, M.P.; Erasmus, L.K.; Ndjeka, N.O.; Mvusi, L.; Vassall, A.; et al. Xpert MTB/RIF versus sputum microscopy as the initial diagnostic test for tuberculosis: A cluster-randomised trial embedded in South African roll-out of Xpert MTB/RIF. *Lancet Glob. Health* **2015**, *3*, e450–e457. [CrossRef]
18. Nwachukwu, N.O.; Onyeagba, R.A.; Nwaugo, V.O.; Ononiwu, H.A.; Okafor, D.C. Diagnostic Accuracy of Xpert MTB/RIF Assay in Diagnosis of Pulmonary Tuberculosis. *J. Infect. Dis. Treat.* **2016**, *2*, 1–3.
19. Van Kampen, S.C.; Tursynbayeva, A.; Koptleuova, A.; Murzabekova, Z.; Bigalieva, L.; Aubakirova, M.; Pak, S.; Hof, S.V.D. Effect of Introducing Xpert MTB/RIF to Test and Treat Individuals at Risk of Multidrug-Resistant Tuberculosis in Kazakhstan: A Prospective Cohort Study. *PLoS ONE* **2015**, *10*, e0132514. [CrossRef] [PubMed]
20. Grandjean, L.; Gilman, R.H.; Martin, L.; Soto, E.; Castro, B.; López, S.; Coronel, J.; Castillo, E.; Alarcón, V.; Lopez, V.; et al. Transmission of Multidrug-Resistant and Drug-Susceptible Tuberculosis within Households: A Prospective Cohort Study. *PLoS Med.* **2015**, *12*, e1001843. [CrossRef] [PubMed]
21. Singla, N.; Singla, R.; Jain, G.; Habib, L.; Behera, D. Tuberculosis among household contacts of multidrug-resistant tuberculosis patients in Delhi, India. *Int. J. Tuberc. Lung Dis.* **2011**, *15*, 1326–1330. [CrossRef] [PubMed]
22. Titiyos, A.; Jerene, D.; Enquselasie, F. The yield of screening symptomatic contacts of multidrug-resistant tuberculosis cases at a tertiary hospital in Addis Ababa, Ethiopia. *BMC Res. Notes* **2015**, *8*, 501. [CrossRef]
23. Chamie, G.; Wandera, B.; Luetkemeyer, A.; Bogere, J.; Mugerwa, R.D.; Havlir, D.V.; Charlebois, E.D. Household ventilation and tuberculosis transmission in Kampala, Uganda. *Int. J. Tuberc. Lung Dis.* **2013**, *17*, 764–770. [CrossRef]
24. World Health Organization. WHO Policy on TB Infection Control in Health-Care Facilities, Congregate Settings and Households. Available online: https://www.who.int/tb/publications/2009/9789241598323/en/ (accessed on 11 October 2019).
25. Puryear, S.; Seropola, G.; Ho-Foster, A.; Arscott-Mills, T.; Mazhani, L.; Firth, J.; Goldfarb, D.M.; Ncube, R.; Bisson, G.P.; Steenhoff, A.P. Yield of contact tracing from pediatric tuberculosis index cases in Gaborone, Botswana. *Int. J. Tuberc. Lung Dis.* **2013**, *17*, 1049–1055. [CrossRef]
26. Amanullah, F.; Ashfaq, M.; Khowaja, S.; Parekh, A.; Salahuddin, N.; Lotia-Farrukh, I.; Khan, A.J.; Becerra, M.C. High tuberculosis prevalence in children exposed at home to drug-resistant tuberculosis. *Int. J. Tuberc. Lung Dis.* **2014**, *18*, 520–527. [CrossRef]

27. Becerra, M.C.; Franke, M.F.; Appleton, S.C.; Joseph, J.K.; Bayona, J.; Atwood, S.S.; Mitnick, C.D. Tuberculosis in Children Exposed at Home to Multidrug-resistant Tuberculosis. *Pediatr. Infect. Dis. J.* **2013**, *32*, 115–119. [CrossRef]
28. Chheng, P.; Nsereko, M.; Malone, L.L.; Okware, B.; Zalwango, S.; Joloba, M.; Boom, W.H.; Mupere, E.; Stein, C.M. Tuberculosis case finding in first-degree relative contacts not living with index tuberculosis cases in Kampala, Uganda. *Clin. Epidemiol.* **2015**, *7*, 411–419.
29. Padmapriyadarsini, C.; Das, M.; Burugina Nagaraja, S.; Rajendran, M.; Kirubakaran, R.; Chadha, S.; Tharyan, P. Is Chemoprophylaxis for Child Contacts of Drug-Resistant TB Patients Beneficial? A Systematic Review. *Tuberc. Res. Treat.* **2018**, *2018*, 3905890. [CrossRef]
30. Seddon, J.A.; Hesseling, A.C.; Finlayson, H.; Fielding, K.; Cox, H.; Hughes, J.; Godfrey-Faussett, P.; Schaaf, H.S. Preventive Therapy for Child Contacts of Multidrug-Resistant Tuberculosis: A Prospective Cohort Study. *Clin. Infect. Dis.* **2013**, *57*, 1676–1684. [CrossRef] [PubMed]
31. Seddon, J.A.; Godfrey-Faussett, P.; Hesseling, A.C.; Gie, R.P.; Beyers, N.; Schaaf, H.S. Management of children exposed to multidrug-resistant Mycobacterium tuberculosis. *Lancet Infect. Dis.* **2012**, *12*, 469–479. [CrossRef]
32. Moore, D.A.J. What can we offer to 3 million MDRTB household contacts in 2016? *BMC Med.* **2016**, *14*, 64. [CrossRef] [PubMed]

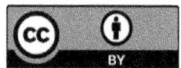

© 2019 by the authors. Licensee MDPI, Basel, Switzerland. This article is an open access article distributed under the terms and conditions of the Creative Commons Attribution (CC BY) license (http://creativecommons.org/licenses/by/4.0/).

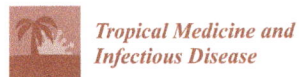 *Tropical Medicine and Infectious Disease*

Article

GeneXpert and Community Health Workers Supported Patient Tracing for Tuberculosis Diagnosis in Conflict-Affected Border Areas in India

Mrinalini Das [1,*], Dileep Pasupuleti [2], Srinivasa Rao [3], Stacy Sloan [2], Homa Mansoor [1], Stobdan Kalon [1], Farah Naz Hossain [1], Gabriella Ferlazzo [4] and Petros Isaakidis [4]

1. Médecins Sans Frontières/Doctors Without Borders, Delhi 110024, India; msfocb-delhi-med@brussels.msf.org (H.M.); Msfocb-India-ops-strategic-advisor@brussels.msf.org (S.K.); msfocb-delhi-medco@brussels.msf.org (F.N.H.)
2. Médecins Sans Frontières/Doctors Without Borders, Bhadrachalam, Telangana 507111, India; 1drdileep1@gmail.com (D.P.); MSFOCB-Bhadrachalam-PMR@brussels.msf.org (S.S.)
3. District TB Office, RNTCP, Bhadrachalam district hospital, Bhadrachalam, Telangana 507111, India; golla.srinivasulu99@gmail.com
4. Southern Africa Medical Unit, Médecins Sans Frontières, Cape Town 7925, South Africa; Gabriella.FERLAZZO@joburg.msf.org (G.F.); Petros.Isaakidis@joburg.msf.org (P.I.)
* Correspondence: msfocb-delhi-epi@brussels.msf.org; Tel.: +91-8010261984

Received: 19 November 2019; Accepted: 11 December 2019; Published: 21 December 2019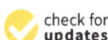

Abstract: Médecins Sans Frontières (MSF) has been providing diagnosis and treatment for patients with tuberculosis (TB) via mobile clinics in conflict-affected border areas of Chhattisgarh, India since 2009. The study objectives were to determine the proportion of patients diagnosed with TB and those who were lost-to-follow-up (LTFU) prior to treatment initiation among patients with presumptive TB between April 2015 and August 2018. The study also compared bacteriological confirmation and pretreatment LTFU during two time periods: a) April 2015–August 2016 and b) April 2017–August 2018 (before and after the introduction of GeneXpert as a first diagnostic test). Community health workers (CHW) supported patient tracing. This study was a retrospective analysis of routine program data. Among 1042 patients with presumptive TB, 376 (36%) were diagnosed with TB. Of presumptive TB patients, the pretreatment LTFU was 7%. Upon comparing the two time-periods, bacteriological confirmation increased from 20% to 33%, while pretreatment LTFU decreased from 11% to 4%. TB diagnosis with GeneXpert as the first diagnostic test and CHW-supported patient tracing in a mobile-clinic model of care shows feasibility for replication in similar conflict-affected, hard to reach areas.

Keywords: sputum; health promotion; operational research; indigenous population

1. Introduction

The management of tuberculosis (TB) is challenging for patients residing in remote and inaccessible areas. The scale of the challenge escalates when inaccessibility to healthcare increases due to conflict. Patients in these hard-to-reach areas need special attention from TB programmes and implementing partners [1].

India is a high-burden TB country, contributing to approximately a quarter of global incident TB cases. In 2018, the estimated number of TB cases in the country was 2,790,000 [2]. The border areas of central India (including four states, i.e., Chhattisgarh, Odisha, Telangana, Andhra Pradesh) have been affected by a long-standing, low-intensity, chronic conflict [3]. The majority of the population residing in these areas belong to various tribes and have limited access to healthcare services, including access to TB diagnosis and treatment facilities [4].

The Revised National TB Control Programme (RNTCP) has been providing TB care to remote and tribal populations [5]; however, these services in conflict-affected areas are often interrupted due to frequent instances of minor clashes. Basic healthcare services are provided at selected primary healthcare centers, but patients need to travel more than 50–100 km to access tertiary care services in district hospitals.

Médecins Sans Frontières (MSF), a nongovernmental, medical humanitarian organization, has been providing primary healthcare services, including diagnosis and treatment for patients with TB, via mobile clinics in the chronic conflict-affected border areas of Chhattisgarh, India since 2009 [6]. A unique model of care in collaboration with RNTCP has been implemented, aiming at offering improved delivery of TB diagnosis and treatment services. GeneXpert in the nearby government hospital (Bhadrachalam district hospital) has been utilized as the first diagnostic test for TB diagnosis since January 2017. Community Health Workers (CHW) are trained in patient tracing (that is, in the follow up of patients) in order to minimize pretreatment loss-to-follow-up (LTFU).

To date, there has been no documentation of this TB model of care in India. The aim of this study is to contribute to the body of evidence related to TB diagnostic delivery in conflict-affected and tribal areas, and to help policy makers and implementers to develop tailor-made, diagnostic strategies for such conflict-affected, hard-to-reach populations.

The specific objectives of the study included determining the number and proportions of (1) patients diagnosed with TB, (2) pretreatment lost-to-follow-up patients (from first presentation for diagnosis up to the date of receipt of TB diagnosis results, and (3) to compare the proportion of bacteriological confirmation and pretreatment LTFU between two time periods: (a) April 2015–August 2016 and (b) April 2017 August 2018 (before and during the utilization of GeneXpert as a first diagnostic test for TB diagnosis).

2. Materials and Methods

2.1. Study Design

This was a retrospective analysis of routinely collected clinical and programmatic data.

2.2. Setting

The state of Chhattisgarh in central India has a population of 26 million [7], including conflict-affected zones in the Sukma, Dantewada, and Bastar districts. Accurate information on the populations residing in the conflict-affected zones is not available [8]. The total number of notified TB cases in the Sukma district (where MSF TB Programme is operational) was 335 in 2018 [2].

TB Model of Care Description

MSF has been providing routine primary healthcare services, including TB care in the conflict-affected border areas with an estimated population of 90,000 since 2009 [6,9,10]. TB diagnosis and treatment is offered by a multidisciplinary team including doctors, nurses, counselors, health promoters, and CHWs. A doctor and nurse are TB focal points for the TB program. The nurses provide support with sample collections for TB diagnosis. The counselors provide information to patients and family members about TB signs/symptoms, treatment regimen, routes of TB transmission, and infection control. Health promoters carry out community sensitization sessions in villages every month on TB, malaria, diarrheal diseases, general hygiene, and sanitation.

A group of local CHWs are trained the identify the symptoms/signs of TB and support the tracing of patients. In case patients miss appointments for two weeks or more, a CHW visits the patient at their residence in the villages. Repeated sensitization of CHWs (once every three months) is carried out by the TB focal points and health promoters. The CHWs are paid a fixed stipend every month.

Since 2017, GeneXpert in the nearest district hospital in Bhadrachalam, Telangana has been utilized as the first diagnostic test for TB diagnosis in patients with presumptive TB. In India, studies have shown that GeneXpert has a sensitivity and specificity of 100% each for pulmonary TB samples and a sensitivity and specificity of 90.7% and 99.6% respectively for extra-pulmonary TB samples, in comparison with composite reference standards [11]. The patients with presumptive TB are requested to provide a spot sample in order to avoid the need to travel 10–15 kms to visit a clinic. Patients are given sputum containers for morning samples to be submitted on the next mobile clinic day (3 days later). The GeneXpert results (using spot samples) are given to patients on the next mobile van visit (the same visit when the morning sample is submitted); in cases whereby the GeneXpert result on the spot sample is negative, microscopy is performed on the morning sample. Patients are referred to the district hospital for a biopsy or chest X-ray, as required. For those with negative TB diagnostic results, a clinical decision is taken by the medical team. As laboratory results become available and are reported to the patient, pretreatment counseling is provided and treatment is initiated.

2.3. Study Site and Population

All patients with presumptive TB who received care in the MSF TB Programme in border areas of Chhattisgarh between 01 April 2015 and 31 August 2018 were included.

2.4. Data Variables and Sources, Data Analysis

The demographic (age, sex) and clinical characteristics (presence of cough, history of previous TB) of patients with presumptive TB, date of presentation, date of sputum collection, and diagnostic results (sputum, GeneXpert, Biopsy, Xray) were extracted from an electronic database and imported into STATA (version 11, StataCorp, College Station, Texas, USA) for analysis. TB diagnosis and pretreatment loss-to-follow up were summarized using frequency and proportions. Continuous variables such as age were summarized using median and inter-quartile range (IQR). Categorical variables (sex, previous history of TB, site of TB) were summarized as frequency and proportions. Associations between demographic and clinical characteristics and diagnosis of TB were assessed using a chi-square test and unadjusted relative risks (RR) with 95% Confidence Intervals (95% CI). A p value of less than 0.05 was considered statistically significant.

2.5. Operational Definitions

1. Presumptive TB: Presumptive TB refers to a patient who presented with symptoms or signs suggestive of TB [12]
2. Bacteriological confirmation: Presence of MTB+ in GeneXpert results; smear microscopy or culture evaluation was considered as a means of bacteriological confirmation
3. Clinically-diagnosed TB case: Patient diagnosed with active TB by a clinician on the basis of X-ray abnormalities and/or clinical evaluation. This includes smear-negative pulmonary TB and extra-pulmonary TB cases without laboratory confirmation.
4. Confirmed TB case: Patients with bacteriological confirmation or clinically-diagnosed TB
5. Error: Failure to test for diagnosis of TB was termed as error, which included poor-quality of sputum, technical error of equipment, machine malfunction, etc.
6. Prediagnosis loss-to-follow-up: If the patients with presumptive TB, after the first consultation, did not visit the clinic to provide a sample for TB diagnosis, it was considered a prediagnosis loss-to-follow-up.
7. Diagnosed TB loss-to-follow-up: If the patients were diagnosed with TB but did not visit the clinic for receipt of results within 1 month of THE initial consultation date, it was termed as diagnosed TB loss-to-follow-up.
8. Pretreatment loss-to-follow-up: The prediagnosis loss-to-follow-up and diagnosed TB loss-to-follow-up patients were together termed as pretreatment loss-to-follow-up.

2.6. Ethics

This research fulfilled the exemption criteria set by the Médecins Sans Frontières Ethics Review Board for a posteriori analyses of routinely-collected clinical data. and thus, did not require MSF ERB review. It was conducted with permission from Medical Director, Operational Centre Brussels, Médecins Sans Frontières. Since it is a record-based study, we obtained a waiver from obtaining informed consent. Permission for conducting the study was sought from the National TB Programme of India (RNTCP).

3. Results

Among 1042 patients with presumptive TB identified in the program during April 2015 to August 2018, 376 (36%) were diagnosed with TB. The demographic and clinical characteristics of the patients with presumptive TB and those diagnosed with TB are shown in Table 1. The proportion of patients diagnosed with TB was largest (44.8%) in children aged 0–14 years compared to other age groups; it was similar in males (37.7%, 216/573) and females (34.1%, 160/469). Diagnosis of Pulmonary TB (PTB) was much more common than extra-pulmonary TB (82.9% versus 17.1%); however, a larger proportion of extra-pulmonary presumptive TB patients had confirmation of TB diagnosis than pulmonary TB patients (60.0% versus 32.4%). The younger age group [(0–14 years RR (95% CI): 1.5 (1.2–1.9); 15–24 years: 1.4 (1.1–1.8)] and extra-pulmonary TB [1.9 (1.6–2.1)] had a higher risk of developing TB.

Table 1. Demographic and clinical characteristics of patients with presumptive TB and those diagnosed with TB in conflict-affected border areas in India, 2015–2018.

Characteristic	Patients with Presumptive TB * n (%)	Patients Diagnosed with TB ** n (%)	Unadjusted RR (95% CI)	Chi-Square (*p*-Value)
Total	1042	376 (36.1)		
Age group (years) (N = 1038)				
0–14	134 (12.9)	60 (44.8)	1.5 (**1.2–1.9**)	12.01 (**0.02**)
15–24	117 (11.2)	49 (41.9)	1.4 (**1.1–1.8**)	
25–34	197 (19.0)	75 (38.1)	1.3 (0.9–1.6)	
35–44	231 (22.3)	84 (36.4)	1.2 (0.9–1.5)	
45 and above	359 (34.6)	108 (30.1)	1	
Sex				
Male	573 (55.0)	216 (37.7)	1.1 (0.9–1.3)	1.43 (0.23)
Female	469 (45.0)	160 (34.1)	1	
TB site (N = 997)				
Pulmonary	827 (82.9)	268 (32.4)	1	46.0 (**<0.01**)
Extra-pulmonary	170 (17.1)	102 (60.0)	1.9 (**1.6–2.1**)	
Previous TB (N = 995)				
Yes	201 (20.2)	75 (37.3)	1.0 (0.8–1.2)	0.01 (0.9)
No	794 (79.8)	293 (36.9)	1	

* Column percentage, ** Row percentages, Unadjusted RR: Unadjusted Relative Risk; CI: Confidence Intervals.

A total of 60 (5.8%) out of 1042 patients with presumptive TB were prediagnosis LTFU, while one died before providing sample for TB diagnosis. Of those who were diagnosed with TB (with bacteriological or clinical confirmation, n = 376), nine (2.4%) did not come back to receive the test results (termed as 'diagnosed TB LTFU') and did not initiate treatment during the study period. Thus, 69 (6.6%) of 1042 patients were pretreatment LTFU. Of those for whom a diagnosis of TB was made, 217 (57.7%), 49 (13%), and 110 (29.2%) had sputum-positive pulmonary TB, sputum-negative pulmonary TB, and extra-pulmonary TB, respectively (nontabulated).

Upon comparing the "before–after" time periods (Figure 1), bacteriological confirmation increased from 20% (67/342) to 33% (109/335). Errors in TB diagnoses decreased from 9% (34/376) to 0.1% (1/336). The pretreatment LTFU decreased from 11% (45/417) to 4% (13/346) during the study period.

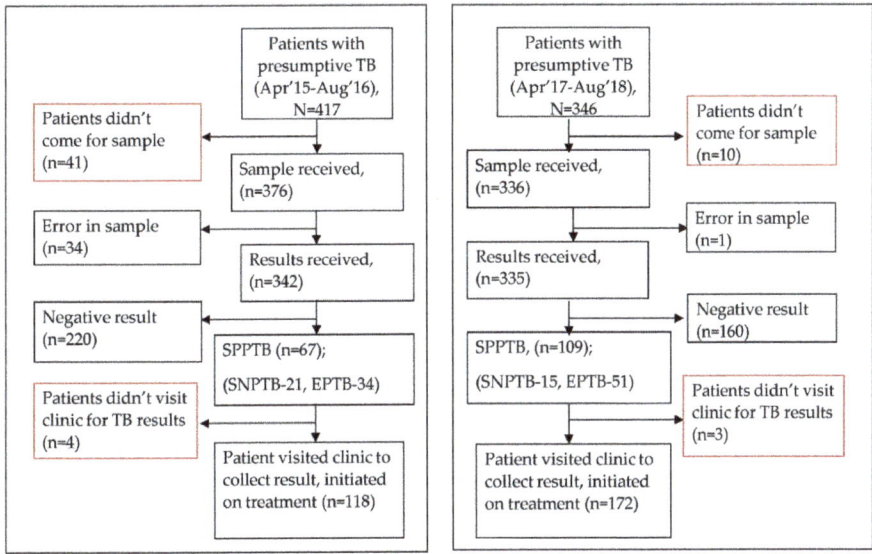

SPPTB: Smear-positive pulmonary tuberculosis; SNPTB: Smear negative pulmonary tuberculosis; EPTB: Extra-pulmonary tuberculosis

Figure 1. Bacteriological confirmation and pretreatment loss-to-follow-up during two time periods: (1) Apr. 2015–Aug. 2016 (Before GeneXpert was used as first diagnostic tool for TB-diagnosis), (2) Apr. 2017–Aug. 2018 (GeneXpert used for TB-diagnosis) in conflict-affected border areas in India.

4. Discussion

A model for TB diagnosis with the use of GeneXpert as a first test and CHW-supported patient tracing resulted in a 66% reduction of pretreatment loss-to-follow-up during 2015–2018 in a conflict-affected tribal area in India.

More than one-third of patients identified with presumptive TB were diagnosed with active TB; this is higher than other studies reported in similar tribal areas (6.5% in the Bharia tribe of Madhya Pradesh, 12.5% in Maharashtra, and 21% in the Sahariya tribe of central India) [13–15]. This could be due to the availability of a trained medical team for supporting TB diagnosis. Further, the availability of GeneXpert as a first diagnostic test for presumptive TB patients in government district hospitals likely contributed to the increased number of detected cases [16,17], some of which may have been missed earlier. Investments for the continuous operation of GeneXpert must be considered by TB programs. The availability and accessibility of diagnostic tools like GeneXpert [17] and the implementation by a trained team [18] help in early and appropriate TB diagnoses in these hard-to-reach areas.

Studies in conflict areas across the globe have reported multiple challenges of access to healthcare services [19–21]. Few TB programs have been successful in delivering treatment in conflict areas by adapting to local needs [22]. Other than direct medical care under the National TB Programme, intersectoral measures such as access to a public distribution system, nutritional support, social welfare schemes, and security measures at the central and state levels will help to minimize the TB burden.

The proportion of children and young adults was low in this group of patients with presumptive TB; however, the proportion of diagnosed TB was high compared to other age groups. As children are considered proxy indicators of TB transmission [23], it may be noted that the burden of TB is high in this tribal population, as it is in other tribal populations in the country [15]. The national TB program in country, with the involvement of other NGOs and stakeholders, must devise tailored approaches for the provision of improved diagnoses and treatment in children [24,25].

The proportion of diagnosed EPTB cases among presumptive EPTB cases was higher than expected. This may hint at the late arrival of EPTB cases for diagnosis [26] and lower awareness about extrapulmonary signs of TB among the community [27]. EPTB is often considered low priority by TB programs, as it does not lead to the transmission of infection [28]. Strategies must be proposed to improve access to diagnostics for EPTB (fine needle aspiration cytology, biopsy) in the nearest healthcare facilities [29].

The proportion of pretreatment loss-to-follow-up is lower than in other studies in the country [16,30]. This could be due to the dedicated and trained CHW personnel who were responsible for tracing the patients, in case they missed mobile clinic appointments. The CHW were from the same communities, and therefore, were likely to be more accepted by the population [31,32]. However, the uncertain security situation and the movements among the population to nearby cities during nonharvest seasons (for work) posed major challenges in tracing patients.

The study had several limitations. The mobile clinics often faced limitations in routine activities in case of security issues. It was difficult for CHWs to trace patients from far off villages, deep in forest areas. The study results may not be generalized to other tribal areas, as the study is based on a resource-intensive TB program of a medical humanitarian NGO, working in the same area for about a decade. Most of the authors of the study were employees of the NGO, though the research team was not involved in the implementation of the program in the field. We believe that this might have moderated the potential bias in reporting on the implementation of the program. Despite the limitations, this is one of the first studies from a conflict-affected, tribal area in India, describing a unique diagnostic TB model of care based on a routine, mobile clinic-based TB program of an NGO, and thereby documenting the reality on the ground.

5. Conclusions

A mobile-clinic model of care for TB shows feasibility for replication in similar 'hard to reach' (namely conflict-affected and tribal) areas for improved access to quality TB diagnosis and care. Improved diagnostics such GeneXpert and utilizing CHWs from the communities for tracing and following the patients would be beneficial for early TB diagnoses.

Author Contributions: Conceptualization and protocol writing: M.D., H.M., S.K., G.F., P.I.; Data collection: M.D., D.P.; Data analysis: M.D., D.P., S.R., S.S.; Drafting the paper: M.D., D.P., S.R., S.S., S.K.; Critical review and approval for submission: M.D., D.P., S.R., S.S., H.M., S.K., F.N.H., G.F., P.I. All authors have read and agreed to the published version of the manuscript.

Funding: This research received no external funding.

Acknowledgments: We would like to acknowledge the time and efforts of patients with TB and their families, health care providers and project team involved in providing care to patients with TB.

Conflicts of Interest: The authors declare no conflict of interest.

References

1. Corninx, R. *Tuberculosis in Complex Emergencies [Internet]*; World Health Organization: Geneva, Switzerland, 2011; Available online: https://www.who.int/bulletin/volumes/85/8/06-037630/en/ (accessed on 18 September 2019).
2. Central TB Division. *India TB Annual Report—2018*; Directorate General of Health Services, Ministry of Health & Family Welfare: Nirman Bhawan, New Delhi, India, 2018.
3. Guha, R. Adivasis, Naxalites and Indian Democracy. *Econ. Polit. Wkly.* **2007**, *42*, 3305–3312.
4. Thomas, B.E.; Adinarayanan, S.; Manogaran, C.; Swaminathan, S. Pulmonary tuberculosis among tribals in India: A systematic review & meta-analysis. *Indian J. Med. Res.* **2015**, *142*, 614–623.
5. Central TB Division. *National Strategic Plan for Tuberculosis Elimination 2017–2025*; Directorate General of Health Services Ministry of Health & Family Welfare: Nirman Bhawan, New Delhi, India, 2017.

6. Das, M.; Isaakidis, P.; Armstrong, E.; Gundipudi, N.R.; Babu, R.B.; Qureshi, I.A.; Claes, A.; Mudimanchi, A.K.; Prasad, N.; Mansoor, H.; et al. Directly-observed and self-administered tuberculosis treatment in a chronic, low-intensity conflict setting in India. *PLoS ONE* **2014**, *9*, e92131. [CrossRef] [PubMed]
7. Raipur News—Times of India. 47% Tuberculosis Cases in Chhattisgarh Go Unreported. 25 March 2013 [Internet]. Available online: https://timesofindia.indiatimes.com/city/raipur/47-tuberculosis-cases-in-Chhattisgarh-go-unreported/articleshow/19188197.cms (accessed on 18 September 2019).
8. Kundu, D.; Katre, V.; Singh, K.; Deshpande, M.; Nayak, P.; Khaparde, K.; Moitra, A.; Nair, S.A.; Parmar, M. Innovative social protection mechanism for alleviating catastrophic expenses on multidrug-resistant tuberculosis patients in Chhattisgarh, India. *WHO South-East Asia J. Public Health* **2015**, *4*, 69. [CrossRef] [PubMed]
9. Armstrong, E.; Das, M.; Mansoor, H.; Babu, R.B.; Isaakidis, P. Treating drug-resistant tuberculosis in a low-intensity chronic conflict setting in India. *Confl. Health* **2014**, *8*, 1–6. [CrossRef] [PubMed]
10. Corrêa, G.; Das, M.; Kovelamudi, R.; Jaladi, N.; Pignon, C.; Vysyaraju, K.; Yedla, U.; Laxmi, V.; Vemula, P.; Gowthami, V.; et al. High burden of malaria and anemia among tribal pregnant women in a chronic conflict corridor in India. *Confl. Health* **2017**, *11*, 1–9. [CrossRef]
11. Singh, U.B.; Pandey, P.; Mehta, G.; Bhatnagar, A.K.; Mohan, A.; Goyal, V.; Ramachandran, R.; Sachdeva, K.S.; Samantaray, J.C. Genotypic, Phenotypic and Clinical Validation of GeneXpert in Extra-Pulmonary and Pulmonary Tuberculosis in India. *PLoS ONE* **2016**, *11*, e0149258.
12. WHO. *Definitions and Reporting Framework for Tuberculosis—2013 Revision*; World Health Organization: Geneva, Switzerland, 2014; pp. 1–47.
13. Rao, V.G.; Bhat, J.; Yadav, R.; Gopi, P.G.; Selvakumar, N.; Wares, D.F. Prevalence of pulmonary tuberculosis among the Bharia, a primitive tribe of Madhya Pradesh, central India. *Int. J. Tuberc. Lung Dis.* **2010**, *14*, 368–370.
14. Purty, A.J.; Mishra, A.K.; Chauhan, R.C.; Prahankumar, R.; Stalin, P.; Bazroy, J. Burden of Pulmonary Tuberculosis among Tribal Population: A Cross-sectional Study in Tribal Areas of Maharashtra, India. *Indian J. Community Med.* **2019**, *44*, 17–20.
15. Rao, V.G.; Bhat, J.; Yadav, R.; Sharma, R.K.; Muniyandi, M. Declining tuberculosis prevalence in Saharia, a particularly vulnerable tribal community in central India: Evidences for action 11 Medical and Health Sciences 1117 Public Health and Health Services. *BMC Infect. Dis.* **2019**, *19*, 180.
16. Subbaraman, R.; Nathavitharana, R.R.; Satyanarayana, S.; Pai, M.; Thomas, B.E.; Chadha, V.K.; Rade, K.; Swaminathan, S.; Mayer, K.H. The Tuberculosis Cascade of Care in India's Public Sector: A Systematic Review and Meta-analysis. *PLoS Med.* **2016**, *13*, e1002149. [CrossRef] [PubMed]
17. Raizada, N.; Sachdeva, K.S.; Sreenivas, A.; Vadera, B.; Gupta, R.S.; Parmar, M.; Kulsange, S.; Babre, A.; Thakur, R.; Gray, C.; et al. Feasibility of Decentralised Deployment of Xpert MTB / RIF Test at Lower Level of Health System in India. *PLoS ONE* **2014**, *9*, e89301. [CrossRef] [PubMed]
18. Shewade, H.D.; Gupta, V.; Satyanarayana, S.; Sahai, K.N.; Murali, L.; Kamble, S.; Deshpande, M.; Kumar, N.; Kumar, S.; Pandey, P. Active case finding among marginalised and vulnerable populations reduces catastrophic costs due to tuberculosis diagnosis. *Glob. Health Action* **2018**, *11*, 1494897. [CrossRef] [PubMed]
19. Hassanain, S.A.; Edwards, J.K.; Venables, E.; Ali, E.; Adam, K.; Hussien, H.; Elsony, A. Conflict and tuberculosis in Sudan: A 10-year review of the National Tuberculosis Programme, 2004–2014. *Confl. Health* **2018**, *12*, 18. [CrossRef] [PubMed]
20. Gele, A.A.; Bjune, G.A. Armed conflicts have an impact on the spread of tuberculosis: The case of the Somali Regional State of Ethiopia. *Confl. Health* **2010**, *4*, 2–7. [CrossRef]
21. Ismail, M.B.; Rafei, R.; Dabboussi, F.; Hamze, M. Tuberculosis, war, and refugees: Spotlight on the Syrian humanitarian crisis Armed conflicts and forced population displacements markedly increase TB risk and selection of TB-resistant forms. *PLoS Pathog* **2018**, *14*, e1007014.
22. Munn-Mace, G.; Parmar, D. Treatment of tuberculosis in complex emergencies in developing countries: A scoping review. *Health Policy Plan.* **2018**, *33*, 247–257. [CrossRef]
23. Marais, B.J. Childhood tuberculosis: Epidemiology and natural history of disease. *Indian J. Pediatr.* **2011**, *78*, 321–327. [CrossRef]
24. Raizada, N.; Khaparde, S.D.; Salhotra, V.S.; Rao, R.; Kalra, A.; Swaminathan, S.; Khanna, A.; Chopra, K.K.; Hanif, M.; Singh, V.; et al. Accelerating access to quality TB care for pediatric TB cases through better diagnostic strategy in four major cities of India. *PLoS ONE* **2018**, *13*, e0193194. [CrossRef]

25. Jain, S.K.; Ordonez, A.; Kinikar, A.; Gupte, N.; Thakar, M.; Mave, V.; Jubulis, J.; Dharmshale, S.; Desai, S.; Hatolkar, S.; et al. Pediatric tuberculosis in young children in India: A prospective study. *Biomed. Res. Int.* **2013**, *2013*, 7. [CrossRef]
26. Pawar, S.; Jadhav, H.; Pagar, V.; Radhe, B.; Behere, V. Performance and treatment outcome of tuberculosis among patients on Revised National Tuberculosis Control Programme in Urban and Tribal areas of a district in Maharashtra. *Med. J. Dr. DY Patil Univ.* **2017**, *10*, 46. [CrossRef]
27. Purohit, M.R.; Purohit, R.; Mustafa, T. Patient Health Seeking and Diagnostic Delay in Extrapulmonary Tuberculosis: A Hospital Based Study from Central India. *Tuberc. Res. Treat.* **2019**, *2019*, 1–8. [CrossRef] [PubMed]
28. Ade, S.; Harries, A.D.; Trébucq, A.; Ade, G.; Agodokpessi, G.; Adjonou, C.; Azon, S.; Anagonou, S. National Profile and Treatment Outcomes of Patients with Extrapulmonary Tuberculosis in Bénin. *PLoS ONE* **2014**, *9*, e95603. [CrossRef] [PubMed]
29. Sharma, S.K.; Ryan, H.; Khaparde, S.; Sachdeva, K.S.; Singh, A.D.; Mohan, A.; Sarin, R.; Paramasivan, C.N.; Kumar, P.; Nischal, N.; et al. Index-TB guidelines: Guidelines on extrapulmonary tuberculosis for India. *Indian J. Med. Res.* **2017**, *145*, 448–463.
30. Thomas, B.E.; Subbaraman, R.; Sellappan, S.; Suresh, C.; Lavanya, J.; Lincy, S.; Raja, A.L.; Javeed, B.; Kokila, S.; Arumugam, S.; et al. Pretreatment loss to follow-up of tuberculosis patients in Chennai, India: A cohort study with implications for health systems strengthening. *BMC Infect. Dis.* **2018**, *18*, 142. [CrossRef]
31. Sharma, B.V. WHO Global Tuberculosis Programme. In *Community Contribution to TB Care: An Asian Perspective*; WHO: Geneva, Switzerland, 2002; p. 63. Available online: http://whqlibdoc.who.int/hq/2002/WHO_CDS_TB_2002.302.pdf (accessed on 20 September 2019).
32. Garg, S.; Nanda, P.; Dewangan, M. Role of Community Health Workers in Improving Tb Detection on Scale: A Case Study From the Mitanin Programme in Chhattisgarh, India. *BMJ Glob. Health* **2016**, *1* (Suppl. 1), A2–A43.

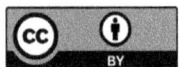

© 2019 by the authors. Licensee MDPI, Basel, Switzerland. This article is an open access article distributed under the terms and conditions of the Creative Commons Attribution (CC BY) license (http://creativecommons.org/licenses/by/4.0/).

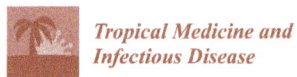 *Tropical Medicine and Infectious Disease*

Article

The Impact of Funding on Childhood TB Case Detection in Pakistan

Amyn A. Malik [1,2,3,]*, Hamidah Hussain [2], Jacob Creswell [4], Sara Siddiqui [1], Junaid F. Ahmed [1], Falak Madhani [1], Ali Habib [5], Aamir J. Khan [2] and Farhana Amanullah [6]

1. Global Health Directorate, Indus Health Network, Karachi 75190, Pakistan; sara.siddiqui@ghd.ihn.org.pk (S.S.); junaid.fuad@ghd.ihn.org.pk (J.F.A.); falak.madhani@ghd.ihn.org.pk (F.M.)
2. Interactive Research and Development (IRD) Global, Singapore 189677, Singapore; hamidah.hussain@ird.global (H.H.); aamir.khan@ird.global (A.J.K.)
3. Emory University Rollins School of Public Health, Atlanta, GA 30329, USA
4. Stop TB Partnership, 1218 Le Grand-Saconnex, Switzerland; jacobc@stoptb.org
5. Interactive Health Solutions, Karachi 75350, Pakistan; ali.habib@ihsinformatics.com
6. The Indus Hospital, Karachi 75190, Pakistan; farhana.maqbool@ird.global
* Correspondence: amyn.malik@ghd.ihn.org.pk

Received: 15 November 2019; Accepted: 13 December 2019; Published: 15 December 2019

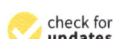

Abstract: This study is a review of routine programmatically collected data to describe the 5-year trend in childhood case notification in Jamshoro district, Pakistan from January 2013 to June 2018 and review of financial data for the two active case finding projects implemented during this period. The average case notification in the district was 86 per quarter before the start of active case finding project in October 2014. The average case notification rose to 322 per quarter during the implementation period (October 2014 to March 2016) and plateaued at 245 per quarter during the post-implementation period (April 2016 to June 2018). In a specialized chest center located in the district, where active case finding was re-introduced during the post implementation period (October 2016), the average case notification was 218 per quarter in the implementation period and 172 per quarter in the post implementation period. In the rest of the district, the average case notification was 160 per quarter in the implementation period and 78 during the post implementation period. The cost per additional child with TB found ranged from USD 28 to USD 42 during the interventions. A continuous stream of resources is necessary to sustain high notifications of childhood TB.

Keywords: pediatric TB; verbal screening; contact tracing; resources

1. Introduction

Childhood TB diagnosis can be difficult and hence many children who develop TB are missed. Of the 10 million people who develop TB each year, 10% or 1 million are children. While national TB programs (NTP) do not report 34% of all incident cases, more than half of children with TB are believed to be missed, resulting in 233,000 deaths each year [1,2]. Modeling studies suggest that 96% of these deaths occur in children who do not access TB treatment [3].

Children with TB are often not diagnosed and reported because of limited capacity of frontline health providers [4,5], lack of dedicated child health services with experienced and appropriately trained clinicians [4], non-specific symptoms overlapping with other common childhood diseases [6], complex diagnostic algorithms [6,7], lack of a sensitive point of care test and technical resources [8], and minimal contact tracing activities [2].

In Pakistan, the estimated TB incidence in 2018 was 265 cases per 100,000 population with approximately 62,000 cases in children. Of the estimated childhood cases, about one in four cases were not notified to the national program [1].

Successful interventions to improve case detection among children have included systematic screening at outpatient departments of hospitals and general practitioners with studies from Pakistan showing that this can increase the case notification among children between 2.5 and 7 times [9,10].

In many high TB burden countries, the response to the epidemic is highly donor dependent. Periodic funding of targeted interventions can lead to increases in diagnosis and notification [11] with a hope that the increase will be sustained given the strengthened health system and capacity building. Recently, the United Nations held a High-Level Meeting on Ending TB (UNHLM), where heads of states committed to mobilize at least 13 billion dollars annually by 2022 for the sufficient and sustainable financing of the global TB response, and to diagnose and treat 3.5 million children with TB between 2018 and 2022 [12].

Our objective is to describe the 5 years trend in childhood case notification in a rural district in Sindh province of Pakistan before, during and after focused active case finding and contact tracing efforts with injection of resources. We sought to understand the impact and cost of finding a child with TB during periodic funding from external sources.

2. Materials and Methods

2.1. Setting and Study Design

This study is a review of programmatically collected case notification data to describe the 5 year trend in childhood case notification in Jamshoro district, Pakistan from January 2013 to June 2018.

As part of the Stop TB Partnership's TB REACH wave 4 funding, an active case finding and contact tracing project in a district in rural Sindh was conducted between October 2014 and March 2016. The detailed methodology of this project and results are reported elsewhere [10]. Briefly, the intervention systematically screened all children in outpatient departments of four large public sector hospitals in Jamshoro district for symptoms of TB and conducted household contact tracing of adults and children diagnosed with TB at these facilities. Three of these four hospitals had pediatric TB specialists as part of their medical staff and were already reporting pediatric TB cases. No other center reported pediatric TB cases regularly. One of the four hospitals is a specialized chest treatment center, which treats both drug-susceptible and drug-resistant TB. Community health workers were recruited from the catchment area and trained to administer questionnaires to assess TB symptoms using a custom-built mHealth data collection application with decision support. All individuals with a high likelihood of TB disease were referred to a TB medical officer for free evaluation and testing. Adults with TB and guardians of children diagnosed with TB were also asked to bring their family members to the health facility for TB screening.

At the specialized chest center, active case finding was re-started through a Global Fund initiative in October 2016 by adding one doctor and one nurse and providing support for data collection. The nurse was trained to administer questionnaires to assess TB symptoms in children in outpatient department using a custom-built mHealth data collection application with decision support. All children with a high likelihood of TB were referred to the medical officer for further evaluation and free testing.

There were no other notable changes in the district during the five-year period being analyzed.

2.2. Data Collection

Age-disaggregated TB case notification data were extracted from the registers of the provincial TB program (PTP) from quarter 1, 2013 to quarter 2, 2018.

Financial data from the TB REACH project was extracted from the accounting system maintained by the finance department. We calculated the operational cost per child verbally screened and cost per TB patient diagnosed through active case finding at the specialized chest center during the implementation period. It included human resources, design, deployment and maintenance of electronic data collection systems and the laboratory tests. We employed two community health workers and one field supervisor exclusively for the intervention and a government employed doctor was incentivized to screen and treat additional children found through the project. The project bore the costs of chest X-rays, Xpert MTB/RIF, Acid Fast Bacilli (AFB) smear and other laboratory and radiological tests as required. Costs were incurred in Pakistani Rupees (PKR) and were converted to US dollars (USD) using the average 2015 exchange rate of 1 USD to 103.1 PKR.

Financial data from the Global Fund project for the support provided to the specialized chest center was extracted from the accounting system from October 2016 to June 2018. During this period, the facility employed one doctor and one nurse. A dedicated doctor was only employed for half of the time period. Chest x-rays, Xpert MTB/RIF, AFB smear and other laboratory and radiological tests as required were done free of charge for the patients. Costs were incurred in Pakistani Rupees (PKR) and were converted to US dollars (USD) using the average 2017 exchange rate of 1 USD to 105.3 PKR.

2.3. Analysis

We analyzed the changes in quarterly notifications of childhood TB in the district through three periods: (1) a baseline period when no resources for active TB case finding and contact tracing interventions were in place with only passive case finding with no questionnaire-based screening and contact tracing happening (January 2013 to September 2014); (2) an implementation period when active TB case finding and contact tracing interventions were deployed (October 2014 to March 2016); and (3) a post-implementation period when the project ended and additional resources for active case finding and contact tracing were withdrawn (April 2016 to June 2018) (Figure 1). We adjusted for trend in our analysis extrapolating from the baseline period. We used linear regression to calculate the effect of intervention period, a proxy for additional resources, on case notification adjusting for time.

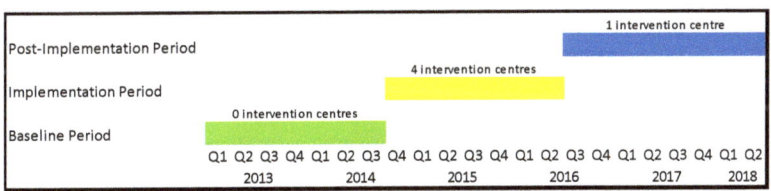

Figure 1. Figure enumerating the details of different intervention periods Jamshoro District, Sindh, Pakistan between Q1 2013 and Q2 2018.

We analyzed the changes at the specialized chest center through the baseline January 2013 to March 2015 (27 months) and implementation May 2015 to March 2016 (11 months) periods for the specialized chest center as we had phased in the implementation of the TB REACH project. Because active case finding was re-started in October 2016 at this center through Global Fund resources, the results from this center includes a post-implementation period of two quarters (Q2, 2016–Q3, 2016), and subsequent intervention quarters (Q4, 2016–Q2, 2018) that we refer to as 'New Active Case Finding Project'.

As the specialized chest center received additional resources in the post-implementation period, a more nuanced approach is required to fully understand the trends in notification in relation to available resources. We stratified the data by center type to analyze the trends, separating the specialized chest center from the other centers in the district. We also compared the proportion of TB patients diagnosed and yield of patients diagnosed per child screened across centers during the implementation period to assess the impact by center type.

For financial analysis, we calculated the overall cost of the active case finding during the two different intervention phases at the specialized chest center. This cost did not take into account the existing government infrastructure in place. We calculated the additional cost per additional patient found by dividing our overall cost by the trend-adjusted cumulative increase in the case notifications (additional patients) at the center. All analyses were conducted using Microsoft Excel 2019 and Stata version 15 (StataCorp, College Station, TX, USA).

2.4. Ethical Approval

As this study used de-identified aggregated numbers from existing data sources, this study was exempted from full-review by the Institutional Review Board (IRB) of Interactive Research and Development (IRD). The TB REACH funded project was approved by the same IRB.

3. Results

The average childhood TB case notification rate in the district was 86 a quarter between quarter 1, 2013 and quarter 3, 2014 (seven quarters). It rose to an average of 322 per quarter during the six intervention quarters (quarter 4, 2014 to quarter 1, 2016), a trend-adjusted increase of 2 times ($p < 0.01$). During the nine post-implementation quarters, the average case notification was 245 per quarter, a trend-adjusted increase of 0.9 times ($p < 0.01$) (Figure 2a).

At the specialized center, the average case notification was 50 per quarter during the baseline period. In 2014, the center had screened 762 household contacts of all ages through passive contact screening with 21 contacts diagnosed with TB disease. The case notification rose steadily throughout the project implementation at the center reaching a peak of 354 children with TB in the first quarter of 2016 with an average of 218 a quarter during this period, a trend-adjusted increase of 2.6 times ($p < 0.01$). There was a fall in the case notification in quarters 2 and 3 of 2016 when no additional resources were available. Starting from quarter 4, 2016 when the new funding for active case finding started, the case notification rose again and reached 207 children with TB in quarter 1 of 2018 with an average of 172 children with TB notified a quarter during this period, a trend-adjusted increase of 1.4 times ($p < 0.01$) (Figure 2b).

The notifications in the remaining facilities in the district are depicted in Figure 2c. The average case notification was 36 a quarter during the baseline period rising to an average of 160 per quarter during the implementation period, a trend-adjusted increase of 3.9 times ($p < 0.01$). Notifications declined to an average of 78 per quarter during the post-implementation period when additional funding ceased, a trend-adjusted increase of 0.8 times ($p = 0.07$).

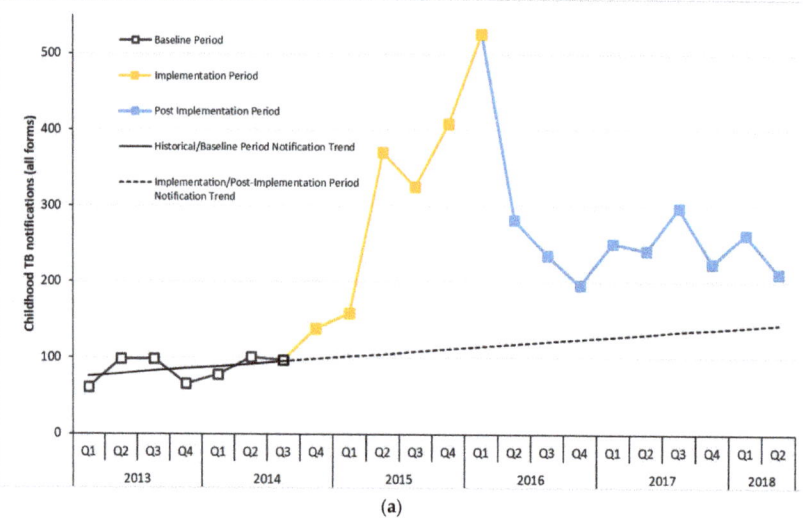

(a)

Figure 2. *Cont.*

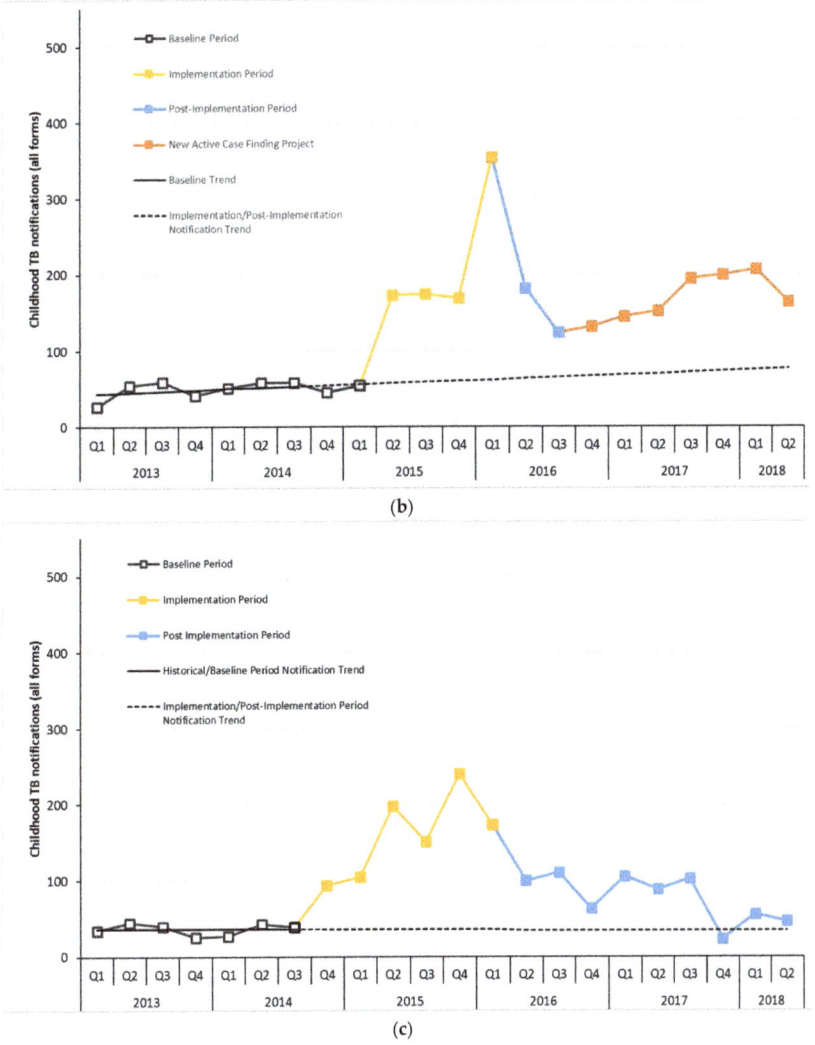

Figure 2. (**a**) Trend in childhood TB case notification before, during and after active case finding and contact tracing implementation in Jamshoro District, Sindh, Pakistan between Q1 2013 and Q2 2018. (**b**) Trend in childhood TB case notification before, during and after active case finding and contact tracing implementation at a specialized chest center in Jamshoro District, Sindh, Pakistan between Q1 2013 and Q2 2018. (**c**) Trend in childhood TB case notification before, during and after active case finding and contact tracing implementation at rest of the centers, in Jamshoro District, Sindh, Pakistan between Q1 2013 and Q2 2018.

During the implementation period, a total of 1807 children were diagnosed with TB in the four hospitals with the specialized chest center contributing 820 (45%) of them including 188 children detected through contact tracing. The other three centers contributed 987 (55%) TB cases including 202 through contact tracing (Table 1). The yield of TB cases diagnosed per child screened from the specialized chest center was 7.5 times higher as compared to the other three centers.

Table 1. (a) Yield of Active Case Finding in Children by Center type in Jamshoro District, Sindh, Pakistan between Q4 2014 and Q1 2016. (b) Yield from household contact investigation by Center type in Jamshoro District, Sindh, Pakistan between Q4 2014 and Q1 2016.

	Specialized Chest Center (%)	General Centers (%)	Total
(a)			
Number of children verbally screened	10,534	94,804	105,338
Children with presumptive TB	3411 (32)	2469 (3)	5880 (6)
Children tested/investigated for TB	2852 (84)	2287 (93)	5139 (87)
Children diagnosed with Bac + TB	26 (1)	16 (1)	42 (1)
Children diagnosed with All Forms TB	632 (22)	785 (34)	1417 (28)
Children with All Forms TB started on treatment	626 (99)	778 (99)	1404 (99)
(b)			
Number of child contacts screened	1129	1885	3014
Child contacts with presumptive TB	802 (71)	1034 (55)	1836 (61)
Child contacts/investigated for TB	707 (88)	900 (87)	1607 (88)
Child contacts diagnosed with Bac+ TB	4 (1)	1 (0.1)	5 (0.3)
Child contacts diagnosed with All Forms TB	188 (27)	202 (22)	390 (24)
Child contacts with All Forms TB started on treatment	183 (97)	202 (100)	385 (99)

Table 2 summarizes all costs incurred at the specialized chest center for the active case finding from May 2015 till March 2016 (11 months). The majority of the cost incurred (70%) was for salaries of the medical officer and community health workers hired at the center. The next biggest contributor to the cost was development of clinical decision support system (CDSS) with 18% of the total funds expended being used for it. The additional cost per additional child diagnosed was USD 41.8.

Table 2. Cost categories at specialized chest center in Kotri through active case finding (May 2015 to June 2018).

Cost Categories	Cost for May 2015 to March 2016 in USD (%)	Cost for October 2016 to June 2018 in USD (%)
Salaries for staff at center	18,551 (70)	6649 (35)
Diagnostic tests	1344 (5)	2810 (15)
Equipment (laptop and phones)	987 (4)	798 (4)
Clinical Decision Support System development (android based application)	4658 (18)	8424 (44)
Telephone and Internet cost	572 (2)	329 (2)
Stationery and Data Management	154 (1)	100 (1)
Training of staff	142 (1)	45 (0.2)
Total Cost	**26,409**	**19,155**

Conversion rate for May 2015–March 2016: 1 USD = 103.1 PKR. Conversion rate for October 2016–June 2018: 1 USD = 105.3 PKR.

Costs incurred from October 2016 to June 2018 at the specialized chest center for active case finding in the post implementation period are also summarized in Table 2. The major cost incurred was CDSS development and maintenance cost (44%) followed by salaries of additional staff hired (35%). The additional cost per additional child diagnosed was USD 27.7.

4. Discussion

Studies from Pakistan, India, Nepal and Nigeria have shown that intensified case finding can result in large increases in childhood TB case notification [9,13–15]. Our study indicates that injection of new resources through focused active TB case finding and contact tracing efforts can substantially raise the baseline TB case notification among children. The peak case notification was reached when all aspects of the project, active case finding and contact tracing, were fully functional. Once funding for activities ceased, the district saw a marked decrease in childhood TB case notification although a residual effect of the intervention persisted with somewhat elevated notifications despite the removal of funding for new resources. Once funding for active case finding activities started again, a second increase in childhood TB case notification was observed, but the increase was smaller, likely due to limited resources available. Our findings suggest that activities that go above the routine work of the NTP require additional funding to show impact on childhood TB case diagnosis and notification.

Actively screening children for TB resulted in more than doubling of the case notification in the district during the implementation period [10] with the yield from the specialized chest center being 7.5 times higher as compared to the other three centers in this project. We believe the increased yield was due to the profile of the children presenting at the specialized center being a select population with respiratory symptoms. The cost incurred per additional child with TB found through active case finding was less than USD 42. The cost incurred per additional child with TB found through active case finding in the post implementation period was less than USD 28. The lower costs were due to the absence of active contact tracing involving greater costs from home visits.

The three non-specialized centers saw a slow decline in the case notification after the project ended, returning to baseline after almost two years. This slow decline is likely the combined result of establishment of referral behaviors, transfer-out of health center staff, programmatic and health systems strengthening and a modest communication campaign that the TB REACH project implemented. However, with time the institutional memory eroded, trained health staff left for other jobs and things returned to baseline [16,17].

Although we did not setup the evaluation as a strictly controlled trial, our results strongly point to the role that additional funding and resources play in improving performance of case detection. While not all case finding approaches will have an impact on the numbers of people being notified, a combination of different approaches including strengthening of existing systems are needed in order to improve on the status quo [9,10,18]. Most of the time, additional work will cost more money, but if the interventions are impactful, continued support must be sought [19]. As there were no notable changes in the district and the time frame is relatively short, we do not believe that external factors confound our findings.

Active TB screening in outpatient departments requires resources that NTPs do not always have. The cost of active case finding ranges from USD 72 to 963 per patient found depending on the screening algorithm used and the population being screened [20,21]. However, it will always cost more to increase the number of people offered TB services. It is estimated that in 2020 there will be a shortfall of approximately USD 6 billion globally for TB prevention, diagnosis and treatment services given the current available funding of USD 6.8 billion per year [1,22]. A significant portion of the current funding in low- and middle-income countries with high TB burdens outside of the BRICS countries is through large international donors. For example, in 19 of the 30 high burden countries more than 50% of the TB program-specific budget is through international funding [1].

Recently, the United Nations held a High-Level Meeting on Ending TB (UNHLM) where a political declaration on grounds of human rights with a target of successfully diagnosing and treating 40 million people with tuberculosis including 3.5 million children by 2022 was adopted [22]. To achieve these milestones, a greater commitment by the countries to public policies and practices related to TB will need to be realized including additional domestic funding. Increases in domestic funding has been responsible for the progress in BRICS and other European and Latin American countries in their efforts to end the TB epidemic [23]. India provides a good example where domestic funding for TB increased almost four times between 2015 and 2018 and accounts for 77% of the total TB budget of the country with no funding gap in 2019. India has seen case notifications increase by 24% nationally between 2015 and 2018 [1].

In the context of our case study, the budget for Pakistan's national program for the year 2019 is USD 135 million with only approximately 3% of the budget funded through domestic sources and

67% of the budget remaining unfunded [1]. The proportion of domestic funding for TB Pakistan will need to increase dramatically to meet its baseline provision of services as well as provide TB screening and testing facilities at high patient-volume centers, including contact management and follow-up in all districts.

5. Conclusions

Children have been a historically neglected population in the TB community as they have not been sources of transmission nor can they be diagnosed with the basic tools promoted in the early years of the TB response. Global leaders, including those of Pakistan, have signed the UNHLM for TB political declaration which mandates that countries hold themselves accountable for reaching their targets. Successful, low cost, interventions such as this one that resulted in finding large numbers of missing children with TB should be scaled up with domestic funding to include health centers where patients with respiratory symptoms seek care.

Author Contributions: A.A.M., H.H. and F.A. conceptualized the study. A.A.M., S.S., J.F.A., F.M. and A.H. collected the data. A.A.M., H.H., J.C., F.M., A.H., A.J.K. and F.A. performed the analysis. A.A.M., J.C., H.H. and F.A. wrote the initial draft of the manuscript. All authors helped interpret the findings, read and approved the final version of the manuscript.

Funding: Active case finding during October 2014 to March 2016 was supported through Stop TB Partnership's TB REACH initiative. TB REACH is generously supported by Global Affairs Canada. Active case finding during October 2016 to March 2018 was supported through The Global Fund funding.

Acknowledgments: The authors would like to acknowledge Manzoor Brohi and Provincial TB Program Sind for providing the routinely collected programmatic data used for the analysis and Salman Khan.

Conflicts of Interest: J.C. is employed by Stop TB Partnership, but had no role in the decision to fund the active case finding and contact tracing project described; F.A. is the Chair of the WHO's Child and Adolescent TB Working Group. All other authors declare no conflict of interest.

References

1. WHO. *Global Tuberculosis Report 2019*; WHO: Geneva, Switzerland, 2019.
2. WHO. *Roadmap towards Ending TB in Children and Adolescents*; WHO: Geneva, Switzerland, 2018.
3. Dodd, P.J.; Yuen, C.M.; Sismanidis, C.; Seddon, J.A.; Jenkins, H.E. The global burden of tuberculosis mortality in children: A mathematical modelling study. *Lancet Glob. Health* **2017**, *5*, e898–e906. [CrossRef]
4. André, E.; Lufungulo Bahati, Y.; Mulume Musafiri, E.; Bahati Rusumba, O.; Van der Linden, D.; Zech, F. Prediction of Under-Detection of Paediatric Tuberculosis in the Democratic Republic of Congo: Experience of Six Years in the South-Kivu Province. *PLoS ONE* **2017**, *12*, e0169014. [CrossRef] [PubMed]
5. Bjerrum, S.; Rose, M.V.; Bygbjerg, I.C.; Mfinanga, S.G.; Tersboel, B.P.; Ravn, P. Primary health care staff's perceptions of childhood tuberculosis: A qualitative study from Tanzania. *BMC Health Serv. Res* **2012**, *12*, 6. [CrossRef] [PubMed]
6. Hesseling, A.; Schaaf, H.; Gie, R.; Starke, J.; Beyers, N. A critical review of diagnostic approaches used in the diagnosis of childhood tuberculosis. *Int. J. Tuberc. Lung. Dis.* **2002**, *6*, 1038–1045. [PubMed]
7. Hatherill, M.; Hanslo, M.; Hawkridge, T.; Little, F.; Workman, L.; Mahomed, H.; Tameris, M.; Moyo, S.; Geldenhuys, H.; Hanekom, W. Structured approaches for the screening and diagnosis of childhood tuberculosis in a high prevalence region of South Africa. *Bull. World Health Organ.* **2010**, *88*, 312–320. [CrossRef] [PubMed]
8. Kumar, M.K.; Kumar, P.; Singh, A. Recent advances in the diagnosis and treatment of childhood tuberculosis. *J. Nat. Sci. Biol. Med.* **2015**, *6*, 314–320. [CrossRef] [PubMed]
9. Khan, A.J.; Khowaja, S.; Khan, F.S.; Qazi, F.; Lotia, I.; Habib, A.; Mohammed, S.; Khan, U.; Amanullah, F.; Hussain, H. Engaging the private sector to increase tuberculosis case detection: An impact evaluation study. *Lancet Infect. Dis.* **2012**, *12*, 608–616. [CrossRef]
10. Malik, A.A.; Amanullah, F.; Codlin, A.J.; Siddiqui, S.; Jaswal, M.; Ahmed, J.F.; Saleem, S.; Khurshid, A.; Hussain, H. Improving childhood tuberculosis detection and treatment through facility-based screening in rural Pakistan. *Int. J. Tuberc. Lung. Dis.* **2018**, *22*, 851–857. [CrossRef] [PubMed]

11. Creswell, J.; Sahu, S.; Blok, L.; Bakker, M.I.; Stevens, R.; Ditiu, L. A Multi-Site Evaluation of Innovative Approaches to Increase Tuberculosis Case Notification: Summary Results. *PLoS ONE* **2014**, *9*, e94465. [CrossRef] [PubMed]
12. Stop TB Partnership. *Un High-Level Meeting on Tb Key Targets & Commitments for 2022*; Stop TB Partnership: Geneva, Switzerland, 2018.
13. Joshi, B.; Chinnakali, P.; Shrestha, A.; Das, M.; Kumar, A.; Pant, R.; Lama, R.; Sarraf, R.; Dumre, S.; Harries, A. Impact of intensified case-finding strategies on childhood TB case registration in Nepal. *Public Health Action.* **2015**, *5*, 93–98. [CrossRef] [PubMed]
14. Oshi, D.C.; Chukwu, J.N.; Nwafor, C.C.; Meka, A.O.; Madichie, N.O.; Ogbudebe, C.L.; Onyeonoro, U.U.; Ikebudu, J.N.; Ekeke, N.; Anyim, M.C. Does intensified case finding increase tuberculosis case notification among children in resource-poor settings? A report from Nigeria. *Int. J. Mycobacteriol.* **2016**, *5*, 44–50. [CrossRef] [PubMed]
15. Pathak, R.R.; Mishra, B.K.; Moonan, P.K.; Nair, S.A.; Kumar, A.M.; Gandhi, M.P.; Mannan, S.; Ghosh, S. Can intensified tuberculosis case finding efforts at nutrition rehabilitation centers lead to pediatric case detection in Bihar, India? *J. Tuberc. Res.* **2016**, *4*, 46. [CrossRef] [PubMed]
16. Dolea, C. *Increasing Access to Health Workers in Remote and Rural Areas through Improved Retention: Global Policy Recommendations*; World Health Organization: Geneva, Switzerland, 2010.
17. Van Camp, J.; Chappy, S. The Effectiveness of Nurse Residency Programs on Retention: A Systematic Review. *AORN J.* **2017**, *106*, 128–144. [CrossRef]
18. Barry, R.; Bloom, R.A.; Ted, C.; Christopher, D.; Hamish, F.; Gabriela, B.G.; Gwen, K.; Megan, M.; Edward, N.; Eric, R.; et al. Tuberculosis. In *Major Infectious Diseases*, 3rd ed.; King, K., Holmes, S.B., Barry, R.B., Prabhat, J., Eds.; The International Bank for Reconstruction and Development/The World Bank: Washington, DC, USA, 2017. [CrossRef]
19. The Global Fund. Catalytic Investments. Available online: https://www.theglobalfund.org/en/funding-model/before-applying/catalytic-investments/ (accessed on 1 October 2019).
20. James, R.; Khim, K.; Boudarene, L.; Yoong, J.; Phalla, C.; Saint, S.; Koeut, P.; Mao, T.E.; Coker, R.; Khan, M.S. Tuberculosis active case finding in Cambodia: A pragmatic, cost-effectiveness comparison of three implementation models. *BMC Infect. Dis.* **2017**, *17*, 580. [CrossRef] [PubMed]
21. Zhang, C.; Ruan, Y.; Cheng, J.; Zhao, F.; Xia, Y.; Zhang, H.; Wilkinson, E.; Das, M.; Li, J.; Chen, W.; et al. Comparing yield and relative costs of WHO TB screening algorithms in selected risk groups among people aged 65 years and over in China, 2013. *PLoS ONE* **2017**, *12*, e0176581. [CrossRef] [PubMed]
22. United Nations General Assembly. *Political Declaration of the High-Level Meeting of the General Assembly on the Fight Against Tuberculosis*; United Nations General Assembly: New York, NY, USA, 2018.
23. Floyd, K.; Fitzpatrick, C.; Pantoja, A.; Raviglione, M. Domestic and donor financing for tuberculosis care and control in low-income and middle-income countries: An analysis of trends, 2002–2011, and requirements to meet 2015 targets. *Lancet Glob. Health* **2013**, *1*, e105–e115. [CrossRef]

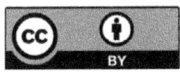

© 2019 by the authors. Licensee MDPI, Basel, Switzerland. This article is an open access article distributed under the terms and conditions of the Creative Commons Attribution (CC BY) license (http://creativecommons.org/licenses/by/4.0/).

MDPI
St. Alban-Anlage 66
4052 Basel
Switzerland
Tel. +41 61 683 77 34
Fax +41 61 302 89 18
www.mdpi.com

Tropical Medicine and Infectious Disease Editorial Office
E-mail: tropicalmed@mdpi.com
www.mdpi.com/journal/tropicalmed

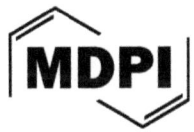

www.ingramcontent.com/pod-product-compliance
Lightning Source LLC
LaVergne TN
LVHW070427100526
838202LV00014B/1544